T0331718

THE STRESSED HEART

DEVELOPMENTS IN CARDIOVASCULAR MEDICINE

Lancee, C.T., ed.: Echocardiology. 1979. ISBN 90-247-2209-8.
Baan, J, Arntzenius, A.C., Yellin, E.L., eds.: Cardiac dynamics. 1980. ISBN 90-247-2212-8.
Thalen, H.J.T., Meere, C.C., eds.: Fundamentals of cardiac pacing. 1970. ISBN 90-247-2245-4.
Kulbertus, H.E., Wellens, H.J.J., eds.: Sudden death. 1980. ISBN 90-247-2290-X.
Dreifus, L.S., Brest, A.N., eds.: Clinical applications of cardiovascular drugs. 1980. ISBN 90-247-2295-0.
Spencer, M.P., Reid, J.M., eds.: Cerebrovascular evaluation with Doppler ultrasound. 1981. ISBN 90-247-2348-1.
Zipes, D.P., Bailey, J.C., Elharrer, V., eds.: The slow inward current and cardiac arrhythmias. 1980. ISBN 90-247-2380-9.
Kesteloot, H., Joossens, J.V., eds.: Epidemiology of arterial blood pressure. 1980. ISBN 90-247-2386-8.
Wackers, F.J.T., ed.: Thallium-201 and technetium-99m-pyrophosphate myocardial imaging in the coronary care unit. 1980. ISBN 90-247-2396-5.
Maseri, A., Marchesi, C., Chierchia, S., Trivella, M.G., eds.: Coronary care units. 1981. IBSN 90-247-2456-2.
Morganroth, J., Moore, E.N., Dreifus, L.S., Michelson, E.L., eds.: The evaluation of new anti-arrhythmic drugs. 1981. ISBN 90-247-2474-0.
Alboni, P.: Intraventricular conduction disturbances. 1981. ISBN 90-247-2483-X.
Rijsterborgh, H., ed.: Echocardiology. 1981. ISBN 90-247-2491-0.
Wagner, G.S., ed.: Myocardial infarction. Measurement and intervention. 1982. ISBN 90-247-2513-5.
Meltzer, R.S., Roelandt, J., eds.: Contrast echocardiography. 1982. ISBN 90-247-2531-3.
Amery, A., Fagard, R., Lijnen, R., Staessen, J., eds.: Hypertensive cardiovascular disease; pathophysiology and treatment. 1982. ISBN 90-247-2534-8.
Bouman, L.N., Jongsma, H.J., eds.: Cardiac rate and rhythm. 1982. ISBN 90-247-2626-3.
Morganroth, J., Moore, E.N., eds.: The evaluation of beta blocker and calcium antagonist drugs. 1982. ISBN 90-247-2642-5.
Rosenbaum, M.B., ed.: Frontiers of cardiac electrophysiology. 1982. ISBN 90-247-2663-8.
Roelandt, J., Hugenholtz, P.G., eds.: Long-term ambulatory electrocardiography. 1982. ISBN 90-247-2664-8.
Adgey, A.J., ed.: Acute phase of ischemic heart disease and myocardial infarction. 1982. ISBN 90-247-2675-1.
Hanrath, P., Bleifeld, W., Souquet, eds.: Cardiovascular diagnosis by ultrasound. Transesophageal, computerized, contrast, Doppler echocardiography. 1982. ISBN 90-247-2692-1.
Roelandt, J., ed.: The practice of M-mode and two-dimensional echocardiography. 1983. ISBN 90-247-2745-6.
Meyer, J., Schweizer, P., Erbel, R., eds.: Advances in noninvasive cardiology. 1983. ISBN 0-89838-576-8.
Morganroth, Joel, Moore, E.N., eds.: Sudden cardiac death and congestive heart failure: Diagnosis and treatment. 1983. ISBN 0-89838-580-6.
Perry, H.M., ed.: Lifelong management of hypertension. ISBN 0-89838-582-2.
Jaffe, E.A., ed.: Biology of endothelial cells. ISBN 0-89838-587-3.
Surawicz, B., Reddy C.P., Prystowsky, E.N., eds.: Tachycardias. 1984. ISBN 0-89838-588-1.
Spencer, M.P., ed.: Cardiac Doppler diagnosis. ISBN 0-89838-591-1.
Villareal, H.V., Sambhi, M.P., eds.: Topics in pathophysiology of hypertension. ISBN 0-89838-595-4.
Messerli, F.H., ed.: Cardiovascular disease in the elderly. 1984. ISBN 0-89838-596-2.
Simoons, M.L., Reiber, J.H.C., eds.: Nuclear imaging in clinical cardiology. ISBN 0-89838-599-7.
Ter Keurs, H.E.D.J., Schipperheym, J.J., eds.: Cardiac left ventricular hypertrophy. ISBN 0-89838-612-8.
Sperelakis, N., ed.: Physiology and pathophysiology of the heart. ISBN 0-89838-615-2.
Messerli, F.H., ed.: Kidney in essential hypertension. 1983. ISBN 0-89838-616-0.
Sambhi, M.P., ed.: Fundamental fault in hypertension. ISBN 0-89838-638-1.
Marchesi, D., ed.: Ambulatory monitoring: Cardiovascular system and allied applications. ISBN 0-89838-642-X.
Kupper, W., Macalpin, R.N., Bleifeld, W., eds.: Coronary tone in ischemic heart disease. ISBN 0-89838-646-2.
Sperelakis, N., Caulfield, J.B., eds.: Calcium antagonists: Mechanisms of action on cardiac muscle and vascular smooth muscle. ISBN 0-89838-655-1.
Godfraind, T., Herman, A.S., Wellens, D., eds.: Entry blockers in cardiovascular and cerebral dysfunctions. ISBN 0-89838-658-6.
Morganroth, J., Moore, E.N., eds.: Interventions in the acute phase of myocardial infarction. ISBN 0-89838-659-4.
Abel, F.L., Newman, W.H., eds.: Functional aspects of the normal, hypertrophied, and failing heart. ISBN 0-89838-665-9.
Sideman, S., and Beyar, R., eds.: Simulation and imaging of the cardiac system. ISBN 0-89838-687-X.
van de Wall, E., Lie, K.I., eds.: Recent views on hypertrophic cardiomyopathy. ISBN 0-89838-694-2.
Beamish, R.E., Singal, P.K., Dhalla, N.S., eds.: Stress and heart disease. ISBN 089838-709-4.
Beamish, R.E., Panagia, V., Dhalla, N.S., eds.: Pathogenesis of stress-induced heart disease. ISBN 0-89838-710-8.
Morganroth, J., Moore, E.N., eds.: Cardiac arrhythmias: New therapeutic drugs and devices. ISBN 0-89838-716-7.
Mathes, P., ed.: Secondary prevention in coronary artery disease and myocardial infarction. ISBN 0-89838-736-1.
Stone, H. Lowell, Weglicki, W.B., eds.: Pathology of cardiovascular injury. ISBN 0-89838-743-4.
Meyer, J., Erbel, R., Rupprecht, H.J., eds.: Improvement of myocardial perfusion. ISBN 0-89838-748-5.
Reiber, J.H.C., Serruys, P.W., Slager, C.J.: Quantitative coronary and left ventricular cineangiography. ISBN 0-89838-760-4.
Fagard, R.H., Bekaert, I.E., eds.: Sports Cardiology. ISBN 0-89838-782-5.
Reiber, J.H.C., Serruys, P.W., eds.: State of the art in quantitative coronary arteriography. ISBN 0-89838-804-X.
Roelandt, J., ed.: Color doppler flow imaging. ISBN 0-89838-806-6.
van der Wall, E.E., ed.: Noninvasive imaging of cardiac metabolism. ISBN 0-89838-812-0.
Liebman, J., Plonsey, R., Rudy, Y., eds., Pediatric and fundamental electrocardiography. ISBN 0-89838-815-5.
Hilger, H., Hombach, V., eds., Invasive cardiovascular therapy. ISBN 0-89838-818-X.

THE STRESSED HEART

EDITED BY MARIANNE J. LEGATO, M.D.
Associate Professor of Clinical Medicine
Columbia University College of Physicians and Surgeons

MARTINUS NIJHOFF PUBLISHING
A Member of the Kluwer Academic Publishers Group
Boston/Dordrecht/Lancaster

Distributors

for the United States and Canada: Kluwer Academic Publishers, 101 Philip Drive, Assinippi Park, Norwell, MA 02061

for the UK and Ireland: Kluwer Academic Publishers, MTP Press Limited, Falcon House, Queen Square, Lancaster LAI IRN, UK

for all other countries: Kluwer Academic Publishers Group, Distribution Centre, P.O. Box 322, 3300 AH Dordrecht, The Netherlands

Library of Congress Cataloging-in-Publication Data

The Stressed heart.

   (Developments in cardiovascular medicine; (62)
   Includes index.
   1. Heart—Hypertrophy—Etiology. 2. Stress
(Physiology) 3. Heart—Diseases. 4. Physiology,
Pathological. I. Legato, Marianne J., 1935–
II. Series: Developments in cardiovascular medicine;
v. 62. [DNLM: 1. Heart—physiopathology. 2. Heart
Enlargment—physiopathology. W1 DE997VME v. 62/
WG 200 S914]
RC685.H9S77 1987   616.1'2071   86-28474
ISBN 0-89838-849-X

For Michael R. Rosen, M.D.

In recognition of his lively intelligence, his unswerving integrity, and his qualities of leadership. They have illuminated and expanded investigative cardiology for us all.

CONTENTS

CONTRIBUTING AUTHORS

Page Anderson, M.D.
  Professor of Pediatrics
  Duke University School of Medicine
  Durham, NC 27710

Natalio Banchero, M.D.
  Professor of Physiology
  University of Colorado Health Sciences Center
  4200 East 9th Avenue
  Denver, Colorado 80262

Claude R. Benedict, M.D.
  Assistant Professor of Medicine
  University of Texas Medical Branch
  Galveston, Texas 77550

Craig A. Canby, M.D.
  Graduate Student
  Department of Anatomy
  University of Iowa Cardiovascular Center
  Iowa City, Iowa 52242

William M. Chilian, Ph.D.
  Department of Medical Physiology
  Texas A & M University College of Medicine
  College Station, Texas 77843

George Cooper, IV, M.D.
  Professor of Medicine and Physiology
  Medical University of South Carolina
  Cardiology Section, Department of Medicine
  VA Medical Center
  109 B Street
  Charleston, South Carolina 29403

Edward M. Dwyer, Jr., M.D.
  Professor of Clinical Medicine
  Columbia University College of Physicians and Surgeons
  St. Luke's-Roosevelt Hospital Center
  428 West 59th Street
  New York, New York 10019

Stephen Factor, M.D.
  Professor of Pathology and Associate Professor of Medicine
  Albert Einstein College of Medicine
  1300 Morris Park Avenue
  Bronx, New York 10461

John Fenoglio, Jr., M.D.
  Professor and Chairman, Department of Pathology
  Columbia University College of Physicians and Surgeons
  622 West 168th Street
  New York, New York 10032

Anthony P. Goldman, M.D.
  Assistant Professor of Medicine
  Temple University School of Medicine
  Albert Einstein Medical Center
  York and Tabor Roads
  Philadelphia, Pennsylvania 19141

Graeme L. Hammond, M.D.
  Professor of Cardiothoracic Surgery
  Acting Chief, Cardiothoracic Surgery
  Yale University School of Medicine
  New Haven, Connecticut 06510

Morris N. Kotler, M.D.
  Professor of Medicine
  Temple University School of Medicine
  Albert Einstein Medical Center
  York and Tabor Roads
  Philadelphia, Pennsylvania 19141

Melvin L. Marcus, M.D.
  Professor of Medicine
  University of Iowa Cardiovascular Center
  Iowa City, Iowa 52242

Barry M. Massie, M.D.
  Associate Professor of Medicine
  University of California, San Francisco
  Cardiology Division (111 C)
  VA Hospital
  4150 Clement Street
  San Francisco, California 94121

Jean Marie Moalic, Ph.D.
  INSERM U 127
  Hôpital Lariboisière
  41 Boulevard de la Chapelle
  75010
  Paris, France

Karel Rakusan, M.D., Ph.D.
  Professor of Physiology
  University of Ottawa College of Medicine
  Ottawa, Ontario Canada

Thomas F. Robinson, Ph.D.
  Associate Professor of Medicine and Physiology and Biophysics
  Albert Einstein College of Medicine
  1300 Morris Park Avenue
  Bronx, New York 10461

Bernard Swynghedauw, M.D.
  INSERM U 127
  Hôpital Lariboisière
  41 Boulevard de la Chapelle
  75010
  Paris, France

Louis A. Sordahl, Ph.D.
  Professor of Biochemistry
  University of Texas Medical Branch
  Galveston, Texas 77550

Robert J. Tomanek, Ph.D.
  Professor of Anatomy
  University of Iowa Cardiovascular Center
  Iowa City, Iowa 52242

FOREWORD

The Stressed Heart is truly unique in concept and will provide an exciting adventure to the reader no matter what his or her field of expertise and interest. The title, although quite appropriate, does not adequately indicate the range of topics considered or the rational interrelationships among them. Indeed, perhaps the most important point to be learned from the book is that a serious consideration of the response of the heart to mechanical overload, ischemia, or excessive humoral stimuli must include evaluation of each of the topics in the table of contents.

The heart responds to stress through alterations in both structure and function. How these changes are brought about is the subject of the initial chapters. These consider first the normal regulation of gene expression in the heart, the rapid response to mechanical overload that leads to both quantitative and qualitative changes in the contractile proteins, and our current understanding of the signals that might be elicited by stress and alter gene expression. One chapter emphasizes the fact that, regardless of the nature of the stress, the common denominator is a discrepancy between energy requirements and expenditure. The central role of cellular acidosis in initiating the sequence of responses to stress and the possible roles of peptide regulators of transcription and protein regulators of translation are considered in detail.

Next, we are provided with a clear summary of the subcellular adaptations to stress that lead to cell growth and cardiac hypertrophy. This chapter emphasizes the fact that the response to stress is uniquely determined by the nature of the stress. Thus, an increase in afterload leads to a greater increase in myofibrils than in mitochondria whereas anemia and thyroxine excess have the opposite effect. Interestingly, the volume fractions of both myofibrils and mitochondria may increase proportionally, as during volume overload. The compensatory nature of the adaptations to stress are clearly emphasized.

To understand the changes in cardiac perfusion that result from different forms of stress, one must understand the capillarity of the normal heart, its development and regulation, and the differences between normal growth and hypertrophy. Three chapters are devoted to these topics and provide a detailed summary of the changes in coronary vessel anatomy during hypertrophy, the factors associated with hypertrophy that elicit changes in the coronary vasculature and, once again, the dependence of the nature of the response of the vasculature on the stimulus for change. In relation to the crucially important area of microcirculation, emphasis is placed on the almost invariant pattern of decreased capillary density and increased intercapillary distances in the hypertrophied adult heart. Differences between responses of immature and, adult hearts are emphasized for both the cardiac myocyte and the vasculature and suggest that, if we understood more about the regulation of gene expression, we might be able to induce a more effective pattern of response in adult hearts stressed by mechanical overload or ischemia by increasing capillarity.

These chapters provide an essential introduction to what follows: clear and authoritative expositions of the pathology and pathophysiology of the coronary circulation in ischemia, biochemical alterations associated with heart failure and the relationships between hypertrophy and failure. Once again, emphasis is placed on a number of interesting and important topics not usually included in considerations of the effects of stress on the heart. One chapter considers the changes in cardiac connective tissue during cardiac hypertrophy and two chapters emphasize the anatomical and functional changes associated with regression of hypertrophy and their clinical consequences.

A final topic not often considered in relation to effects of stress on the heart is the change in cardiac cell function and structure that results from aging per se. This subject is explored and data cited to indicate that, in spite of some consistent alterations in function and structure, there is no convincing evidence of significant degeneration of cardiocytes during senescence. The diminished response of the senescent heart to stress is best attributed to a diminished ability of the heart to respond to increased work requirements imposed for prolonged periods. The final chapter is devoted to relationships between stress and sudden cardiac death and evaluates available data and concepts. It is emphasized that both emotional and physical stress are important triggers of sudden death in certain subsets of patients and that improved means to identify such patients are needed to assist in prevention.

The authors of the sixteen chapters have all excelled in clarity of exposition and illustration, and avoidance of excessive detail. All write with real enthusiasm but at the same time fairly evaluate current limits on experimental method and interpretation. References are selected with care. All in all this is an excellent book that will provide new insights as well as new information to the reader. The investigator will become aware of many new avenues of productive research and the clinician will better understand how and why different forms of stress lead to the cardiovascular abnormalities with which he is familiar. This book is one we all should read and one all will want to own.

Brian F. Hoffman, M.D.

PREFACE

The heart's remarkable ability to meet changing demands allows it to adapt during the normal growth of the organism and to survive stress during adult life. As data about how the individual cells of the myocardium grow and modify their composition to do specific kinds of work, it is more and more apparent that there are important parallels between normal cardiac development and compensatory hypertrophy of the adult heart.

This is the second of a pair of books I have edited to illustrate some of these parallels. The important and, in most cases, quite recently appreciated characteristics of the young, growing myocyte were discussed in *The Developing Heart*, the companion piece to this volume. This second book emphasizes the adaptations of the adult myocardium to stress—adaptations which are basically the same as those used by the myocyte during normal growth.

The tailoring of the myocardium is adapative; as more information accumulates, it is apparent that the type, intensity, and duration of the demand for work imposed on the heart determine the ultimate structural and functional features of the myocardium. The pressure-overloaded heart is modified for slower, more efficient contraction; the heart of the thyrotoxic animal can beat much more rapidly (albeit less efficiently) than the normal heart but responds to a sudden demand for work against increased pressure very poorly indeed.

I have asked some of the leading scientists in the field of compensatory hypertrophy to contribute to this volume, which begins with the work of

xvi

Swynghedauw and his colleagues, who address the fact that the proteins produced in the overloaded myocardium are qualitatively different than those of the normal heart. In this way, the hypertrophying myocardium equips itself for a specific type of work. Swynghedauw's group has devoted itself to understanding the way the genes controlling the synthesis of proteins of the desired type are activated and regulate the production of these new molecules in the cell. This capacity of the myocyte to modify its protein composition is reminiscent of the ability of the neonatal cell to tailor and modify its constituent proteins to meet the changing hemodynamic demands of the first days and weeks of life. In his elegant and complementary chapter, Graeme Hammond expands our view of what regulates protein synthesis in the stressed heart, discussing the importance and effect on the myocyte of the triggering "stress proteins," which translate a physiologic impulse, such as pressure overload, into the biochemical signal that initiates protein synthesis in compensatory hypertrophy.

Tomanek and Canby examine the parallels and differences between normal cardiac growth and compensatory hypertrophy in terms of the population of myocyte organelles and how their proportions change during myocardial enlargment. The type, duration, and intensity of the stimulus influence the final composition of the hypertrophied cell.

Banchero's chapter begins an exploration of the myocardial circulation. He reviews the numbers and distribution of capillaries in the growing heart, particularly as they relate to the volume and distribution of mitochondria in the myocytes themselves. Chilian, Tomanek, and Marcus have authored a discussion of the behavior of the circulation in the hypertrophied myocardium and Rakusan focuses attention on the microcirculation in compensatory enlargement of the heart, whether due to pressure or volume overload, exercise, or hypoxia. Finally, Factor's chapter discusses the pathology and pathophysiology of the coronary microcirculation in myocardial ischemia.

The molecular basis for the failure of the stressed heart is explored by Louis Sordhal and Claude Benedict; the elements in the response of the myocardium to stress are reviewed and described, including decreased myosin ATP utilization, enhanced synthesis of myosin isoenzyme V3, and "downtuning" of calcium transport in the individual cell. In a complementary chapter, Anderson discusses some of the functional consequences of hypertrophy, exploring its effects on the modulation of activator calcium by examining the force/velocity relationship in myocardial hypertrophy and congestive failure.

John Fenoglio, Jr. and Tuan Duc Pham review some of the responses of atrial tissue to stress and discuss their work on the ultrastructure of that chamber in ischemic heart disease. Thomas Robinson writes of still another component of myocardium, the connective tissue matrix in which the myocytes are embedded, discussing the changes in the collagen network in the hypertrophied heart.

Barry Massie outlines the relationship between hypertrophy and myocardial decompensation. It is his view that the two states actually represent a "dynamic continuum" and he reviews the literature providing evidence for his hypothesis. Chapters by George Cooper, IV and Morris Kotler consider the details of the regression of hypertrophy: Cooper addresses functional, anatomic and hemodynamic considerations, referring to the extensive work he has done on the cat ventricle, while Kotler discusses primarily the regression of left ventricular hypertrophy, with particular reference to the patient.

Finally, Tomanek describes the aging process of the heart in senescence and Edward M. Dwyer, Jr., reviews the phenomenon of sudden cardiac death in patients with intrinsic myocardial disease and/or exposure to overwhelming stress.

ACKNOWLEDGMENTS

I would like to thank my research associate, Gloria McCord, who helped immeasurably to facilitate the preparation of this volume, and my editor, Jeff Smith, whose encouragement and thoughtful advice were invaluable in assembling the final product.

This work was supported by HL 28958 and HL 33727 from the National Institutes of Health and by funds from the Morris Lamer Fund of the St. Luke's Roosevelt Institute for Health Sciences.

THE STRESSED HEART

1. REGULATION OF GENE EXPRESSION
IN THE NORMAL AND OVERLOADED HEART

JEAN MARIE MOALIC AND BERNARD SWYNGHEDAUW

Mechanical overload is usually tolerated over a long period because of the development of several adaptational factors. At the fiber level, the reaction of myocardium to chronic overload is basically the same as that of skeletal muscle [1]. Two fundamental processes help striated muscle to adapt to a chronic enhancement of work: a decrease in the maximum shortening velocity for an unloaded muscle which in turn improves efficiency, and a hypertrophy which adapts the tissue to the new requirements both by multiplying the contractile units and, for the heart, by lowering the wall stress [2].

Both processes involve a change in gene expression, a quantitative change for hypertrophy and a qualitative one for the improvement of efficiency since it has been shown for rats that the latter, at least in part, is related to isoform modifications of myosin [3, 4, 5], creatine kinase [6], lactate dehydrogenase [7], and very likely other proteins [8].

An overview of gene expression in nucleated cells has previously been published [9]. The present review will focus on three particular aspects of the subject: the time course of the process, cardiac contractile protein synthesis, and gene structure and regulation. This third topic in fact concerns only the normal heart but we have done a detailed review because the new techniques of molecular biology will soon be used to study pathology and will very likely change our present understanding of that field.

TIME-COURSE OF THE EVENTS

The stimulation of gene expression in the heart is a rapid process. As initially shown by P.Y. Hatt [10] the stimulation of protein synthesis is almost

Table 1-1. Cardiac overload. Time course of the events. The data are recalculated from several papers from our laboratory [3, 4, 5, 6, 12, 13, 15, 17, 21].

	Control values	Days (d) or weeks (w.) after aortic stenosis							
		1d.	2d.	3d.	4d.	1w.	2w.	3w.	4w.
Degree of hypertrophy (in %)	0					10	30	55	55
Max. shortening velocity (unloaded, Vmax, muscle 1/sec)	3					2			1
Myosin ATPase (in %)	100						85		75
Isomyosin shift (% of V_3, electrophoresis)	10			10			20		70
Isomyosin shift (% of myocytes label anti V_3)	2			10	15	35	60		
Creatine kinase shift (B in % of total)	7						10		14
Rate of synthesis (%)									
total proteins	0	35	87		57	44			5
myosin H.C.	0		79						
actin	0		96						
28 S rRNA	0	35	55		52	38			
Total RNA (%)									
concentration	0	41			47	22	7		
per heart	0	42			70	55	60		
Poly A mRNA (%)									
per heart	0	30			50	50	46		
Densification of microtubules (% of total cells)	1		1	10	17	32	20	10	

immediate and can be observed by electron microscopy 30 minutes after an acute pressure overload. Other methods, using radioactive precursors, have confirmed this both in vivo and in vitro on an isolated working heart preparation [11, 12, 13, 14]. It was also shown that qualitative changes, i.e., the isoenzymatic shift of myosin from the high ATPase form, V_1 (containing the α-myosin heavy chain) to the low ATPase form, V_3 (containing the β-myosin heavy chain), occur as early as the quantitative changes. Indeed, using double immunolabeling of isolated myocytes with specific antibodies, Samuel et al. [15] showed such an isozyme transformation as early as three days after an abdominal aortic stenosis in the rat (table 1-1). These changes precede by a week or two the modifications of heart weight and shortening velocity. The situation is different for diastolic overload where it has been shown both in vivo [12] and on an isolated working heart preparation [16] that a volume overload did not stimulate protein synthesis as early as a pressure overload.

The mass of total RNA, as well as its concentration and rate of synthesis, increased by 30-80% within one to four days. This increase in synthesis occurs in parallel with the augmentation of protein synthesis suggesting that there is an excess of preexisting ribosomal RNA. In addition, both the mass and the concentration of total poly-A-containing messenger RNA [17] as well as specific messengers such as that of myosin heavy chain [18] increase simultaneously without any change in the ratio of poly-A mRNA to total RNA (table 1–1). The stimulation of RNA polymerase is also an early event [19] as is the enhancement of polyamines concentration [20].

More recently other possible candidates for a specific signal have been reported. Using immunofluorescence Samuel et al. [15] showed that tubulin, but not desmin, was redistributed in arrays parallel to the long axis of the myocytes, and became denser around the nuclei. This alteration was observed a few days after a stenosis, in circumstances where there are no mitoses, and was transitory, since it disappeared after a week or two. Simultaneous labeling of myocytes with specific antiisomyosin sera showed that the microtubular change precedes the isomyosin shift suggesting that this type of filament served as a sort of guideline for sarcomere rearrangement [15]. This is probably the first indisputable signal really reported as a true primary event in the development of the hypertrophic process.

PROTEIN SYNTHESIS

We will focus only on sarcomeric proteins and on the heterogeneity of sarcomeric protein turnover, function-related differences in turnover, and turnover during mechanical overload.

Heterogeneity of Contractile Protein Turnover

There are well-established differences between the fractional turnover rate of the different contractile proteins in both cardiac and skeletal muscle (tables 1–2 and 1–3): (i) the fractional turnover rate of myosin heavy chain is approximately twice as fast as that of actin. In ventricular cardiac muscle of the rat, 23% of myosin is renewed every day compared to 11% of the actin [13, 22]. The values for fast skeletal muscle are lower, at 7% for myosin and 3% for actin. These values have been obtained by using the continuous infusion flow technique of Waterlow, Garlick and Millward [23] and using free amino acids of the plasma or tissue as precursors [13, 22]. Data obtained using the specific precursor radioactivity of plasma-free aminoacids are close to that obtained with the more sophisticated determination of amino acyl tRNA [11]. The half-lives of MHC and actin in normal rat ventricles, the tissue in which these values have been most accurately determined, are five and ten days respectively. Different absolute values have been obtained by single pulse experiments or using the double isotope technique, but even with these techniques the turnover rate of myosin heavy chain is approximately twice as rapid as that of actin. This has also been shown in vitro in cardiac cell cultures [25]. These differences are not easily explained but they do reflect the well-known correlation between the molecular weight (M.W. or log M.W.) of protein subunits, and the degradation rate—with the largest molecules showing the

Table 1-2. Half-lives of contractile proteins in fast skeletal muscles (t ½ in days). Relative turnover rates. A > B means that A turns over faster than B. t ½ has been recalculated according to Zilversmit. Proteins are arranged according to the M.W. of their subunits; M.W. are from (1). Note that the M.W. of MLC and TN components are nearly identical. M, MHC, MLC₃, MLC₂ and MLC₁: myosin, myosin heavy and light chains. A: actin. TM: tropomyosin. TNT, I, C: troponin components. LMM and HMM: light and heavy meromyosin.

Reference	MHC	Actin	TM	TNT	MLC$_1$	TNI	MPLC$_2$	TNC	MLC$_3$	Relative turnover rates
42	20 (?)	67	27							LMM = HMM (?) TM > A
43	30									
44	20									
45	165									
46	13	13								
47										TN > TM > A = M
48										MLC$_3$ > MPIC$_2$ > MHC > MLC$_1$
36										TM > MLC > A > MHC
										M > A
49	(20)	52	15	8		8		11		TNT = TNI > TNC >TM > MHC = MLC > A
50										MHC > MLC
24	27									
31										A = M
22	10	25								MHC > A

Table 1–3. Half-lives of contractile proteins in ventricles. See table 1–2 for further explanation.

Reference	MHC	Actin	TM	TNT	MLC_1	TNI	$MPLC_2$	TNC	Relative turnover rates
45	7								
38									
51	17	10							
52	11		11		8		8		MLC > MHC
50									
40	5.9	7.7			9		9		MHC > MLC
53	3 to 6								MHC > A > MLC_1 = MLC_2 depending of the precursor used
54	11								
36									
24	8.6								M > A
55	5.4	10.3	5.5	3.5	8.7	3.2	7.5	5.3	TNI = TNT > TNC > M = TM > MLC_2 > MLC_1 > A
25	2.0	4.7	1.9		1.8		1.6		MLC_2 > MLC_1 ≥ TM ≥ MHC > A
56									TM > MHC > A > MLC_2 > MLC_1
13	3 to 5	4 to 8							MHC > A

fastest rates. [26]. (ii) The turnover of tropomyosin usually approximates that of myosin heavy chains. (iii) Concerning the myosin light chains (MLC), the problem is still unresolved. In fast skeletal myosin, MLC_{3f} and $MPLC_{2f}$ seem to turn over more rapidly than myosin heavy chain while the rate of synthesis of MLC_{1f} appears slower. In the heart, myosin light chains turn over more slowly than heavy chain. (iv) For troponin components the situation has recently been clarified, and in both cardiac and skeletal muscles the tropomyosin binding factor and the inhibitory factor (TNT and TNI) have the same rate of synthesis, which is faster than that of the calcium binding factor, TNC. This corresponds to the instability of TNI and TNT as opposed to the stability of TNC [55].

The turnover rate of the different myosin isoforms has also been measured in rabbit heart. Both α- and β-myosin heavy chain (corresponding to V_1 and V_3 respectively) had the same fractional turnover rate in normal animals (14% per day) [27]. Indirect evidence suggests that the synthesis of the fast isoform of skeletal myosin heavy chain is slower than that of the slow isoform. The skeletal slow form is, according to molecular cloning data, the same as the cardiac β form.

How the entire sarcomere is renewed is a question which has been largely unexplored. Newly synthesized myofilaments are located at the periphery of glycerinated muscle fibers [28, 29]. This was determined by lightly washing labeled myofibrils and determining the specific activity of myosin heavy and light chains, actin, troponin, and tropomyosin [30]. These "easily releasable myofilaments" can be obtained from both cardiac and skeletal muscles, and come apparently from an intermediate pool of free molecules. Kinetic studies suggest that this pool is not a precursor, but more likely represents molecules being degraded. This has been confirmed by others [31, 32].

Turnover of Contractile Proteins in Different Striated Muscles

The heterogeneity of turnover of the different contractile proteins is accompanied by a heterogeneity of turnover of myosin and actin in different striated muscles. As shown in table 4, the renewal of myosin is twice that of actin for a given muscle, and the turnover of each of these proteins is twice as rapid in the ventricles than it is in fast muscle. This has been determined using the same techniques and the same animal to estimate the rate of synthesis [33, 34, 35, 36]. Those differences have been shown for the "easily releasable myofibrils" described above [32]. Earl [24] used the continuous infusion procedure or pulse labelling on dogs, fowl, and rats and found, for example, in the fast posterior latissimus dorsi skeletal muscle of chicken a half-life of 35 days for total proteins compared to values of 14 days in the slow anterior latissimus dorsi and 8 in the cardiac ventricles. As shown by these authors the rate of synthesis correlates with the total RNA concentration. Although a more accurate estimation of the turnover of a well-characterized protein is needed, it is already possible to suggest that a relationships exists between the function of the muscle and its protein turnover rate. It is possible to attribute this relationship to the duration of stimulus [24], (table 1–4). For example the cardiac proteins turn over more rapidly than skeletal muscles whether they are contracting at a rapid rate as in rats [13, 24, 53], or at a slow rate, as in dogs [24] or rabbits [45]. Soleus, a predominantly slow postural muscle, has a rapid turnover and is also working continuously. (The existence of continuous impulses in postural muscles is well-documented.) Smooth muscle, which is also continuously contracting, turns over faster than the heart [24]. These differences are also accompanied by differences in RNA concentration, which is higher in muscles which turn over rapidly [23], and in myosin concentration, which is higher in the heart, suggesting that the enhanced turnover rate leads to net accumulation.

Effect of Increased Work

Mechanical overload stimulates protein synthesis in both the heart and skeletal muscles. This occurs rapidly and leads to hypertrophy which confers an adaptational advantage to skeletal muscle by multiplying the contractile units, and to the heart by multiplying contractile units and normalizing wall stress. Nearly all measurements have been carried out on total proteins, even for heart tissue which, because of its clinical importance, has received the most attention. While there is reason to think that data obtained with total proteins are applicable to myosin and actin, it is of course hazardous to extrapolate.

It was originally shown, by the decay method, that hypertrophy is due both to increased synthesis and decreased breakdown of total proteins. Using the constant infusion method, where the problem of amino acid reutilization can be largely overcome, most of the models of mechanical overload for both heart and skeletal tissue reveal that work-induced striated muscle hypertrophy is associated with an increased synthesis and a paradoxically enhanced lysis, the so-called "wastage effect" [12, 23, 37]. Another important feature, presumably common to all proteins, is the rapidity of the induction process [11]. In fact, as new techniques appear, earlier events have been discovered.

One reasonably complete study dealing with individual contractile proteins is that of Morkin [37], who studied cardiac overload obtained by banding the aorta of rabbits. The labeling of cardiac myosin by lysine four hours after a single injection of tritiated amino acid was used to estimate the rate of synthesis at several time intervals after surgery. The decay curve obtained after an injection given one day before surgery was used to calculate lysis. The results were analyzed by a computerized simulation of myosin metabolism, allowing the rate constant for degradation to be calculated on successive days after coarctation. The best fit is obtained when degradation is either increased [37] or unchanged [38], and the conclusion is that hypertrophy is primarily a consequence of a twofold increase in synthesis.

Whether this activation of synthesis affects the myosin heavy chains (MHC)

Table 1–4. Myosin turnover rates in relation to the speed of shortening, the fiber type, and the myosin content in striated muscles. Fast ventricles: in pigs, humans, dogs. Slow ventricles: in rodents. t ½: see table 1–2 [24, 57, 23].

	Fast skeletal muscle	Slow skeletal muscle	Atria	Slow ventricles	Fast ventricles
t ½ in days					
actomyosin in rats	19	9			
actomyosin in fowls	12	4			
myosin in dogs	27			8	
myosin in rats	165	148			3 to 6
myosin in rabbits				7	1.5
RNA (mg/g f.t.) in fowls	0.8	1.2			
in dogs	0.95	1.18		1.15	
Myosin concentration (mg/g f.t.) in rabbits	27	36		48	
Speed of shortening	fast	slow	fast	slow	fast
Type of activation	discontinuous	± permanent	permanent	permanent	permanent

and the myosin light chain (MLC) equally is controversial [39, 40] but it has been shown [13] that the ratio between the turnover of MHC and actin, normally around 2, remains unchanged. The rates of synthesis (in percent per day) of total protein (ks), as well as myosin heavy chains (ke HC), and actin (ke A), isolated by preparative electrophoresis from myofibrils from which the "easily releasable myofibrils" have been removed, are normally 19% for ke, 23% for ke HC, and 11% for ke A. Four days after an abdominal aortic stenosis, rate of synthesis increased to 37% for ks, 41% for ke HC, and 21% for ke A. The ratio ke HC/ke A, therefore, remained unchanged. The normal heterogeneity in the rates of synthesis of the main contractile proteins was therefore unmodified by cardiac overload, although both of these rates were stimulated [13].

Protein synthesis is stimulated in response to new requirements, but in fact most information on this topic refers to total protein rather than to specific contractile proteins. One important fact is that sarcomere structure is respected [41] and that the stimulation of synthesis and the probable acceleration of breakdown with which it is associated, are most likely harmonious and may apply to all the contractile proteins.

CONTRACTILE PROTEIN GENES

This section is still mainly a catalog more than a comprehensive discussion of regulation, but it appears necessary at this time to review the main data published in this rapidly developing field.

Cardiac Myosin Heavy Chain (MHC) (table 1–5)

The myosin heavy chains are encoded by a multigene family which can be divided into two groups: the sarcomeric and the nonmuscle/smooth muscle myosin heavy chain. Eight to ten sarcomeric MHC genes with highly conservative sequences have been reported in vertebrates [58, 59, 60]. In man, at least three genes coding for this peptide have been assigned to the short arm of chromosome 17. Several skeletal sarcomeric MHC genes in mice are on chromosome 11 [61, 62, 63] while the cardiac genes are found on chromosome 14 [Weydert et al., Proc. Natl. Acad. Sc. USA November 85]. Using different cDNA clones containing cardiac MHC inserts, Mahdavi et al. [60] identified two different MHC genes in rats, α and β, coding for two different MHC, α which is the MHC of the fast isomyosin V_1, and β which is the MHC of the slow isomyosin V_3. Analysis of approximately 50 kb of chromosomal DNA showed that the two genes are organized in tandem, the β gene being 4 kb upstream. The sequence of these genes is very similar in the region coding for the rod part of myosin. The overall sequence is 90–95% homologous. At the 3' end of the genes, sequences are highly divergent and this in fact corresponds to a specific exon.

Some data [60, 64] suggest that in both atria and ventricles two MHC

Table 1–5. Myosin genes. "Tissue" indicates the tissue where the isoform is predominant. Adult tissues except as indicated.

	Main genes	Protein encoded	Tissue	Mode of regulation
Myosin heavy chains (MHC)	MHC_{emb}	MHC_{emb}	embryonic sk. muscle	
	MHC_{neo}	MHC_{neo}	neonatal sk. muscle	
	MHC_f	MHC_f	fast sk. muscle	
	MHC_β	MHC_β	slow sk. muscle and ventricles	MHC_α and β are in tandem and regulated on an antithetic fashion
	MHC_α	MHC_α	atria, ventricles of rodents	differential splicing
	MHC_α	?		differential splicing
Myosin light chains (MLC)	ML_{1f+3f}	MLC_{1f}, MLC_{3f}	fast sk. muscle	
	MLC_{1s}	$MLC_{1s} = MLC_{1v}$	slow sk. muscle and ventricles	
	MLC_{1emb}	$MLC_{emb} = MLC_{1a}$	embryonic sk. muscle, embryonic heart, atria	
			slow sk. muscle	
Myosin phosphorylatable light chains (MPLC)		MLC_{2s}	atria	
	$MPLC_{2a}$	$MPLC_{2a}$	fast sk. muscle	
	$MPLC_{2f}$	$MPLC_{2f}$	slow sk. muscle	
		$MPLC_{3s}$		

mRNAs could exist having a common coding region but differing in sequences located at the 3' terminal and resulting from differential splicing of the above-mentioned exon.

Actin Genes (table 1-6)

At least six isoforms of actin have been reported in mammals (65). Recent studies indicate however that the genome contains more than six different genes. In mice for example, Minty et al. [66] identified specific genes coding for the α skeletal and the α cardiac actin together with genes coding for nonmuscle and smooth muscle actins. In addition, they found a subfamily of sequences resembling those of the actins and very likely resulting from duplications of the original gene(s). Several of these sequences are probably nonfunctional genes, the so-called pseudogenes [67]. More than 20 actin or actin-like genes have been reported in the human genome [68]. Four different subfamilies of actin genes were described by Ponte et al. [68] who showed that in humans the α skeletal and α cardiac actin genes were not repetitive, while the sequences homologous to the nonmuscle cell actin probes were present in multiple copies and are frequently pseudogenes.

Hamada et al. [69] have isolated the human cardiac actin gene. Most of the sequence corresponds to the known protein sequence with one exception: a cysteine located just after the initiation codon. This suggests the existence of a processing mechanism. This gene contains five different introns and a 3' non-coding region of 160-200 bases in length. The human cardiac actin gene's similarity to that of chickens and rats suggests that muscle actin genes in mammals have the same ancestor.

The different actin genes are located on different chromosomes in humans (chromosome 1 for α skeletal, and chromosome 15 for α cardiac [69]) and in mice. In addition it has been shown by genetic back-cross experiments and polymorphism analysis that the different functional actin genes are not linked [66].

Myosin Light Chains (table 1-5)

Using a chicken genomic library, Nabeshima et al. [70] demonstrated that the two nonphosphorylated light chains of skeletal myosin are encoded by the same 18 kb gene made up of nine exons, with exons 1 and 4 being specific for light chain 1, while exons 2 and 3 represent the specific part of the light chain 3. Both light chains have 5 exons in common, exons 5 to 9; and the gene contains two different transcription initiation sites from which the two different precursors are transcribed and then processed by differential splicing. A similar situation has been found in mice and in rats, and genetic linkage analysis demonstrated that the mouse gene is on chromosome 1 [71].

A group of myosin light chain-like sequences has been isolated from a mouse cDNA library [72], one of which—the clone pA29—was specific for the adult ventricular nonphosphorylated myosin light chain 1. This clone contains an insert of 540 bp, which is approximately half the length of the messenger RNA. Subsequent Northern blot analysis showed that this clone also hybridizes with a mRNA in the soleus in skeletal muscle and that in fact ventricular and slow skeletal muscle myosin light chain 1 mRNA are identical. Genomic analysis using R-loop hybridization confirms the existence of a single gene made up of three introns of 1300, 1300, and 250 bp. This gene is located on chromosome 9.

Atrial myosin light chains are different from those of the ventricles, and Arnold et al. [73] have published the sequence of a cDNA clone covering nearly the entire coding region as well as the 3' non-coding regions of the mRNA of chicken atria light chain 2. As in the case of other genes, including actin, putative regulatory sequences have been found, and one of them, AATAAA, which sequences 17 nucleotides upstream from the poly A segment, is a possible polyadenylation signal. Based on secondary structure analysis, the stop codon was found near the 3' end of the noncoding sequence in a stable loop structure. The corresponding mRNA is 727 nucleotides long in its coding region and 69 in the 5' noncoding sequence.

Troponin (table 1–6)

Among the three troponin components, TNT (tropomyosin binding factor), TNI (troponin inhibitory factor), and TNC (troponin calcium binding factor), the TNT gene has been more extensively studied than the others [74, 75]. A cDNA clone was isolated from a cDNA library, which was prepared from adult rat skeletal muscle. This clone does not cross-react with the corresponding slow skeletal- and cardiac-TNT genes and this result confirms other studies showing no immunological cross-reactivity between the different proteins. In addition it was shown that the adult skeletal TNT gene is in fact able to code for at least two different mRNAs, α and β. The corresponding proteins differ by an internal 13 amino acid oligopeptide which is encoded by one of two different exons. Once again, a differential splicing mechanism seems to be an important regulatory process.

Tropomyosins (table 1–6)

Tropomyosin is a dimeric protein, and usually a heterodimer composed of two subunits, α and β. cDNA clones specific for α- and β-tropomyosin subunits have been reported [76 to 81] but one of the most interesting findings of the molecular biology approach is that in fact at least α tropomyosin is heterogeneous. In rats, cDNA clones coding for both tropomyosin from smooth muscle (uterus) and from striated muscle (adult hind leg) have been isolated. The tropomyosins of the two different muscles can be differentiated using a DNA fragment specific for each of them and coding for a so-called isotype-switch peptide. Further studies using S_1 nuclease mapping showed the existence of three different mRNAs. Alpha-1 and α-2 are specific for skeletal muscle, with α-2 being present only in adults; α-3 is specific for smooth

Table 1–6. Thin filament contractile protein genes.

	Main genes	Protein encoded	Tissue	Mode of regulation
Actin	α skeletal	α skeletal	sk. muscle	genes not repetitive, located on several different chromosomes
	α cardiac	α cardiac	ventricles	
	α smooth	α smooth	smooth muscle	
	β smooth	β smooth	nonmuscle cell	
	γ smooth	γ smooth		
	actin	other coding sequences have been reported but protein is unknown		
	pseudogenes			
Tropomyosin	α ⎡ α1 ⎢ α2 ⎣ α3	α subunit	fetal and adult sk. muscle adult sk. muscle (fast) smooth muscle	differential splicing
	β	β subunit	adult (slow) and fetal sk. muscle	
Troponin	TNI TNC TNT TNT ⎡ α ⎣ β	although these proteins exist as isoforms, no corresponding isogenes have so far been reported proteins encoded? no tissue specificity differential splicing		

muscle. Such a situation is also highly suggestive of a differential splicing mechanism using one or several exons in common and three isotype-specific exons.

Regulation of the Expression of the α and β MHC Genes

These two genes are organized in tandem, β being upstream. In the case of rats, this is the order of developmental expression since it is expressed in the fetal heart and is predominant in adult life [82]. Moreover these genes are apparently under hormonal control. It was shown by Lompré et al. [64] that thyroxine stimulates expression of the α MHC gene while that of β MHC is repressed. Conversely hypothyroidism activates β and inhibits α. In these conditions, there is a good correlation between the level of the messenger expressed and the amount of the proteins [64, 83].

Dillman [84] used a different approach, and carried out two-dimensional gel electrophoresis of the proteins, or of their peptide maps, expressed in an in vitro reticulocyte translation system. They found an enhanced synthesis of MHC β and a parallel drop in MHC α in a rat model of experimental diabetes—indirectly suggesting that insulin is also capable of regulating the expression of these genes.

Other data based on protein analysis (electrophoresis, mapping, and various immunological methods), also strongly suggest that the two heavy chain sequences derive from a common ancestral gene, and that they always respond in an antithetic [64] fashion to a given stimulus. The best example, extensively analyzed in another chapter of this book, is cardiac overload in rats. In this model, overload induces a progressive shift from MHC α to MHC β, and this change parallels both the drop in myosin ATPase and the decrease in the shortening velocity [21]. This process is reversible. A more curious example is overload in fast skeletal muscle, where a shift from MHC α to MHC β has been consistently observed in all experimental models studied so far [1].

Coexpression

Alpha-skeletal and α cardiac actin genes differ in both their coding and their noncoding sequences. Several laboratories have shown that, during development, these two genes are coexpressed (table 1–7), for example, in mouse or avian skeletal muscle [85, 88] or in rat fetal heart [86]. Unpublished data from our laboratory show the same situation in adult heart during cardiac overload. In adult human skeletal muscle, 5% of actin mRNA is in cardiac form while 50% of actin messenger in the heart is of the skeletal type. This coexpression is unrelated to chromosomal location since the α skeletal gene in man is on chromosome 1 and α cardiac is on chromosome 15.

Differential Splicing

Currently, this appears to be a rather general mechanism for controlling contractile protein gene expression since it occurs in several groups of genes:

Table 1–7. Coexpression of α skeletal and α cardiac actin genes during development.

		skeletal muscles		Heart	
		fetal	adult	fetal	adult
Mouse	(85)				
	cardiac	+	0	+	+
	skeletal	+	+	0	0
Rat	(86)				
	skeletal		+	+	0
Human	(87)				
	cardiac		+		+
	skeletal		+++		+
Avian	(88)				
	cardiac	+++	0		
	skeletal	+	+++		

troponins [74, 75], the α tropomyosins [76], the non phosphorylated myosin light chains [70], and possibly MHC α [60].

SUMMARY

Mechanical overload is usually tolerated for a long period because of the development of quantitative and qualitative adaptational factors. The stimulation of gene expression is rapid and, within hours after aortic constriction, increases in incorporation of radioactive amino acids and in both total and poly-A-containing RNA become significant. Within several days, isomyosin changes can be observed together with a possible signal in the form of an increased density of the microtubular network. In normal muscles, contractile protein turnover is definitely heterogeneous, and the rate of synthesis of myosin is more rapid than that of actin. The turnover of these proteins is also faster in the heart than in skeletal muscle, and faster in the slow than in the fast skeletal muscle. This is probably related to the permanency of the contractile stimulus. Mechanical overload stimulates synthesis but a paradoxical increased lysis is also well documented. This activation is harmonious and involves all proteins. Contractile protein genes are reviewed in order to point out future directions of research. The myosin heavy chains (MHC) are encoded by at least eight to ten different genes, among which the MHC α and MHC β are organized in tandem and are regulated in an antithetic fashion. The MLC_{1f} and MLC_{3f} proteins are products of differential splicing from a common unique gene. The same process apparently occurs for TNT α and β mRNA and for α tropomyosin isoforms $α_1$, $α_2$, and $α_3$. Actin genes are numerous, and genes coding for the six known isoforms have been described together with a number of pseudogenes. Alpha-skeletal and α cardiac genes are frequently coexpressed in adult muscles or during development.

REFERENCES

1. Swynghedauw, B. Developmental and functional adaptation of contractile proteins in cardiac and skeletal muscles. 1986 *Physiol. Reviews.* 66:210–221.
2. Swynghedauw, B., and Delcayre, C. 1982. Biology of cardiac overload. *Pathobiol. Ann.* 12:137–183.
3. Lompré, A.M., Schwartz, K., d'Albis, A., Lacombe, G., Thiem, N.V., and Swynghedauw, B. 1979. Myosin isozymes redistribution in chronic heart overloading. *Nature.* 282:105–107.
4. Mercadier, J.J., Lompré, A.M., Wisnewsky, C., Samuel J.L., Bercovici, J., Swynghedauw, B., Schwartz, K. 1981. Myosin isoenzymic changes in several models of rat cardiac hypertrophy. *Circ. Res.* 49:525–532.
5. Mercadier, J.J., Bouveret, P., Gorza, L., Schiaffino, S., Clark, W.A., Zak, R., Swynghedauw, B., and Schwartz, K. 1983. Myosin isoenzymes in normal and hypertrophied human ventricular myocardium. *Circ. Res.* 53:52–62.
6. Younes, A., Schneider, J.M., Bercovici, J., and Swynghedauw, B. 1985. Creatine kinase isoenzymes redistribution in chronically overloaded myocardium. *Cardiovasc. Res.* 19:15–19.
7. Revis, N.W., Thomson, R.Y., Cameron, A.J.V. 1977. Lactate dehydrogenase isoenzymes in the human hypertrophic heart. *Cardiovasc. Res..* 11:172–176.
8. Charlemagne, D., Mansier, P., Preteseille, M., Swynghedauw, B., and Lelievre, L.G. 1984. Hypertrophied rat heart. New Na+, K+−ATPase-ouabain interactions in sarcolemnal vesicles. *Europ. Heart J.* 5 suppl. F, 315–322.
9. Zak, R. 1985. The role of protein synthesis and degradation in cardiac growth. In *The Developing Heart.* M.J. Legato, ed. Boston; Martinus Nijhoff Publishing, pp. 191–204.
10. Hatt, P.Y., Ledoux, C., and Bonvalet, J.P. 1965. Lyse et synthèse des protéines myocardiques au cours de l'insuffisance cardiaque experimentale. *Arch. Mal. Coeur* 58:1703–1721.
11. Everett, A.W., Sparrow, M.P., and Taylor, R.R. 1979. Early changes in myocardial proteins synthesis in vivo in response to right ventricular pressure overload in the dog. *J. Mol. Cell Cardiol.* 11:1253–1263.
12. Moalic J.M., Bercovici, J., and Swynghedauw, B. 1981. Protein synthesis in systolic and diastolic overloading in rat. A comparative study. *Cardiovasc. Res.* 15:515–521.
13. Moalic J.M., Bercovici, J., and Swynghedauw, B. 1984. Myosin heavy chain and actin fractional rate of synthesis in normal and overloaded rat heart ventricles. *J. Mol. Cell. Cardiol.* 16:875–884.
14. Schreiber, S.S., Oratz, M., Rothschild, M.A. 1967. Effects of acute overload on protein synthesis in cardiac muscle microsomes. *Am. J. Physiol.* 213:1552–1555.
15. Samuel, J.L., Bertier, B., Bugaisky, L., Marotte, F., Swynghedauw, B., Schwartz, K., and Rappaport, L. 1984. Different distributions of microtubules, desmin filaments, and isomyosins during the onset of cardiac hypertrophy in the rat. *Eur. J. Cell Biol.* 34:300–306.
16. Schreiber, S.S., Evans, C.D., Oratz, M, and Rothschild, M.A. 1981. Protein synthesis and degradation in cardiac stress. *Circ. Res.* 48:601–611.
17. Swynghedauw, B., Moalic, J.M., Bouveret, P., Bercovici, J., de la Bastie, D., and Schwartz, K. 1984. Messenger RNA content and complexity in normal and overloaded rat heart. *Eur. Heart J.* 5 (suppl. F):211–218.
18. Cutilletta A.F. 1984. Myosin heavy chain mRNA during the development and regression of myocardial hypertrophy. *Eur. Heart J.* 5 (suppl F):193–198.
19. Cutilletta A.F. 1981. Muscle and non-muscle cell RNA polymerase activities in early myocardial hypertrophy. *Am. J. Physiol.* 240:H901–H907.
20. Caldarera C.M., Orlandini, G., Casti, A., and Moruzzi, G. 1974. Polyamine and nucleic acid metabolism in myocardial hypertrophy of the overloaded heart. *J. Mol. Cell Cardiol* 6:95–104.
21. Schwartz, K., Lecarpentier, Y., Martin, J.L., Lompré, A.M., Mercadier, J.J., and Swynghedauw, B. 1981. Myosin isoenzymic distribution correlates with speed of myocardial contraction. *J. Mol. Cell Cardiol* 13:1071–1075.
22. Bates, P.C., Grimble G.K., Sparrow, M.P., and Millward D.J. 1983. Myofibrillar protein turnover. *Biochem. J.* (219):593–605.
23. Waterlow J.C., Garlick, P.J., Millard, D.J. 1978. *Protein turnover in mammalian tissues and in the whole body.* Amsterdam, North Holland.
24. Earl C.A., Laurent, G.F., Everett, A.W., Bonnin, C.M., Sparrow, M.P. 1978. Turnover rates of muscle proteins in cardiac and skeletal muscles of dog, fowl, rat, and mouse:turnover rate related to muscle function. *Aust. J. Exp. Biol. Med. Sci.* 56:265–277.

25. Clark W.A., and Zak, R. 1981. Assessment of fractional rates of protein synthesis in cardiac muscle cultures after equilibrium labelling. *J. Biol. Chem.* 256:4863–4870.
26. Goldberg A.L. and Dice, J.F. 1974. Intracellular protein degradation in mammalian and bacterial cells. *Annual Review of Biochemistry.* 43:835–869.
27. Everett A.W., Prior, G., Zak R. 1981. Equilibration of leucine between the plasma compartment and leucyl-tRNA in the heart, and turnover of cardiac myosin heavy chain. Biochem. J. 194:365–368.
28. Morkin, E. 1972. Postnatal muscle fiber assembly: localization of new synthesis and degradation during development of cardiac hypertrophy in the rabbit. *Circ. Res.* 30:690–702.
29. Westhuyzen, D.R. Matsumoto, K., Etlinger, J.D. 1981. Easily releasable myofilaments from skeletal and cardiac muscle maintained in vitro. *J. Biol. Chem.* 256:11791–11797.
30. Etlinger, J.D., Zak, R., Fischman, D.A., Rabinowitz, M. 1975. Isolation of newly synthetized myosin filaments from skeletal muscle homogenates and myofibrils. *Nature* 255:259–261.
31. Lobley, G.E., Lovie, J.M. 1979. The synthesis of myosin, actin and the major protein fractions in rabbit skeletal muscle. *Biochem. J.* 182:867–874.
32. Aumont, M.C., Bercovici, J., Berson, G., Leger, J., Preteseille, M., Swynghedauw, B. 1980. The incorporation of radioactive lysine or tyrosine into cardiac and skeletal myofibrillar and non-myofibrillar contractile proteins. *Biomedicine* 32:139–143.
33. Biron, P., Dreyfus, J.C., Schapira, F. 1964. Différences métaboliques entre les muscles rouges et blancs chez le lapin. *C.R. Soc. Biol.* 158:1841–1843.
34. Kazaryan, V.A., Goncharova, L.A., Zelina, I.A., Rapoport, E.A. 1975. The biosynthesis of proteins and ribonucleic acids in red and white skeletal muscles of rats. *Biokhimiya* 40: 242–247.
35. Kimata, S., Morkin, E. 1971. Comparison of myosin synthesis in heart and red and white skeletal muscles. *Am. J. Physiol.* 221:1706–1713.
36. Swick, R.W., Song, W. 1974. Turnover of various muscle proteins. *J. Anim. Sci.* 38:1150–1157.
37. Morkin, E., Kimata, S., Skillman, J.J. 1972. Myosin synthesis and degradation during development of cardiac hypertrophy in the rabbit. *Circ. Res.* 30:690–702.
38. Morkin, E., Yazaki, Y., Katagiri, T., Laraia, P.J. 1973. Comparison of the synthesis of the light and heavy chains of adult skeletal myosin. *Biochim. Biophys. Acta* 324:420–429.
39. Evans, C., Schreiber, S.S., Oratz, M., Rothschild, M.A. 1978. Synthesis of myosin heavy and light chains in the after loaded guinea pig right ventricle. *Cardiovasc. Res.* 12:731–734.
40. Zak, R., Martin, A.F., Prior, G., Rabinowitz, M. 1977. Comparison of turnover of several myofibrillar proteins and critical evaluation of double isotope method. *J. Biol. Chem.* 252: 3430–3435.
41. Hatt, P.Y., Berjal, G., Moravec, J., Swynghedauw, B. 1970. Heart failure: and electron microscropic study of the left ventricular papillary muscle in aortic insufficiency in the rabbit. *J. Mol. Cell. Cardiol.* 1:235–247.
42. Velick, S.F. 1956. The metabolism of myosin, the meromyosin, actin and tropomyosin in the rabbit. *Biochim. Biophys. Acta* 20:228–236.
43. Dreyfus, J.C., Kruh, J., Schapira, G. 1960. Metabolism of myosin and life time of myofibrils. *Biochem. J.* 75:574–578.
44. MacManuc, J.R., Mueller, H. 1966. The metabolism of myosin and the meromyosins from rabbit skeletal muscle. *J. Biol. Chem.* 241:5967–5973.
45. Kimata, S., Morkin, E. 1971. Comparison of myosin synthesis in heart and red and white skeletal muscles. *Am. J. Physiol.* 221:1706–1713.
46. Funabiki R., Cassens, R.G. 1972. Heterogeneous turnover of myofibrillar protein. *Nature* 236:249.
47. Morkin, E., Yazaki, Y., Katagiri, T., Laraia, P.J. 1973. Comparison of the synthesis of the light and heavy chains of adult skeletal myosin. *Biochim. Biophys. Acta* 324:420–429.
48. Low, R.B., Golberg, A.L., 1973. Nonuniform rates of turnover of myofibrillar proteins in rat diaphragm. *J. Cell. Biol.* 56:590–595.
49. Koizumi, T. 1974. Turnover rates of structural proteins of rabbit skeletal muscle. *J. Biochem.* Tokyo 76:431–439.
50. Lagrange, B.M., Low, R.B. 1976. Turnover of myosin heavy and light chains in cultured embryonic chick cardiac and skeletal muscle. *Develop. Biol.* 54:214–229.
51. Wikman-Coffelt, J., Zelis, R., Fenner, C., Mason, D.T. 1973. Studies on the synthesis and

degradation of light and heavy chains of cardiac myosin, *J. Biol. Chem.* 248:5206–5207.

52. Rabinowitz, M. 1979. Overview on pathogenesis of cardiac hypertrophy. *Circ. Res.* 35:Suppl II:3–11.
53. Martin, A.F., Rabinowitz, M., Blough, R., Prior, C. Zak, R. 1977. Measurement of half-life of rat cardiac myosin heavy chain with leucyl-t RNA as precursor pool. *J. Biol. Chem.* 252:3422–3429.
54. Wyborny, L.E., Kritcher, E.M., Luchi, R.J. 1978. Synthesis of guinea pig cardiac myosins as measured by constant infusion. *Biochem. J.* 170:189–192.
55. Martin, A.F. 1981. Turnover of troponin subunits. *J. Biol. Chem.* 256:964–968.
56. Evans, C.D., Schreiber, S.S., Oratz, M., Rothschild, M.A. 1981. Relative synthesis of cardiac contractile proteins. Evidence for synthesis from the same precursor pool. *Biochem. J.* 194:673–678.
57. Everett, A.W., Prior, G., Clark, W.A., Zak, R. 1983. Quantitation of myosin in muscle. *Anal. Biochem.* 130:102–107.
58. Nguyen, H.T., Gubits, R.M., Wydro, R.M., Nadal-Ginard, B. 1982. Sarcomeric myosin heavy chain is coded by a highly conserved multigene family. *Proc. Natl. Acad. Sci. USA* 79:5230–5234.
59. Mahdavi, V., Periasamy, M., Nadal-Ginard B. 1982. Molecular characterization of two myosin heavy chain genes expressed in the adult heart. *Nature* 297:659–664.
60. Mahdavi, V., Chambers, A.P., Nadal-Ginard B. 1984. Cardiac α- and β-myosin heavy chain genes are organized in tandem. *Proc. Natl. Acad. Sci. USA.* 81:2626–2630.
61. Leinwand, L.A. Saez, L., McNally, E., Nadal-Ginard, B. 1983. Isolation and characterization of human myosin heavy chain genes. *Proc. Natl. Acad. Sci. USA.* 80:3716–3720.
62. Leinwand, L.A., Fournier, R.E.K., Nadal-Ginard, B., Shows, T.B. 1983. Multigene family for sarcomeric myosin heavy chain in mouse and human DNA: localization on a single chromosome. *Science* 221:766–769.
63. Czosnek, H., Nudel, V., Shani, M., Barker, P.E., Pravtcheva, D., Ruddle, F.H., Yaffe, D. 1982. The genes coding for the muscle contractile proteins, myosin heavy chain, myosin light chain 2 and skeletal muscle actin are located on three different mouse chromosomes. *EMBO J.* 1:1299–1305.
64. Lompré, A.M., Nadal-Ginard, B., Mahdavi, V. 1984. Expression of the cardiac ventricular α and β-myosin heavy chain genes is developmentally and hormonally regulated. *J. Biol. Chem.* 259:6437–6446.
65. Vandekerchove, J. Weber, K. 1979. The complete amino acid sequence of actins from bovine aorta, bovine heart, bovine fast skeletal muscle and rabbit slow skeletal muscle. *Differentiation.* 14:123–133.
66. Minty, A.J., Alonso, S., Guenet, J.L., Buckingham, M.E. 1983. Number and organization of actin-related sequences in the mouse genome. *J. Mol. Biol.* 167:77–101.
67. Engel, J., Gunning, P., Kedes, L. 1982. Human actin proteins are encoded by a multigene family. In *Muscle development: molecular and cellular control*, ed. M.L. Pearson, H.F. Epstein. Cold Spring Harbor Lab. p. 107–117.
68. Ponte, P., Gunning, P., Blau, H., Kedes, L. 1983. Human actin genes are single copy for α-skeletal and α-cardiac actin but multicopy for β- and y-cytoskeletal genes: 3' untranslated regions are isotype specific but also conserved in evolution. *Mol. Cell. Biol.* 3:1783–1791.
69. Hamada, H., Petrino, M.G., Kakunaga, T. 1982. Molecular structure and evolutionary origin of human cardiac muscle actin gene. *Proc. Natl. Acad. Sci. USA:* 79:5901–5905.
70. Nabeshima, Y., Fujii-Kuriyama, Y., Muramatsu, M., Ogata K. 1984. Alternative transcription and two modes of splicing result in two myosin light chains from one gene. *Nature* 308:333–338.
71. Robert, B., Barton, P., Minty, A., Daubas, P., Weydert, A., Bonhomme, F., Catalan, J., Chazottes, D., Guenet, J.L., Buckingham, M. 1985. Investigation of genetic linkage between myosin and actin genes using an interspecific mouse back-mouse. *Nature* 314:181–182.
72. Barton, P.J.R., Cohen, A., Robert, B., Fiszman, M.Y., Bonhomme, F., Guenet, J.L., Leader, D.P., Buckingham, M.E. 1985. The myosin alkali light chain of mouse ventricular and slow skeletal muscle are indistinguishable and are encoded by the same gene. *J. Biol. Chem.* 260:8578–8584.
73. Arnold, H.H., Kranskopf, M., Siddiqui, M.A.Q. 1983. The nucleotide sequence of myosin light chain (L-2A) mRNA from embryonic chicken cardiac muscle tissue. *Nucleic Acids Res.* 11:1123–1131.

74. Medford, R.M., Nguyen, H.T., Destree, A.T., Summers, E., Nadal-Ginard, B. 1984. A novel mechanism of alternative RNA splicing for the developmentally regulated generation of troponin T isoform for a single gene. *Cell* 38:409–421.
75. Breitbart, R.E., Nguyen, H.T., Medford, R.M., Destree, A.T., Mahdavi, V., Nadal-Ginard, B. 1985. Intricate combinatorial patterns of exon splicing generate multiple regulated troponin T isoforms from a single gene. *Cell* 41:67–82.
76. Ruiz-Opazo, N., Weinberger, J., Nadal-Ginard, B. 1985. Comparison of α-tropomyosin sequences from smooth and striated muscle. *Nature* 315:67–70.
77. Garfinkel, L.I., Periasamy, M., Nadal-Ginard, B. 1982. Cloning and characterization of cDNA sequences corresponding to myosin light chains 1, 2 and 3 troponin C, troponin T, α-tropomyosin and α-actin. *J. Biol. Chem.* 257:11078–11086.
78. Hastings, K.E.M., Emerson, C.P. Jr. 1982. cDNA clone analysis of six co-regulated mRNAs encoding skeletal muscle contractile proteins. *Proc. Natl. Acad. Sci.* USA 79:1553–1557.
79. MacLeod, A.R. 1981. Separation of the mRNAs coding for α- and β-tropomyosin. *FEBS Lett.* 130:227–229.
80. MacLeod, A.R. 1981. Construction of bacterial plasmids containing sequences complementary to chicken α-tropomyosin mRNA. *Nucleic Acid Res.* 9:2675–2689.
81. MacLeod, A.R. 1982. Distinct α-tropomyosin mRNA sequences in chicken skeletal muscle. *Eur. J. Biochem.* 126:293–297.
82. Lompré, A.M., Mercadier, J.J., Wisnewsky, C., Bouveret, P., Pantaloni, C., d'Albis, A., Schwartz, K. 1981. Species and age-dependent changes in the mammals. *Develop. Biol.* 84: 286–290.
83. Dillmann, W.H., Barrieux, A., Neeley, W.E., Contreras, P. 1983. Influence of thyroid hormone on the in vitro translational activity of specific mRNAs in the rat heart. *J. Biol. Chem.* 258:7738-7745.
84. Dillmann, W.H., Barrieux, A., Reese, G.S. 1984. Effect of diabetes and hypothyroidism on the predominance of cardiac myosin heavy chains synthesized in vivo or in a cell-free system. *J. Biol. Chem.* 259:2035–2038.
85. Minty, A.J., Alonso, S., Caravatti, M., Buckingham, M.E. 1982. A fetal skeletal muscle actin mRNA in the mouse and its identity with cardiac actin mRNA. *Cell* 30:185–192.
86. Mayer, Y., Czonek, H., Zeelon, P.E., Yaffe, D., Nudel, U. 1984. Expression of the genes coding for the skeletal muscle and cardiac actins in the heart. *Nucleic Acid Res.* 12:1087–1100.
87. Gunning, P., Poule, P., Blan, H., Kedes, K. 1983. α-skeletal and α-cardiac actin genes are coexpressed in adult human skeletal muscle and heart. *Mol. Cell. Biol.* 3:1985–1995.
88. Paterson, B.M., Eldridge, J.D. 1984. α cardiac actin is the major sarcomeric isoform expressed in embryonic avian skeletal muscle. *Science* 224:1436–1438.

2. CELL STRESS AND THE INITIATION OF GROWTH

GRAEME L. HAMMOND

The cardiac cell must function in a universe whose very fabric favors disorder over order, disarray over structure. Irresistible forces of nature, true to the second law of thermodynamics, constantly drive the ordered structure of cells to the disordered, random collection of their component elements [1]. Order cannot be maintained, or arise out of chaos, without help. In all systems, physical or biological this help comes only in the form of energy. Consequently cellular structure and function are inextricably interwoven in an inseparable relationship with energy. The energy required to maintain cellular order, however, cannot be used to perform work, and, as nature will have it, the more work that is performed, the more energy must then be diverted to maintain cellular order. The energy-structure relationship is uniquely illustrated by the physical chemistry of covalent bonds.

We remember from elementary chemistry that when hydrogen and oxygen are ignited, energy is liberated as covalent bonds are formed. If the same amount of energy is driven back into the newly formed water molecules, covalent bonds are broken and hydrogen and oxygen reappear. Variations of this simple principle form the basis for all biological energy transfers and explain not only how a cell derives energy but also how and why cellular

This research has been supported by NIH grant HL-25699.

structures must yield and degrade. For example, an energy equivalent of approximately 80 Kcal/mol are required to rupture a C-C bond. Although it is difficult to precisely measure the energy absorbed by cardiac proteins during contraction, force generation can be converted into mcal/g [2] as can the energy derived from oxidative metabolism. At an O_2 consumption of 9 ml/min per 100 g of heart muscle, approximately 8 Kcal/hr of energy is generated by the average adult human heart. Although this seems like a manageable amount of wear and tear, it is well to remember that there is a minimum of 6×10^{23} carbon-carbon linkages per mole of any substance containing two or more carbon atoms, and the rupture of only one linkage renders any protein functionally useless. As a result, the half-life of cardiac proteins is only four to six days for just the normal maintenance of physiologic activity [3]. Therefore, random degradation of proteins, including those at or near the breaking point, is the counterpart to protein synthesis that forms the essential symmetry permeating most, if not all, natural phenomena. On their way from cradle to grave, the contractile protein's short life span consists of performing work, absorbing energy, and becoming the substrate for enzymatic degradation.

Under normal operating conditions, cardiac cells direct energy into work production and order maintenance by adjusting coronary blood flow so that oxidation proceeds aerobically. The key to understanding cardiac stress is to recognize that the heart must adapt to a prolonged alteration in the normal balance between aerobic energy supply and energy expenditure per cell while, simultaneously, maintaining critical cell functions and cellular order. These requirements can only be met by temporarily turning off, or throttling down, many non-imminently essential cell functions. Since all cells must have a mechanism for adjusting to stress, the resulting stress response is not unique to the heart.

In general, the response to a sublethal stress in any organ is growth. For example, a physiologic, or pathophysiologic, stimulus provokes increased heart size after aortic banding, kidney size after unilateral nephrectomy, or restoration of liver size after hepatic lobectomy. Whether the imposed stress is an increase in mechanical work, in active transport of sodium, or in synthesis of albumin, the end result is the same, and all are related to changes in cellular energy requirements induced by altered environmental situations.

Bear in mind, however, that hypertrophy is only the final visible result of a sequence of complex and precisely programmed events that are extremely difficult to unravel. A deeper level of insight into hypertrophy, or the stress response, emerges as one analyzes the immediate cellular events that are produced by stress before cellular changes—such as polyploidization of nuclei, mitochondrial multiplication, and fibroblast proliferation—occur. In this regard, the heart plays a unique role since its need for energy is so clearly tied to mechanical work which, in turn, can be precisely monitored and easily observed.

EARLY RESPONSES TO STRESS OCCUR IN THE NUCLEUS

If the eventual outcome of cellular stress is growth, then an overall increase in protein synthesis must occur. As will be discussed later, however, quantifying protein synthesis is not simple and the rate at which labeled amino acids are incorporated into protein can be interpreted in many ways.

Less controversial is the observation that mRNA synthesis increases in response to stress. It is less controversial, however, only if:

1. measurements do not depend upon scintillation counting of labeled nucleotides administered to intact cells (which raise the same problems that plague interpretation of data from protein synthesis) and,
2. data are obtained from in vivo experiments, thereby avoiding the uncertainty of whether metabolic changes are related to the experimental conditions one wishes to study or to the trauma of extirpation for experiments conducted in vitro. In our experience, the conditions required for retention of normal metabolic function are extremely exacting and it is impossible to reproduce these conditions in any in vitro system.

We have avoided these problems by analyzing translational activity of RNA, extracted from intact, in situ, hearts that were subjected to various forms of stress. Translational activity provides an extremely accurate measurement of the proportion of mRNA in any particular sample of total RNA extracted from cells. Since it is not necessary to extract all mRNA from tissues, one is freed from the errors involved in total extraction. Translational activity therefore represents the ratio between mRNA to other RNA species in the portion of RNA being examined. The disadvantage of this technique is that mRNAs that synthesize proteins of over 80 kD do not translate well in in vitro systems.

Shown in figure 2-1 are SDS gels of proteins translated in vitro by equal amounts of RNA extracted from the right and left ventricle of a dog one hour after producing an 80 mm Hg gradient across the ascending aorta. The increased translational activity of the stressed left ventricle is obvious in comparison to the nonstressed right ventricle.

An alteration in the rate of RNA synthesis, produced by stress, may occur either by changes in chromatin template activity or RNA polymerase activity. This question was addressed by Cutilletta, who used homologous RNA polymerase II to measure chromatin template activity. He found that template activity increased one day after aortic constriction, but the RNA polymerase activity itself did not. However, three days after aortic constriction, RNA polymerase activity did increase [4]. Therefore, it appears that the initial and immediate increase in mRNA is due to a change in template activity, but the sustained increase in RNA synthesis is due to increased polymerase activity.

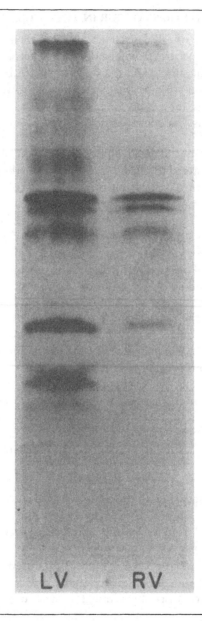

Figure 2–1. Translation products produced by 5 μg of RNA from normal right and hypertrophying left ventricles of a canine heart. (From Hammond, G.L., Wieben, E. and Markert, C.L.: Molecular signals for initiating protein synthesis in organ hypertrophy. *Proc. Natl. Acad. Sci. USA* 76:2455–2459, 1979.)

AN IMMEDIATE AND UNIVERSAL RESPONSE
TO STRESS IS STRESS PROTEIN SYNTHESIS

A considerable volume of literature has appeared recently describing the stress response in a variety of organisms and cells in culture that have been subjected to heat shock. These systems all produce the so-called heat-shock proteins (or, more properly, stress proteins) that have been found in species from bacteria to humans and are produced by many varieties of cellular stress [5]. Studies of cell cultures showed that stress proteins are synthesized following hypoxia [6], uncouplers of oxidative phosphorylation, inhibitors of electron transport, and blockers of hydrogen receptors such as actinomycin A [7], arsenate [7] and cyanide [8].

Figure 2–2 shows two-dimensional autoradiograms of translation products directed by RNAs extracted from tissue samples of canine right ventricle before and after one hour of heat shock [9]. Four newly synthesized stress protein mRNAs (and hence stress proteins) can be seen following stress induction. Otherwise, the autoradiograms are indistinguishable. Our analyses of stress proteins by isoelectric focusing and gel electrophoresis indicate that they have a molecular weight of approximately 70–71 kD (figure 2–3) and that they have acidotic isoelectric points as shown in figure 2–4. Numerous stress proteins have recently been discovered, but by far the most common is the sp 70.

The biological significance of stress proteins is unknown, but the following statements can now be made with a reasonable degree of certainty:

1. The proteins are absolutely essential for growth, both in response to stress and for differentiation and development [10].
2. Stress proteins entail a major redirection of the activities of the cell. During hyperthermia in E. Coli, for example, stress proteins constitute nearly a quarter of the protein mass of the cell [11].
3. The general pattern and time course of heat shock response is similar from bacteria to humans.

The finding of such strong homology from species to species of the stress proteins themselves, is truly unprecedented. Preliminary data of our own gives some idea of the unifying effect stress proteins have had on understanding the stress responses in all species studied so far. Figure 2–5 shows hybridization experiments conducted in our laboratory by P. Havre, Ph.D. using the nick-translated sp 70 DNA from Drosophila (cloned by Schedl) [12] as a probe for identifying sp 70 gene activation in a dog heart. Recently, a high degree of homology between the Drosophila sp 70 gene and human sp 70 gene has been demonstrated [13].

Conservation to this extent portends an importance of this gene, the magnitude of which is still not known. Understanding the regulation of stress protein synthesis, how these proteins function and the role they may play in adaptation will doubtless provide deep insights into the nature of cellular organization.

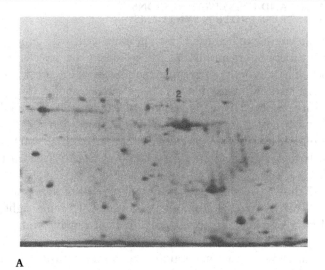

A

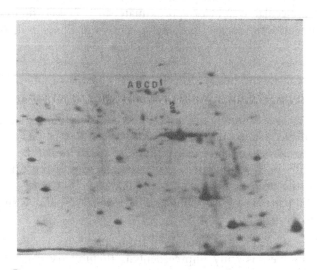

B

Figure 2 **(a)** Two-dimensional autofluorograms of translation products directed by mRNA extracted from canine ventricle before dog was subjected to 1 h of heat shock. Normal occurring reference proteins 1 and 2 labeled.

(b) Two-dimensional autofluorograms of translation products from same heart as in 2a after 1 h of heat shock. Newly synthesized 71 kD stress proteins A, B, C and D appear to the left of reference proteins. Other than the presence of stress proteins, the pre- and post-stress patterns are indistinguishable. (From Lai, Y-K, Havre, P.A., and Hammond, G.L.: Heat shock stress initiates simultaneous transcriptional and translational changes in the dog heart. *Biochem Biophys Res Comm* 134:166–171, 1986.)

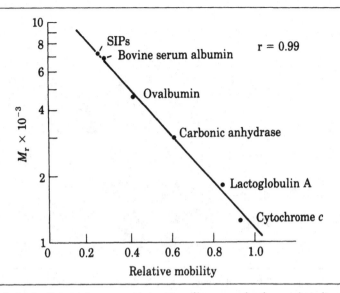

Figure 2–3. Molecular weight curve with proteins of known molecular weight indicates that stress-induced proteins (SIPs) have a molecular weight of 70,000–71,000. (From Hammond, G.L., Lai, Y-K, and Markert, C.L.: Diverse forms of stress lead to new patterns of gene expression through a common and essential metabolic pathway. *Proc. Natl. Acad. Sci. USA* 79:3485–3488, 1982.)

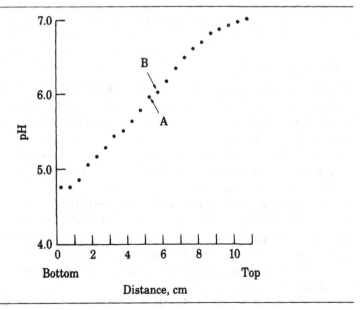

Figure 2–4. Isoelectric point curve indicates that stress proteins have isoelectric points between 5.8 and 6.1 (A & B). (From Hammond, G.L., Lai, Y-K, and Markert, C.L.: Diverse forms of stress lead to new patterns of gene expression through a common and essential metabolic pathway. *Proc. Natl. Acad. Sci. USA* 79:3485–3488, 1982.)

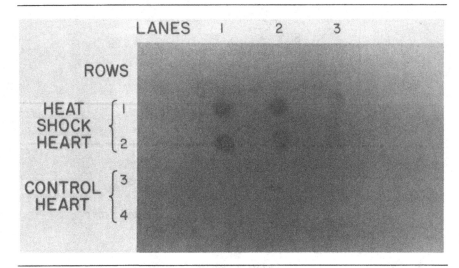

Figure 2–5. Drosophila HSP 70 and canine sp 71 mRNA hybridization. RNA was extracted and mRNA isolated following oligo dT cellulose chromatography. Following glyoxylation, 4 μl of mRNA was spotted onto prewashed nitrocellulose. Lanes 1, 2, and 3 contained 5.2, 2.6, and 1.3 μg of mRNA from heat-stressed canine heart; applied in duplicate (rows 1 and 2). Lanes 1, 2, and 3 contained 6.4, 3.2 1.6 μg of mRNA from control heart, applied in duplicate rows (3 and 4). After a 17 h prehybridization step at 42°, the blot was probed with nick-translated pBR322 with a 2.2 kb insert, containing 95% of the 70 kD heat shock protein mRNA coding sequence (provided by P. Schedl). Following a 22 h hybridization step at 42°, the blot was washed four times in 2 × NaCl-citrate, 0.1% SDS, and two times at 50° in 0.1 × NaCl-citrate, 0.1% SDS. Hybridization can clearly be seen between the probe and canine sp 71 mRNA (rows 1 and 2), whereas mRNA from control canine hearts contains no sp 71 mRNA (rows 3 and 4).

STRESS RECOGNITION

A fundamental question is: how does the heart recognize stress or, in other words, how does the heart translate a physiological impulse such as pressure overload, into a biochemical signal that initiates stress protein synthesis and, subsequently, hypertrophy?

There are two clinical observations that may provide a clue. First is the association of angina with both aortic stenosis and coronary artery disease, and second is the observation that the ventricles of patients with aortic stenosis often resemble those of patients with advanced triple-coronary artery disease. Provided there are no large areas of transmural infarction, the hearts in both clinical conditions may develop fibrotic, noncompliant, hypertrophied ventricles. The observation that ventricular hypertrophy occurs with coronary artery disease, often in the absence of etiological factors such as hypertension, is well documented [14, 15].

The common denominator for both pathological conditions, whether produced by decreased blood supply or increased cardiac work, is a prolonged discordance between energy requirements and energy expenditure per cell. If this discordance is severe, the cell dies; but if intermittent or less severe, the difference between energy requirement and aerobic energy production is made up by glycolysis, resulting in lactic acid synthesis. Alterations in the balance between energy supply and energy expenditure may be the universal mechanism by which cells recognize stress and respond in ways that compensate for environmental changes. We studied the association between cellular acidosis and stress protein synthesis in several ways.

First, we applied four different forms of stress to intact rats, and then analyzed the cardiac RNA-translation products [16]. One group underwent aortic banding for one hour, a second group underwent core hyperthermia to 42° for one hour, a third group was slowly cooled over 90 minutes to 18°, and a fourth group swam to exhaustion which required approximately one hour. In all cases, the cardiac metabolic rate was increased either by swimming, shivering, pressure overload, or hyperthermia. Following termination of the experiments, the RNA was extracted, translated, the proteins resolved by two-dimensional electrophoresis and visualized by autoradiography. Only two stresses provoked cardiac stress protein synthesis: aortic banding and heat shock. Autoradiograms from control hearts and hearts responding to stress are shown in figure 2–6. Two salient features are apparent, first, like those obtained from the dog heart in figure 2–2, the protein patterns are indistinguishable except for the presence of stress proteins in stressed hearts; and, secondly, hearts stressed by heat shock synthesized stress proteins in greater abundance than those stressed by aortic banding.

In order to determine if there was a relationship between these findings and the utilization of energy, we analyzed cardiac lactic acid concentration as an indicator of the metabolic condition of the heart muscle after the four stresses. The findings from these experiments are shown in table 2–1. As can be seen, not only was there an association between lactic acid content and stress protein synthesis, but, the greater the concentration of lactic acid, the greater the concentration of stress protein.

In a second group of experiments, the correlation between stress protein synthesis, arterial pH and lactic acidosis was studied. Dogs were heated to 42° C with a heat exchanger placed between the femoral vessels. At approximately

Table 2–1. Lactic acid content of control and stimulated rat hearts. (From Hammond, G.L., Lai, Y-K, and Markert, C.L.: Diverse forms of stress lead to new patterns of gene expression through a common and essential metabolic pathway. *Proc. Natl. Acad. Sci. USA* 79:3485–3488, 1982.)

Treatment	n	Lactic acid, mg/g
Control	8	0.696 ± 0.090
Banded	4	$1.440 \pm 0.180*$
Heat shock	4	$7.348 \pm 0.510*$
Cold shock	4	0.861 ± 0.125
Swimming	4	0.690 ± 0.191

Results are shown as mean ± SEM.
* $P < 0.01$.

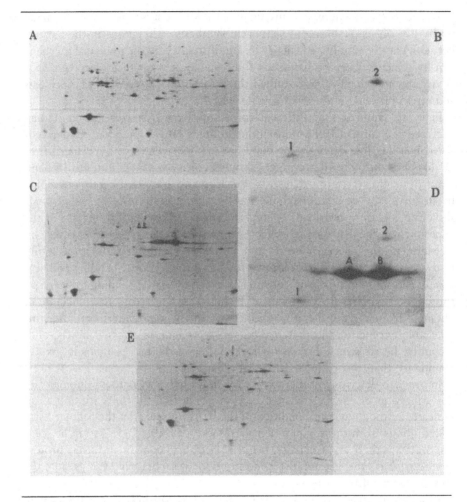

Figure 2–6. Two-dimensional autoradiograms of translation products. (A) From a control heart Proteins 1 and 2 occur normally and are labeled for reference purposes. This autoradiogram is indistinguishable from those from hearts of swimmers or chilled rats. (B) Magnified view of area of reference proteins 1 and 2 in A. (C) From a heat-shocked heart. New Proteins A and B can be seen between reference proteins 1 and 2. (D) Magnified view of area of reference proteins 1 and 2 in C. There was relatively greater synthesis of proteins A and B in hearts from heat-shocked rats than in hearts from rats with banded aortas. This increase corresponds with the increased lactic acid concentration in heat-shocked hearts, which was five times that in hearts from rats with banded aortas. (E) From a heart after aorta banding. Two distinct new proteins, A and B, can be seen between reference proteins 1 and 2. (From Hammond, G.L., Lai, Y-K, and Markert, C.L.: Diverse forms of stress lead to new patterns of gene expression through a common and essential metabolic pathway. *Proc. Natl. Acad. Sci. USA* 79:3488, 1982.)

five-minute intervals, samples of lung were removed, RNA extracted, translated, and visualized by autoradiography. Arterial pH and lactate analyses were simultaneously performed. Figure 2–7 shows pH and lactic acid changes in relation to time at 42° and the point at which stress proteins were syn-

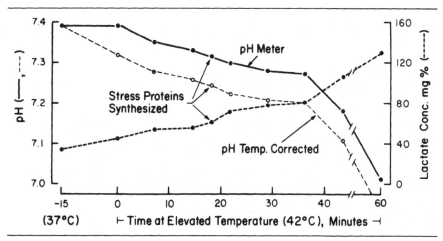

Figure 2-7. Lactate and pH curves in relation to time at 42°. Stress proteins are synthesized at pH 7.24 and lactate concentration of 60 mg%.

thesized. Autoradiograms from the serial lung samples show that a progressive increase in sp 70 mRNA translation products occurs quickly as the pH falls (figure 2-8). The critical point at which stress protein synthesis occurred was at a temperature-corrected pH of 7.24 and lactic acid content of 60 mg %. Figure 2-9 (a subset from figure 2-8) shows that other stress proteins appear as pH decreases, and also reveals that the synthesis of at least one normally occurring protein is inhibited.

A further indication of the ubiquitous nature of stress proteins and their association with acidosis has been reported in yeast cells by Weitzel [17].

Therefore evidence is accumulating that, as in the common occurrence of angina and hypertrophy with both aortic stenosis and coronary artery disease, the underlying trigger that initiates the growth response may be related to pH changes produced by a discordance between energy requirements and energy expenditure per cell. Whether the workload has increased beyond oxidative capabilities, or the blood supply is so diminished that oxidative metabolism is hindered, may make little difference, As far as the cell is concerned, the end result is the same.

WHAT IS THE PURPOSE OF STRESS PROTEIN SYNTHESIS?

The biological significance of stress protein synthesis is unknown except that, in the case of heat shock, they appear to confer a degree of protection against subsequent heat shock exposure [18].

Once synthesized in the cytoplasm, the sp 70, and perhaps other stress proteins, return to the nucleus [19, 20]. In the nucleus, they appear in areas where chromatin is uncondensed and where transcription may be initiated. If in fact stress proteins play a role in gene regulation, many other findings

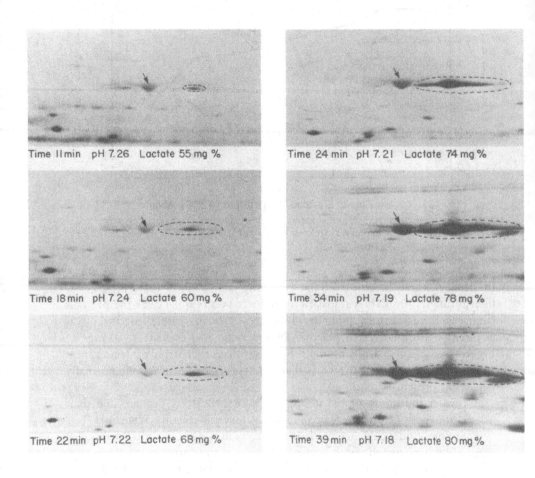

Figure 2–8. Serial examinations of translation products from the lung as the dog becomes progressively acidoti points to normally occurring proteins (NOP) 71 (representing NOP 71 mRNA). Most obvious change is ever-in quantity of sp 70 mRNA, sp 70 is circled.

associated with the response could be explained, particularly isozyme shifts. For example, isozymic forms of cardiac myosin were shown to exist by Hoh [21]. Each molecule is composed of two heavy chains and four light chains. Two different types of heavy chains, α and β, have been found in the ventricles of mammalian laboratory animals. The heavy chains form dimers of $\alpha\alpha$, $\alpha\beta$, or $\beta\beta$ [22]. These correspond to the V_1, V_2, and V_3 myosin isozymes reported by Hoh [21]. The V_3 form predominates in fetal hearts while adult hearts are composed primarily of the V_1 form [23]. In left-ventricular pressure overload, however, Litten [24] has shown that the isozymic pattern in adult

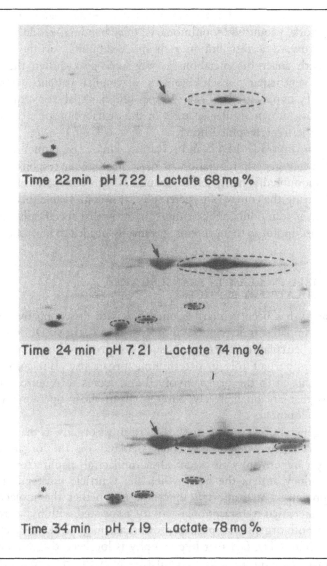

Figure 2-9. Subtle changes also occur in the lung with acidosis. These are three of the same panels that appear in figure 2-8. With increasing acidosis, more genes are activated as other SP mRNAs appear (stress proteins circled) while at least one gene (⋆) is inhibited.

animals shifts to the V_3 form which is adapted for slow tension development. The shift is beneficial for energetic contraction economy since slower shortening velocity improves the efficiency of contraction for equivalent work in much the same way that β blockade lowers myocardial oxygen consumption. There has been some difficulty, however, in showing similar shifts in hypertrophied hearts from human post-mortem specimens [22].

We have examined LDH isozymes and have shown that increased right ventricular work, produced by pulmonary artery banding, produces a shift in the pattern toward a distribution rich in A-subunits, or those that are associated with anaerobic metabolism. We have also shown the identical response in ventricular muscle biopsies of angina patients, undergoing coronary artery bypass grafting [25]. Vatner [26] has analyzed creatine kinase activity and has shown similar changes in the distribution of creatine kinase isozymes in the hypertrophied heart.

Changes in myosin, LDH and creatine kinase isozymic distribution probably indicate genetic regulation of these proteins in response to stress. There are undoubtedly many other changes in protein patterns yet to be discovered during the course of hypertrophy. It is conceivable that the role of stress proteins is to modulate the genome in a way that specifically initiates or represses transcription so that proteins specifically needed to meet the stress are synthesized.

A GENERALIZED INCREASE IN TRANSCRIPTION
MAY BE REGULATED BY PEPTIDES

Our laboratory has been primarily concerned with dissecting the molecular control that initiates transcription in response to stress. During juvenile development, circulating hormones, such as growth hormone, play an obvious and important role in determining organ size. But compensatory growth is localized to the organ involved and seems to require controlling mechanisms that are qualitatively different from those operating in earlier stages of development.

A rather general observation, applicable to most organs, is that growth or regression occurs when the functional demand on the organ changes. Accordingly, hypertrophy is seen after unilateral nephrectomy in the remaining kidney and in the heart when the ventricle must pump against increased pressure. An important question is whether the molecules that regulate the increased transcriptional activity associated with hypertrophy are the same for both organs and, perhaps, for organs in general, or whether they are organ-specific. The fact that hypertrophy is localized to the tissue under stress indicates that the molecules regulating growth arise from within the stressed cells themselves and are not circulating.

To test the hypothesis of specificity versus generality, we obtained water-soluble extracts from control canine kidneys and hearts and those undergoing hypertrophy. The extracts were then perfused through beating but non-working dog hearts in continuity with a support dog's blood supply (figure 2–10). Before and after perfusion, RNA was extracted from tissue samples, translated in vitro, and translational activity quantitated by scintillation counting. We found that extracts from both hypertrophying organs produced an increase in transcriptional activity compared to preperfusion controls or

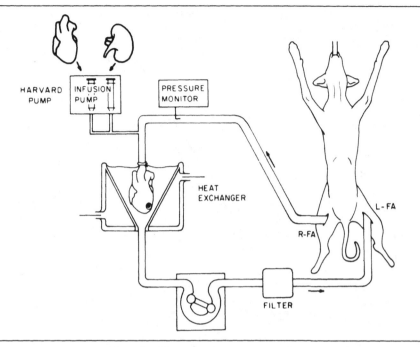

Figure 2-10. Diagram of the isolated heart preparation. Extracts from normal and hypertrophying heart and kidney were infused in separate experiments. (From Hammond, G.L., Wieben, E., and Markert, C.L.: Molecular signals for initiating protein synthesis in organ hypertrophy. *Proc. Natl. Acad. Sci. USA* 76:2455–2459, 1979.)

hearts perfused with control extracts [27]. Furthermore, extracts from hypertrophying canine hearts, when perfused through isolated rat hearts, had a similar effect. In the cross-species experiments, we found increased synthesis of poly A-containing mRNA, as determined by hybridization of total RNA with ³H poly U [28]. Accordingly, data from two separate experiments indicate that factors are present in extracts from hypertrophying organs that affect transcriptional activity. The factors are not organ- or species- specific, are probably basic to cell metabolism, and appear to have been strongly conserved. The evidence that, in response to stress, cells generate factors that alter transcription led us to preliminary steps to characterize those factors.

Crude extracts from control and aortic-banded canine hearts were prepared. The extracts were then filtered through YM 30 and YM 10 membranes. Accordingly, three molecular weight ranges were available for assay: <10 kD, 10–30 kD, and ≥30 kD. Crude extracts were also treated with trypsin to determine if the active molecules were proteins. Finally, the thermostability of active molecules was tested by incubating crude extracts in a boiling water bath for five minutes. Denatured proteins were removed by centrifugation and

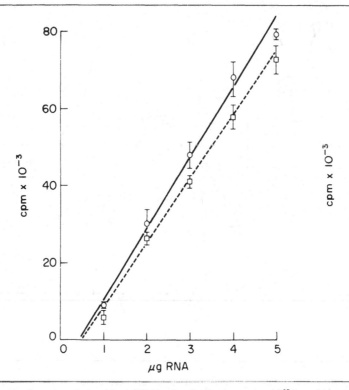

Figure 2–11. Quantity relationships of RNA related to incorporation of ^{35}S-methionine into translation products. Total cytoplasmic RNA was extracted from hearts perfused with control extracts (-----), and extract from stressed hearts (———). (From Hammond, G.L., Lai, Y-K, and Markert, C.L.: Preliminary characterization of molecules that increase cell free translational activity of cardiac cytoplasmic RNA. *European Heart Journal* (Supp. F):225–229, 1984.)

the supernatant proteins were saved for testing. The various fractions were perfused through isolated rat hearts for one hour and the RNA was extracted and translated in vitro with ^{35}S-methionine. Figure 2–11 shows the quantitative relationship and figure 12 shows the time-course relationship for ^{35}S-methionine incorporation into in vitro RNA-translation products of rat hearts perfused for one hour with crude control cardiac extract and crude extract from stressed hearts. Figure 2–13 shows fractionation results and indicates that the active molecules are heat-stable peptides of <10kD.

The problem of fractionation, however, is complex. Current purification experiments demonstrate that the active molecules are excluded by Sephadex G-75 chromatography. They appear in the void volume which is high in nucleic acid content. Accordingly, a large molecular complex of multimeric forms may be present or there may be noncovalent binding to RNA or other proteins. Membrane ultra-filtration suggests that the complex can be disassociated and that essential components of the complex are peptides, since

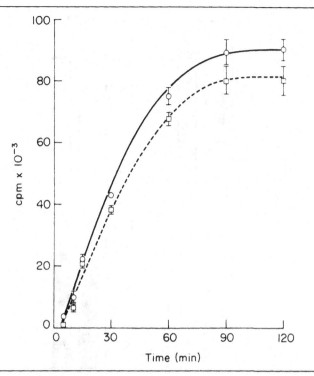

Figure 2–12. Time course for incorporation of ³⁵S-methionine into translation products directed by cytoplasmic RNA extracted from hearts perfused for 1 h with control cardiac extract (-----), and extract from stressed hearts (——). (From Hammond, G.L., Lai, Y-K, and Markert, C.L.: Preliminary characterization of molecules that increase cell-free translational activity of cardiac cytoplasmic RNA. *European Heart Journal* Supp. F:225–229, 1984.)

treatment of the Sephadex G 75-1 fraction with ribonuclease does not inhibit activity. These findings, however, must be interpreted in light of the observation that all perfused hearts examined by two-dimensional electrophoresis showed that stress proteins had been synthesized. Therefore, it is quite likely that the rat heart was responding to the stress of extirpation in addition to any effect that purified extracts may have had on transcriptional activity [29].

AN INITIAL RESPONSE TO STRESS IS ALSO SUPPRESSION OF PROTEIN SYNTHESIS

The process of hypertrophy is a heavy consumer of energy. How an energy-dependent process of this magnitude can be initiated, when the organ itself must function more vigorously, poses a fundamental question concerning the metabolic control of hypertrophy. The acutely-banded heart is acidotic; consequently, it is functioning, at least partially, by anaerobiosis. Therefore,

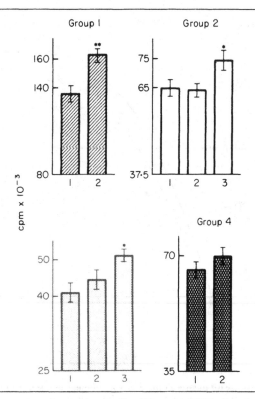

Figure 2–13. Incorporation of counts into perfused hearts (± SEM) of the four experimental groups. Different levels of radioactivity between experimental groups represent different batches of ^{35}S-methionine and lysate:

Group 1: (1) Hearts perfused with control extract (N = 4); (2) hearts perfused with crude extract from stressed hearts (N = 4) 1 vs. 2, P < 0.01.

Group 2: (1) hearts perfused with extract from stressed hearts above 30000 Mr (N − 4); (2) hearts perfused with extract from stressed hearts between 10000–30000 Mr (N = 4); (3) hearts perfused with extract from stressed hearts below 10000 Mr (N = 4), 3 vs. 1 and 2, P < 0.05; 1 vs. 2, NS.

Group 3: (1) hearts perfused with nontrypsinized extract from control hearts (N = 4); (2) hearts perfused with trypsinized extract from stressed hearts (N = 4); (3) hearts perfused with nontrypsinized extract from stressed hearts (N = 4), 3 vs. 1 and 2, P < 0.05; 1 vs. 2, NS.

Group 4: (1) hearts perfused with unheated extracts from stressed hearts (N = 6); (2) hearts perfused with heat treated extracts from stressed hearts (N = 6); 1 vs. 2, NS. (From Hammond, G.L., Lai, Y-K, and Markert, C.L.: Preliminary characterization of molecules that increase cell-free translational activity of cardiac cytoplasmic RNA. *European Heart Journal* Supp. F:225–229, 1984.)

energy must be saved somewhere so that cardiac output can be maintained while hypertrophy is initiated.

A possible answer to this question was published in 1981 by Currie and White [30]. They were the first group to demonstrate conclusively that protein synthesis in acutely stressed cardiac tissue comes almost to a standstill. Their observations were made from two-dimensional autoradiograms of cardiac proteins translated and labeled in vivo by hearts stressed by heat shock and slicing. These experiments showed that a powerful control mechanism was at work in mammalian tissue to inhibit protein synthesis during the acute-stress response. Our studies, shown in figure 2–14, confirm their findings.

Comparison of the autoradiograms in figures 2–2 and 6 with those in figure 2–14 raise an important point. When examining products of RNA, translated in vitro from stressed and control hearts, the only discernible difference is the presence of stress proteins. On the other hand, autoradiograms of proteins, synthesized in vivo by the cardiac cells themselves, show not only the presence of stress proteins in stressed hearts, but also that the synthesis of many normally occurring proteins has ceased. This evidence suggests that the control site for the generalized suppression of protein synthesis operates at the translational, rather than the transcriptional, level, while the control site for stress protein synthesis is clearly at the transcriptional level.

In order to test these observations, we analized polysomes extracted from the right ventricle of dogs before and after heat shock [9]. Sucrose gradient sedimentation of polysomes from control myocardial tissue showed a distribution with the peak at four to five ribosomes per message. The profile obtained from heat-shocked hearts showed a larger monosomal peak and a sharp decline of polysomal material toward the heavier polysomal region as shown in figure 2–15. This and the autoradiographic evidence strongly support the contention that stress-induced suppression of protein synthesis operates through translation inhibition. There are at least three advantages that accrue to the cell by inhibiting protein synthesis:

1. available energy can be diverted to areas more imminently vital to cell function,
2. free ribosomes are available for the rapid synthesis of stress proteins and,
3. free ribosome accumulation inhibits transcription of rRNA genes, thereby saving more energy as has been shown in eukaryotes [31].

Unfortunately, the quantitation of protein synthesis, by scintillation-counting of incorporated precursors, is a complicated and controversial area. Protein turnover is a dynamic process in which extracellular amino acids enter the cell, become part of the intracellular pool, and enter proteins. The proteins are then degraded and their amino acids may either stay in the precursor pool for further protein synthesis, enter a compartmentalized pool, which is not used for protein synthesis, or be excreted from the cell. With present techniques it is almost impossible to provide a reliable indicator of what is happening to the rates of protein synthesis since one cannot be certain where labeled amino acids fit into this picture at any given time. Attempts have been made to solve the precursor pool size problem by determining the specific activity of peptidal tRNA. However, the amount of labeled peptide bound to the specific tRNA is again dependent entirely on the precursor pool size which, in turn, can vary greatly with the type of stress applied to cells. In

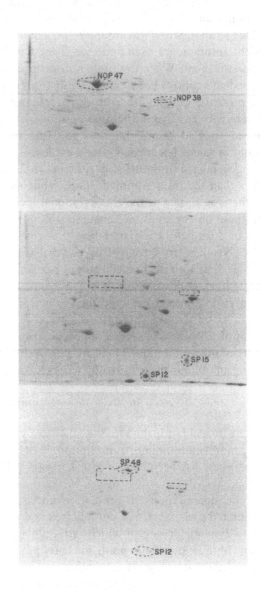

Figure 2–14. Two-dimensional autoradiogram of proteins extracted from rat hearts. a) control; NOPs 47 and 38 are circled; b) heart that underwent aortic banding for 1 h; rectangular boxes show where NOPs 47 and 38 have disappeared while SPs have been synthesized; c) heart from a rat that was heat shocked at 42°C for 1 h; rectangular boxes again show where NOPs 47 and 38 have disappeared while SPs have been synthesized. (From Lai, Y-K, Havre, P.A., and initial suppression of protein synthesis. *Biochem. Biophys. Res. Comm.* 135:857–863, 1986.)

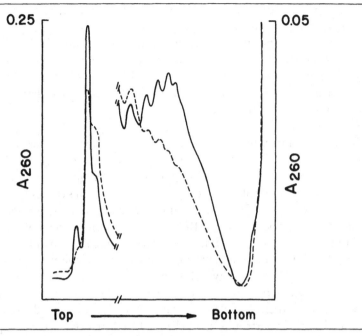

Figure 2–15. Sedimentation distribution of polysomes isolated from control (——) and heat-shocked (-----) canine heart tissue. The ordinate scale is expanded fivefold after the monosome peak. (From Lai, Y-K, Havre, P.A. Hammond, G.L.: Heat shock stress initiates simultaneous transcriptional and translational changes in the dog heart. *Biochem. Biophys. Res. Comm.* 134:166–171, 1986.)

addition, the measurements require a complicated procedure for isolating polysomes, purification of peptidal tRNA and yields which are usually in the ng range requiring HPLC and liquid scintillation counting for determining specific activity. The procedure can be somewhat simplified by calculating aminoacyl tRNA-specific activities, but this is complicated by the fact that aminoacyl tRNA is present in low concentrations and turns over in seconds, as reviewed by Morgan [3].

If one uses high doses of radioactivity and labels for long periods (4 hours or more) in an effort to establish equilibration between extracellular and intra-cellular label concentration, one runs into the possible toxic effect on cells from radioactivity and the possibility, at four hours, that the label may have been a part of many different proteins which have degraded and been resynthesized during the labeling period. On the other hand, if tracer concentrations are used for 30–60 minutes, artifacts resulting from undefined dilution of precursor amino acid-specific activity may occur and pipetting errors are magnified.

Even when the procedure is carefully and repeatedly performed by the same individual, one must make the following assumptions when interpreting data:

1. The labeled amino acid is incorporated in the same manner as the endogenous compound.
2. The measured specific radioactivity of the free amino acid pool reflects the specific radioactivity of the immediate precursor at the site of intracellular protein formation.
3. The free amino acid pool, from which specific activity is derived, provides amino acids for protein synthesis.

There are so many uncertainties about the relationship between amino acid pool sizes and protein synthesis that the results of kinetic analysis should only be seen as a possible indication of qualitative changes in protein synthesis. Happily, there is a simpler way of determining protein synthesis, i.e., directly by protein analysis of two-dimensional autoradiograms, or indirectly by specific DNA probes for the mRNA of the protein under investigation.

With these caveats in mind, it is important to mention the pioneering work of Eugene Morkin in demonstrating that the rate of the protein degradation increases during hypertrophy. Morkin was aware of and, indeed, described many of the problems already mentioned [32]. Morkin's work is particularly relevant since other investigators have reported that the degradation rate associated with hypertrophy is unchanged [33] or even decreased [34].

It is difficult to imagine how there could be anything other than increased degradation, given the fundamental laws of thermodynamics and entropy [35, 36] under which the heart must work. The fact that it has not been universally reported testifies to the difficulty of accurately determining rates of protein synthesis and degradation. Morkin analyzed degradation rates by using a formula that integrated changes in the organ's weight, variations in precursor-specific radioactivity, and the influence of changes in protein synthesis in relation to recycling of amino acids, rather than inference from isotope-decay curves. His experiments showed convincingly that the rate of myosin degradation increased, following pressure overload [37].

ARE MOLECULES THAT REGULATE TRANSCRIPTION AND TRANSLATION COMPARTMENTALIZED?

If factors that regulate transcription are peptides and if, as is suggested from our own preliminary data, factors that regulate translation are proteins, it follows that these molecules must be synthesized prior to stress, are inactive or sequestered during normal cellular activity, but are activated or released during periods of stress. If, as seems inevitable, there is a connection with energy metabolism, then one must ask whether the signals that initiate the appropriate responses arise from the mitochondria. There is little direct evidence to support this idea. However, it is well known that changes occur in mitochondrial DNA during cardiac hypertrophy in the rat [38], and Sin [39] recorded an interesting experiment in which extracts from mitochondria of

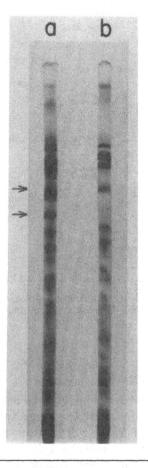

Figure 2–16. Isoelectric-focusing tube gels of proteins extracted from mitochondria from: (a) rat left ventricle which had undergone aortic banding for one hour; and (b) normal rat left ventricle. Proteins are stained with Comassie blue and therefore, do not distinguish new protein synthesis. Protein positions do not reflect relative molecular weights but relative isoelectric points.

heat-shocked Drosophila larvae produced chromosomal puffing when injected into the nonstressed larval salivary glands while control extracts did not.

Preliminary studies from our laboratory, in which we analyzed mitochondrial proteins by isoelectric-focusing gels on isolated mitochondrial preparations from stressed and controlled canine hearts, reveal the changes in protein patterns that occur with stress figure 2–16. The proteins were stained with Comassie Blue and therefore do not necessarily represent newly synthesized proteins. Although the relevance of these findings are entirely unknown, a theoretical pathway, based on impressions, preliminary data, and what is already known, can be made as an aid for planning research protocols to study the stress responses (figure 2–17).

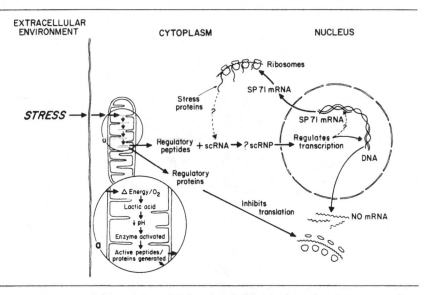

Figure 2–17. Theoretical pathway for the conversion of physiological stimuli into biochemical signals that initiate the stress response. (NO mRNA—normally occurring in RNA; sc—small cytoplasmic.)

AREAS FOR INVESTIGATION

New techniques in molecular biology and refinements in protein chemistry provide many useful tools for studying stress responses. Clinicians who see, touch, and examine stressed organs, and who can approach their specialty from a basic science level, are in a position to ask the critical questions and make the important observations that might advance our understanding of this complicated area. For many years, hypertrophy research was hampered by the lack of a precise biochemical definition of the term and an emphasis on understanding rates of protein synthesis which, though necessary, was problematic, given the many problems in interpreting data. It was also difficult to identify control mechanisms and control molecules that regulate protein synthesis because of the same lack of a simple, sure assay that could quickly identify a response, induced either by physical conditions or application of extracts (under noninducing conditions) that everyone could agree represented the initiation of hypertrophy.

The advent of cDNA probes has vastly simplified the assay problem. Their total response or nonresponse leaves little room for argument as to whether a gene has been activated. The well-recognized shifts in LDH, CPK, and probably myosin isozymes that occur in hypertrophy, allow for the probing of genes that are specific to hypertrophy and, therefore, the isolation and identification of molecules that control the response. Ambiguities about protein degradation could be similarly resolved. Since a myosin molecule under tension does not snap like a cable, but is degraded enzymatically, a control mechanism, tied to the rate at which proteins absorb energy, probably influences lysosomal activity. Using previous experience as a guide, the molecules that regulate this response may also be peptides or proteins.

An observation we have made is that there are far more inhibitors of RNA and protein synthesis present in tissue extracts than there are stimulators. Many factors could account for this, but the cell seems to favor tight control and suppression rather than growth. For example, after considerable difficulty with inhibitors, we have been able to partially purify a factor that promotes transcription in vitro, but we have not been able to selectively activate the sp 70 gene. Does this mean that generalized gene activation can not proceed in vivo until stress proteins have first been synthesized?

What can be said from available data is that the stress response is met by growth and that the initial findings in tissues stressed by work overload, hypoxia, heat shock, or a variety of other conditions, are associated with cellular acidosis, increased transcription, stress protein synthesis, and an initial inhibition of translation. What happens after that cannot be clearly understood until we understand how acidosis is associated with increased transcription, what molecules are involved, where they come from, and what role stress proteins play in the adaptive response.

REFERENCES

1. De Duve, C. 1984. *A Guided Tour of the Living Cell*, Volume One. New York: Scientific American Books, Inc.
2. Alpert, N.R., and Mulieri, L.A. 1982. Increased myothermal economy of isometric force generation in compensated cardiac hypertrophy induced by pulmonary artery constriction in the rabbit. *Circ. Res.* 50:491–500.
3. Morgan H.E., Rannels, D.E., and McKee, E.E. 1979. Protein metabolism of the heart. *The Handbook of Physiology—Section 2, The Cardiovascular System*, eds. Berne, R.M., Sperelakis, N., and Geiger, S.R. pp. 845–868. Bethesda, Maryland: *American Physiological Society*.
4. Cutilletta A.F. 1981. Muscle and nonmuscle cell RNA polymerase activities in early myocardial hypertrophy. *The American Physiological Society* H901–H907.
5. Schlesinger M.J., Ashburner M., and Tissieres A. 1982. *Heat Shock—from bacteria to man*. New York: Cold Spring Harbor Laboratory.
6. Ashburner, M., Bonner, J.J. 1971. The induction of gene activity in Drosophila by heat shock. *Cell* 17:241–254.
7. Leenders H.J., and Berendes, H.D. 1972. The effect of changes in the respiratory metabolism upon genome activity in Drosophila. *I*. The induction of gene activity. *Chromosoma* 37:433–444.
8. Leenders H.J., Kemp, A., Koninkx, J.G., and Rosing, J. 1974. Changes in cellular ATP, ADP, and AMP levels following treatments affecting cellular respiration and the activity of certain nuclear genes in Drosophila salivary glands. *Exp. Cell Res.* 86:25–30.
9. Lai, Y-K, Havre, P.A., and Hammond, G.L. Heat shock stress initiates simultaneous transcriptional and translational changes in the dog heart. *Biochem. and Biophys. Res. Comm.* 134:166–171, 1986.
10. Van de Ploeg, L.H.T., Giannini, S.H., and Cantor, C.R. 1985. Heat shock genes: Regulatory role for differentiation in parasitic protozoa. *Science* 228:1443–1446.
11. Neidhardt F.C., VanBogelen, R.A., and Vaughn, V. 1984. The genetics and regulation of

heat-shock proteins. *Ann. Rev. Genet.* 18:295–329.

12. Schedl, P., Artavenis-Tsakonas, S., Steward, R., Gehring, W., Mirault, M-E, Goldschmidt-Clermont, M., Moran, L., and Tissieres, A. 1978. Two hybrid plasmids with D. melanogaster DNA sequences complementary to mRNA coding for the major heat shock protein. *Cell* 14:921–929.

13. Hunt, C., and Morimoto, R.I. 1985. conserved features of eukaryotic hsp70 genes revealed by comparison with the nucleotide sequence of human hsp70. *P.N.A.S. USA* 81:6455–6459.

14. Gudbjamason, S., Brasch, W., and Bing, R.J. 1968. Protein synthesis in cardiac hypertrophy and heart failure. In *Herzinsuffziena*, Symposium in Hintzerzarten (Schwarzwald). pp. 184–189. Stuttgart: Georg Thieme Verlag.

15. Meerson F.Z. 1974. Development of modern components of the mechanism of cardiac hypertrophy. Circ. Res., Supplement II, 35:58.

16. Hammond, G.L., Lai, Y-K, and Markert, C.L. 1982. Diverse forms of stress lead to new patterns of gene expression through a common and essential metabolic pathway. *P.N.A.S. USA* 79:3485–3488.

17. Weitzel, G., Pilatus, U., and Rensing, L. 1985. Short note: Similar dose response of heat shock protein synthesis and intracellular pH change in yeast. *Exp. Cell Res.* 159:252–256.

18. Li, G.C., and Werb, Z. 1982. Correlation between synthesis of heat shock proteins and development of thermotolerance in Chinese hamster fibroblasts. *Cell Biology* 79:3218–3222.

19. Welch, W.J., and Feramisco, J.R. 1985. Rapid purification of mammalian 70,000-Dalton stress proteins: Affinity of the proteins for nucleotides. *Mol. and Cell Biol.* 5: 1229–1237.

20. Velazquez, J.M., DiDomenico, B.J., and Lindquist, S. 1980. Intracellular localization of heat shock proteins in Drosophila. *Cell* 20:679–689.

21. Hoh, J.F., McGrath, P.A., and Hale, P.T. 1978. Electrophoretic analysis of multiple forms of rat cardiac myosin: Effect of hypophysectomy and thyroxine replacement. *J. of Mol. and Cell. Cardiol.* 10:1053–1076.

22. Mercadier, J-J., Bouveret, P., Gorza, L., Schiaffino, S.C., Clark, W.A., Zak, R., Swynghedauw, B., and Schwartz, K. 1983. Myosin isoenzymes in normal and hypertrophied human ventricular myocardium. *Circ. Res.* 53:52–62.

23. Hoh, J.F.Y., Yeoh, G.P.S., Thomas, M.A.W., and Higginbottom, L. 1979. Structural differences in the heavy chains of rat ventricular myosin isozymes. *FEBS Lett.* 97:330–334.

24. Litten III, R.Z., Martin, B.J., Low, R.B., and Alpert, N.R. 1982. Altered myosin isozyme patterns from pressure-overloaded and thyrotoxic-hypertrophied rabbit hearts. *Circ. Res.* 50:856–864.

25. Hammond, G.L., Nadal-Ginard, B., Talner, N.S., and Markert, C.L. 1976. Myocardial LDH isozyme distribution in the ischemic and hypoxic heart. *Circulation* 53:637–643.

26. Vatner, D.E., and Ingwall, J.S. 1984. Effects of moderate pressure overload in cardiac hypertrophy on the distribution of creatinine kinase isozymes. *Proc. Soc. Exp. Biol. Med.* 175(I):5–9.

27. Hammond, G.L., Wieben, E., and Markert, C.L. 1979. Molecular signals for initiating protein synthesis in organ hypertrophy. *P.N.A.S. USA* 76:2455–2459.

28. Hammond, G.L., Lai, Y-K, and Markert, C.L. 1982. The molecules that initiate cardiac hypertrophy are not species-specific. *Science* 216:529–531.

29. Hammond, G.L., Lai, Y-K, and Markert C.L. 1984. Preliminary characterization of molecules that increase cell free translational activity of cardiac cytoplasmic RNA. *Eur. Heart J.* Supplement F:225–229.

30. Currie, R.W. and White, F.P. Trauma-induced protein in rat tissues: A physiological role for a "heat shock" protein? *Science* 214:72–73, 1981.

31. Nomura, M. 1984. The control of ribosome synthesis. *Science American* 250:102–114.

32. Morkin, E. 1974. Activation of synthetic processes in cardiac hypertrophy. *Circ. Res.*, Supplement II:37–48.

33. Gudbjarnason, S., Telerman, M., Chiba, C., Wolf, P.L., and Bing, R.J. 1964. Myocardial protein synthesis in cardiac hypertrophy. *J. Lab. and Clin. Med.* 63: 245–253.

34. Sanford, C.F., Griffin, E.E., and Wildenthal, K. 1978. Synthesis and degradation of myocardial protein during the development and regression of thyroxine-induced cardiac hypertrophy in rats. *Circ. Res.* 43:688–694.

35. Schimke, R.T. 1976. Protein degradation in vivo and its regulation. *Circ. Res.*, Supplement I 38:131–137.

36. Atkins, P.W. 1984. *The Second Law.* New York: W. H. Freeman and Co.

37. Morkin, E., Kimata, S., and Skillman, J.J. 1972. Myosin synthesis and degradation during development of cardiac hypertrophy in the rabbit. *Circ. Res.* 30:690–702.
38. Rajamanickam, C., Merten, S., Kwiatkowska-Patzer, B., Chuang, C-H, Zak, R., and Rabinowitz, M. 1979. Changes in mitochondrial DNA in cardiac hypertrophy in the rat. *Circ. Res.* 45:505–515.
39. Sin, Y.T. 1975. Induction of puffs in Drosophila salivary gland cells by mitochondrial factor(s). *Nature* 258:159–160.

3. SUBCELLULAR GROWTH OF
CARDIOCYTES DURING HYPERTROPHY

ROBERT J. TOMANEK AND CRAIG A. CANBY

Cardiac enlargement is a biological adaptation which occurs in response to stress. Since hyperplasia of cardiac myocytes (cardiocytes) is limited to the neonatal period, cardiac enlargement in response to increased work or metabolism occurs as a consequence of myocyte hypertrophy [1]. While a variety of stimuli may elicit cardiac hypertrophy, the subcellular growth and architectural reorganization which occur are affected by a variety of factors: the stimulus itself (e.g., volume or pressure overload), the rate of onset (rapid or gradual), age, and the duration and severity of the overload. Thus, cardiac hypertrophies of different origins may differ considerably with regard to their degree of usefulness and liability [2].

In order to gain an insight into adaptive phenomena comprising cardiac hypertrophy, it is essential to understand the structural basis of hypertrophy. This chapter examines the response of the cardiocyte to various stimuli that evoke hypertrophy. During the last 15 years morphometric methods have been employed to quantitate subcellular changes during growth and hypertrophy. Electron microscopic stereology has enabled us to obtain information on volumes and surface densities of various cellular structures. These methods are sufficiently sensitive to detect intergroup differences not evident by descriptive morphology. Point-counting stereology employs a test-point system superimposed on electron micrographs in which the number of test points falling on a specific structure is related to the total number of test points falling on the micrograph. Using this approach, it is possible to accurately

Supported by funds from NIH grants HL-18629 and HL-14388.

estimate densities of various cell components (i.e., the quantity per unit volume, unit area, or unit length). Volume densities of mitochondria (V_{vmito}) and myofibrils (V_{vmyo}) provide a quantitative index of the fraction, or percent, of the cell volume occupied by these organelles, which constitute energy-producing and energy-consuming components, respectively, of the cardiocyte. Surface/volume ratios provide a useful index of the membrane area per unit volume that is available for exchange.

NORMAL CARDIOCYTE GROWTH

Cardiocyte hyperplasia in the neonate accounts for most of the early growth of the heart [3]. Nearly all cardiocytes are mononucleated at birth but many become multinucleated (usually binucleate) during postnatal development [1]. Studies on adult animals indicate that binucleate cardiocytes predominate in most experimental species (e.g., rats, dogs, cats). In human hearts binucleate myocardial cells are less frequent, but polyploidy is common [4].

Consistent with the neonatal transition to aerobic metabolism is a rapid expansion of mitochondria and myofibrils. During the interval of three days before and four days after birth in the rabbit, the relative volume of these organelles increases by about 25% [5]. Moreover, the inner mitochondrial membrane, which is a structural correlate of ATP production, is disproportionately enhanced during this short time period. These changes are consistent with the increased work load and oxygen availability at birth.

Page and colleagues [6] studied organelle growth of left-ventricular cardiocytes in rats between the time of weaning and maturity. Their work established that myofibrillar and mitochondrial growth is proportional and that mitochondrial profile size remains constant. With the great increase in cell size during postnatal growth the T-tubule membrane increases substantially and enables the cell to maintain its surface (cell membrane including T-tubule component) to volume ratio. In cat papillary muscle the percent of the total cell surface contributed by T-tubules triples by the time adulthood is reached [7]. It has also been shown that postnatal growth is associated with a decrease in sarcoplasmic volume density up to six months of age in the rat [8].

DESCRIPTIVE MORPHOLOGY OF HYPERTROPHY

Electron microscopists have described a variety of subcellular changes in cardiocytes in various types of cardiac hypertrophy. These observations are valuable because they may contribute to our understanding of the structural basis of altered ventricular function. However, most nondegenerative subcellular changes are subtle and therefore require quantitative methods for detection. Nevertheless, evidence of increased protein synthesis and subcellular growth is demonstrated by numerical increases in ribosomes, proliferation of the Golgi apparatus, and enlargement of nuclei [9]. During cardiac hypertrophy sarcolemmal alterations have been reported [10, 11] and nuclear pores were found to increase in number in three species undergoing cardiac hypertrophy [12]. Multiple intercalated discs [13] and sarcomereogenesis, or the formation of new sarcomeres [14], are phenomena which may also characterize the developmental stage of hypertrophy. Widening and streaming of Z-bands along with rod-body formation have been described in numerous studies, and their possible significance has been recently reviewed [14, 15].

Other subcellular alterations are not consistent and may be related to early degenerative changes, heart failure, or possibly model-specific phenomena. It has been suggested that the cardiocyte undergoes similar ultrastructural changes during compensatory hypertrophy and normal growth [16].

QUANTITATIVE MORPHOLOGY OF PRESSURE-OVERLOAD HYPERTROPHY

When pressure overload is suddenly introduced, as in experimental aortic constriction, heart weight increases rapidly. During the first day intracellular edema [17] and myocyte hypertrophy [18] are evident, and there is an increase in mitochondrial cytochrome content and respiratory enzyme activity per gram muscle protein [19]. Initially, cytochromes accumulate at a faster rate than mitochondrial DNA [20]. During this initial phase of the hypertrophy process, it has been shown that a 20% increase in myocyte cross-sectional area is due to volume increases of 78% in sarcoplasmic reticulum and matrix, and 36% in mitochondria [18]. Thus, myofibrillar growth is not yet pronounced at this time and the increased V_{mito}/V_{myo} ratio may persist up to seven days [21]. Individual mitochondrial profiles are 16–20% larger than normal during this initial stage of hypertrophy. Recently it has been shown that microtubular reorganization in cardiocytes, as visualized with specific antibody staining, occurs as early as three days following aortic banding [22]. Since this study showed that the intermediate filament desmin was unchanged, it was concluded that microtubules may constitute a structural regulator of early cellular hypertrophy.

Subsequent subcellular characteristics stand in contrast to the early responses to pressure overload. Following the first week of pressure overload, growth of myofibrils exceeds that of the mitochondria, as characterized by a decrease in V_{vmito} and an increase in V_{vmyo}. Thus, V_{mito}/V_{myo} is lower in hypertrophic cells of hypertensive animals compared to nonhypertrophic cells or to those undergoing normal growth. These conclusions are based on several species and several models of pressure overload. Numerous studies have employed constriction of either the ascending, or descending, aorta as a model of pressure overload in rats [23–28], cats [29], and rabbits [30, 31]. Table 3–1 summarizes the relative volumetric changes of these organelles in relation to the duration and magnitude of the hypertrophy. Even though the magnitude of left ventricular hypertrophy (LVH) in these studies was quite variable, myofibrillar volume increased more than did mitochondrial volume. Thus, the magnitude of hypertrophy does not appear to be a factor which determines

Table 3–1. Effects of pressure overload induced by aortic-constriction (AC) on the relative volume of mitochondria and myofibrils comprising myocardial cells

Reference	Species	Duration of AC	Magnitude of hypertrophy	V_{vmito}	V_{vmyo}	V_{mito}/V_{myo}
25	rat	21 days				↓ or normal
23	rat	10–50 days	12–40% (LV dry weight)	↓	↑	
28	rat	3–21 days	4–73% (cell volume)	NS	NS	NS
		35 days	78% (cell volume)	NS	↑	↓
24	rat	35 days	51% (tissue volume)	↓	↑	↓
26	rat	8 weeks	30% (LVW/BW★)	↓	↑	↓
27	rat	3 months	48% (LVW/BW)	NS	NS	NS
30	rabbit	2–4 months	20–89% (LVW/BW★)	↓	↑	↓
31	rabbit	7–142 days	68% (LVW/BW)	↓	↑	↓
29	cat	30 days	53% (LVW/BW)	↑	NS	NS
		120 days	44%	↓	↑	↓
		248 days	46%	↓	↑	↓

★ based on actual LVW—predicted LVW; the latter obtained by a regression line for LVW and BW.

the growth of these organelles. In contrast, the point in time when V_{mito}/V_{myo} ratio becomes significantly reduced may vary. Anversa and colleagues [32] found that this reduction was significant as early as eight days after aortic banding, while Dammrich et al. [28] noted no change through the twenty-first day. In cats the initial increase in V_{vmito} was still evident 30 days after banding but by 120 days the V_{mito}/V_{myo} ratio was significantly reduced [29].

A disproportionate organelle growth is also characteristic of other models of LV pressure overload. In spontaneously hypertensive rats (SHR), arterial pressure increases gradually as does cardiocyte hypertrophy. LV mass is greater in SHR than their WKY controls even prior to the development of hypertension but this difference is due to a greater number of cells in SHR since myocyte dimensions are similar for both groups [1, 33]. The characteristic increase in V_{vmyo} and decreases in the V_{vmito} and V_{mito}/V_{myo} ratio become evident by about four months of age [26, 33, 34]. As illustrated in figure 3–1, this ratio continues to decline not only as hypertrophy peaks (7 mos.), but even during a period of stabilized hypertrophy, which occurs between 7–15 months. [33]. However, in old age (22–23 mos.), the V_{mito}/V_{myo} ratio increases to the level of the control, age-matched, WKY. In the posterior papillary muscle of SHR a normalization of this ratio was observed at one year [34]. We considered transmural differences in hypertrophy and found that during the first four months of life in SHR, endomyocardial myocytes undergo a more marked hypertrophy than their epimyocardial counterparts. This more rapid cell growth is reflected by a lower V_{mito}/V_{myo} ratio in the former than in the latter.

Renovascular hypertension has also been used as a model of pressure overload to study subcellular changes in cardiocytes. Several studies have shown that V_{vmito} is less, and V_{vmyo} greater, in rats during renovascular

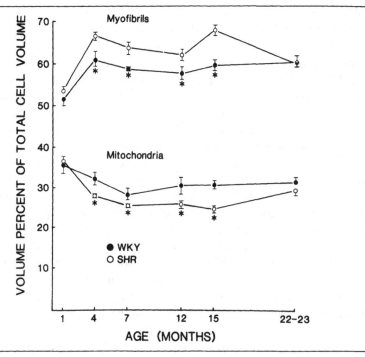

Figure 3–1. Volume densities of myofibrils and mitochondria of SHR and WKY during their life span. *, significant differences between SHR and age control WKY (P ≤ 0.05). [Based on data from reference 33.]

hypertension than in the normotensive controls [35–37]. We have also found mitochondrial volume density to be less in rats with hypertrophy due to renovascular hypertension [38]. Poche et al. [39] demonstrated that V_{mito}/V_{myo} volume ratio in rats is markedly depressed after three months of renovascular hypertension but continues to decrease up to 12 months even though cardiocytes are no longer undergoing hypertrophy. Based on this study as well as the data from SHR, it appears that the fall in the V_{mito}/V_{myo} volume ratio is not dependent upon cardiocyte enlargement but on some factor associated with the persistence of pressure overload.

Alterations in mitochondrial profile size during pressure-overload LVH have also been reported. Mitochondrial surface-to-volume ratio was found to increase in cardiocytes from rat hearts overloaded by aortic constriction [27]. Yet another study reported an increase in mitochondrial size [21] which usually leads to a decrease in the surface-to-volume ratio. This morphological change has been found during heart failure [41]. In SHR we were not able to document an increase in the number of mitochondrial profiles reported by Takatsu and Kashii [40] except during senescence [33]. In view of these inconsistent findings, it appears that mitochondrial size and the surface/volume ratio are parameters which cannot be generalized to LVH. Importantly, mitochondrial function appears to remain unaltered even during congestive heart failure [42].

The surface: volume ratio of the hypertrophic myocardial cell is maintained primarily because of a substantial growth of T-tubules. Both T-tubule surface area [43] and volume [30, 32] are increased relative to cell volume. In rabbits with aortic constriction [30] and twenty-one-week-old SHR [34], the relative volume of T-tubules was found to increase approximately twofold. Thus, in hypertrophy due to either renovascular hypertension or aortic constriction the total myocyte surface area/cell volume ratio is normal [44]. In cats with LVH, however, the surface area of T-tubules/cell volume was unchanged up to 120 days post-banding and then decreased by 248 days [29]. Growth of the sarcoplasmic reticulum appears to be rapid as evidenced by an increase in its volume density eight days following aortic constriction [32]. During this rapid growth its surface/volume ratio is maintained [24]. If sarcoplasmic reticulum area is expressed per myofibril volume, this ratio is higher in left ventricular hypertrophy, induced by either aortic constriction or renovascular hypertension, than it is in the nonoverloaded ventricle [45]. Enhancement of sarcoplasmic reticulum may represent an adaptation aimed at maintaining contractile function, since calcium uptake of this membrane system is reported to be depressed in pressure-overload hypertrophy [46].

Long-term pressure overload is associated with a variety of ultrastructural changes. We have noted that, after one year of life in SHR, cardiocytes show focal changes including increased numbers of caveolae, cell membrane invaginations, honeycombed T-tubules [33] and mitochondrial and myofibril disruptions. Since these alterations are not typical of developing hypertrophy, we have suggested that they are the consequence of long-term hypertension. In addition, we have shown that the accumulation of residual bodies (lipofuscin granules), a characteristic of aging cardiocytes, is more rapid in SHR than in WKY [33]. A more recent cytochemical study indicates that lysosomal structures, associated with degenerative intracellular components, become more numerous in SHR than in WKY as hypertension persists, for 12 months and longer [47]. These data suggest that long-term hypertension generates ultrastructural features indicative of degeneration, as well as adaptations not evident during earlier stages.

In cats with right ventricular pressure overload of 2 weeks [48] or 7–10 weeks [49], volume densities of mitochondria and myofibrils of papillary muscles were not significantly different from the controls. These data imply that subcellular growth after pressure overload in the right ventricle is normal and provides a contrast from the left ventricle responding to a similar stimulus. When the right ventricle hypertrophies, as a consequence of myocardial infarction in the left ventricle, mitochondrial and myofibrillar expansion is also proportional [50]. While the mechanism involved in this growth process has not been demonstrated, the hypertrophy is concentric and probably develops because of an enhanced afterload [50].

The important question regarding altered subcellular growth in LVH due to pressure overload concerns the functional correlates. While impaired left ventricular function may occur with the persistence of hypertension, functional abnormalities are not necessarily evident. In the SHR, peak cardiac output is the same or even greater than that of WKY [51–53]. Thus, the adaptations occurring in the cardiocyte appear to compensate for the increased afterload, at least when the hemodynamic overload increases gradually. In fact, the contractile properties of left ventricular papillary muscles in SHR or DOCA-hypertensive rats show few abnormalities even with long-term hypertension [54, 55]. However, it has yet to be demonstrated whether the energy reserves of the enlarged cells are sufficient to meet the demands of conditions requiring substantial increases in metabolism or hypoxia.

QUANTITATIVE MORPHOLOGY OF OTHER MODELS OF HYPERTROPHY

Volume Overload

Acute volume overload (two hours) causes an increase in mitochondrial volume density [56], a change which is also characteristic of the early response to pressure overload. However, subsequent growth of mitochondria and myofibrils appears to be proportional. Two and ten weeks following induction of volume overload by complete AV block (by injection of formaldehyde into the AV node) volume densities of mitochondria and myofibrils were normal, despite an increase of heart mass approximating 50% at 10 weeks [57]. Biopsies from patients with volume overload LVH due to mitral valve insufficiency also indicate that these organelles grow proportionally [58]. Thus, the subcellular growth pattern during enhanced preload differs from that characteristic of increased afterload. These models also differ in another important dimension: cell length as well as width increases in volume overload [59] but not in pressure overload. Accordingly volume overload leads to eccentric hypertrophy while pressure overload results in concentric hypertrophy.

Hypxoia

Cardiac hypertrophy due to chronic hypoxic exposure in rats is associated with bradycardia, a lowering of arterial pressure and an increased hematocrit [60]. One might predict that hypoxia would preferentially stimulate mitochondrial growth. However, after six weeks of hypoxic exposure, left ventricular myocyte diameter increased 20% but mitochondrial volume density and V_{mito}/V_{myo} were lower than the controls [60]. The number of mitochondrial profiles per unit area increased while their size decreased. In another study, where the duration of hypoxia was 30 days, an increase in the number of small mitochondria was noted and the mitochondrial/myofibril volume ratio was increased [61]. A decrease in the number of mitochondria with an enlargement of profile size [62], no change in mitochondrial profile size, and an increase in the number of profiles/unit area [63] have also been reported. Since the data from this model of hypertrophy are not consistent, no firm conclusion can be drawn at this time.

Exercise Training

LVH due to exercise training facilitates subcellular adaptations, which differ markedly from those of pressure overload. Guski and associates [62] showed that moderate swim-training in rats caused a 21% increase in absolute LV weight and a significant increase in mitochondrial volume density but no change in myofibrillar volume density. Thus, the V_{mito}/V_{myo} ratio increased solely as a consequence of a disproportional growth of mitochondria. Sarcoplasmic reticulum volume density also was enhanced. Treadmill exercise-training in mice [64] and rats [65], associated with mild cardiac hypertrophy, did not alter mitochondrial or myofibrillar volume densities. Right ventricular hypertrophy, induced by treadmill exercise, was also characterized by a proportional expansion of myofibrils and mitochondria [65] even when the regimen was strenuous enough to produce a 31% increase in right ventricular weight [66]. However, in the LV, strenuous treadmill training caused a 29% enhancement of myocyte mass and led to a greater growth of mitochondria (38%) than myofibrils (23%) [67]. A decrease in LV mitochondrial surface density [64] is consistent with a higher total number and higher frequency of small mitochondrial profiles after training [62, 68]. These studies support the supposition that exercise-training facilitates subcellular structural adaptations, which are more akin to normal growth, or which may favor the development of an oxidative reserve.

Thyroid Hormone

Two other models of hypertrophy, which clearly differ from pressure overload in their subcellular responses, are thyroxine treatment and chronic anemia. When adult rats were injected with L-thyroxine (25 mg/kg/day) for nine days, heart weight/body weight ratio increased by 33%, and mitochondrial volume density increased by 34% [69]. These data indicate that mitochondrial growth was substantially in excess of that required to keep pace with cellular enlargement. Interestingly, tri-iodothyronine treatment in rats caused a decrease in myofibril volume density [70]. The role of thyroxine on subcellular growth has also been investigated in thyroidectomized rats that received thyroxine (180 µg/Kg, s.c.) every fourth day over a thirty-day period [71]. Thyroidectomy was associated with 1) arrest of somatic growth, 2) a decrease in the volume density of myocardial mitochondria, but 3) no change in the relative proportion of other cell components. In contrast, the rats that received thyroxine during the experimental period experienced a progressive body weight gain, an unchanged myofibrillar volume density, and growth of plasma and sarcotubular membrane areas which were proportional to the volume increase of cardiocytes. However, mitochondrial volume density was higher than that of the hypothyroid controls, and was evident between 48 and 96 hours after the first injection of thyroxine. These data provide evidence that mitochondrial volume is dependent upon thyroxine.

Anemia

Cardiac enlargement, associated with chronic anemia in young rats, has also been shown to cause an increased volume density of mitochondria [27, 72]. In this model, characterized by low hemoglobin values, mitochondria may undergo progressive deterioration of their cristae [72].

Human Hearts

Ultrastructural morphometric studies on human hearts are few [73–75] owing to the difficulty in biopsying patients with similar stages of a common cause of cardiac hypertrophy. Schaper [75], who compared patients with predominant aortic stenosis, severe regurgitation, and aortic stenosis and regurgitation, found that myofibril volume density was decreased in these groups compared to controls. This decrease, which was accompanied by an increased sarcoplasmic volume density, was associated with a significant reduction in LV ejection fraction. She found that the group with both severe regurgitation and aortic stenosis had the greatest heart weights but the lowest ejection fraction and concluded that myocardial function declines, despite increases in cell size and heart mass. These data imply that impending heart failure in hypertrophied human hearts may be related to the relative loss of contractile filaments. This finding is consistent with data on experimental animals in which the contractile elements expand during volume or pressure overload in order to compensate for an enhanced pre- or after-load. In these models left ventricular function is usually normal.

By comparing various models of cardiac hypertrophy, one can conclude that the stimulus for hypertrophy dictates the subcellular growth patterns of the cardiocyte, and that the specific subcellular adaptations may underlie cardiac function during cardiac hypertrophy of specific origins.

FACTORS REGULATING ORGANELLE GROWTH
DURING MYOCARDIAL HYPERTROPHY

Myocardial hypertrophy is stimulated by extrinsic factors which differ with regard to their functional effects on the ventricle. Therefore, it is not surprising that the subcellular architecture may undergo specific adaptations depending on the factors and mechanisms brought into play under a given condition. In reviewing the various stimuli for cardiac growth, Zak [76] discusses six possibilities: contractile activity, ATP depletion, stretch, humoral factors, hypoxia, and cell degradation products. All of these possibilities provide interesting theories or hypotheses but none can, by itself, explain normal or compensatory growth of the cardiocyte. Thus, a single growth-regulating signal has not yet been established. Likewise, the specific stimuli for the growth of mitochondria and myofibrils are uncertain. We have addressed some interventions in spontaneously hypertensive rats which modify the growth of these organelles and which add further support to the hypothesis that their growth is influenced by different factors. The findings from these studies are summarized in figure 3–2.

When SHR's were chronically treated with either α-methyldopa [77] or hydralazine, chlorothiazide, and reserpine in combination [78] from the time of weaning, myocardial hypertrophy was modified. However, these two studies provided a sharp contrast since arterial pressure was maintained at low-normotensive levels with the three antihypertensive agents in combination, but was similar to the nontreated SHR after α-methyldopa treatment. Thus, hypertrophy was attenuated with the latter despite the presence of unequivocal hypertension. V_{mito}/V_{myo} was normalized after both treatments even in cells from the subendocardium that were mildly hypertrophic.

To evaluate the long-term effects of α-methyldopa on cellular hypertrophy, we treated rats aged 1–12 months, and in order to determine the reversibility of hypertrophy and cellular changes, we treated another group aged 12–15 months [79]. Blood pressure was similar in both treated groups (151 ± 1 and 157 ± 5 mmHg) and slightly lower than in the nontreated, age-matched controls. However, the cellular responses of the two groups were markedly different. Cell size and ventricular weight were attenuated after early, long-term treatment, but not after delayed treatment. In contrast, V_{mito}/V_{myo} was not affected by early, long-term treatment, but showed a slight reduction after delayed treatment. These findings suggest that V_{mito}/V_{myo} ratio is independent of cell size and that factors associated with the development or stabilization of hypertrophy and/or age influence the effects of α-methyldopa on the myocardial cell.

That α-methyldopa may normalize the V_{mito}/V_{myo} ratio in the SHR is consistent with the supposition that the adrenergic system is involved in cardiac hypertrophy (80–82). While sympathectomy is ineffective in preventing left ventricular hypertrophy in SHR [83, 84], it is associated with normalization of V_{mito}/V_{myo} [84]. In order to determine the role of catecholamines on cardiac hypertrophy in this genetic model of hypertension, we performed adrenal demedullations in the young SHR [85]. Even when this procedure was done in combination with chemical sympathectomy, cardiocyte cross-sectional area was not affected despite a moderate reduction in arterial pressure. However, V_{mito}/V_{myo} increased to values characteristic of the normotensive control (WKY) group. The normalization of this ratio was due to a decrease in the volume density of myofibrils; mitochondrial volume density was not affected. Accordingly, catecholamines appear to modulate the disproportional growth of myofibrils characteristic of pressure-overload hypertrophy. Consistent with these data is our finding that chronic β-adrenoceptor blockade with atenolol has similar effects on myofibrillar

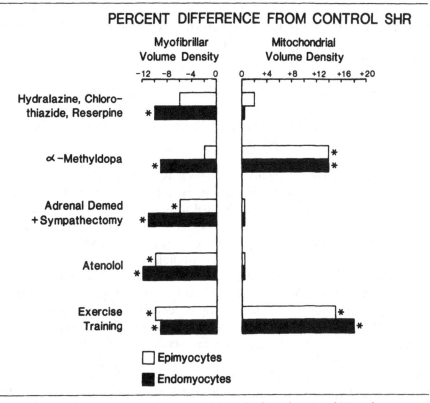

Figure 3-2. Changes in myofibrillar and mitochondrial volume densities of SHR subject to various interventions. *, significantly different from nontreated SHR (P ≤ 0.05) [Based on data from references 77, 78, 85, 86, 88.]

volume ratio [86]. However, unlike sympathectomy and adrenal demedullation, treatment with this β_1-antagonist attenuates LVH.

Since exercise training is associated with beneficial adaptations in the presence or absence of cardiac hypertrophy [87] we tested the hypothesis that exercise brings into play a mechanism(s) which could normalize subcellular growth in a hypertensive model of LVH [88]. We trained SHRs on a motorized treadmill for ten weeks commencing at the age of six weeks. The trained SHR did not differ from their controls in regard to body, heart and ventricular weights, or blood pressure, but they exhibited bradycardia and increased $\dot{V}O_2$. In both epimyocardial and endomyocardial myocytes, training normalized mitochondrial and myofibrillar volume densities, i.e., mitochondrial volume density was higher and myofibrillar volume density was lower than in the control SHR, and these were similar to the normotensive WKY. These findings demonstrate that some factor(s) related to exercise stress facilitate a proportional growth of energy-producing and energy-consuming organelles, even in the presence of hypertension and LVH associated with pressure overload. Thus, it was shown that, at least in this model of hypertrophy, organelle growth can be modified without altering either arterial blood pressure or the magnitude of hypertrophy. This finding is consistent with the idea that blood pressure and LVH in the SHR can be dissociated [89].

These studies imply that:

1. the magnitude of cellular enlargement and organelle growth are not closely linked and
2. specific subcellular adaptations may be influenced by factors other than the primary stimulus for hypertrophy.

The view that an increase in humoral factors is associated with myocardial cell growth in various models of hypertrophy cannot be reconciled with the fact that cardiac hypertrophy is usually limited to one ventricle and may vary in magnitude from one layer of the ventricle to another. Thus, any chemical mediator of any aspect of hypertrophy must act selectively within the myocardium. While we suggest that catecholamines do play a role in subcellular selective growth during LVH, we have also shown that they are not a determinant of the magnitude of cardiac hypertrophy. This view is consistent with experimental data on right ventricular hypertrophy in cats [90]. Papillary muscle mass and cardiocyte cross-sectional area were shown to be dependent upon loading conditions independent of innervation or β- or α-adrenoceptor blockade.

To more completely understand the control of subcellular adaptations during cardiac hypertrophy, future studies need to consider the permissive role of hormones. Thyroxine has been shown to be a requisite for cardiac hypertrophy [91]. When hypothyroidism was induced in rats by propylthiouracyl, subsequent hypertension in response to aortic constriction failed to produce an increase in LV mass. Treatment with propylthiouracyl has a marked effect subcellularly, in that all ventricular myosin is converted to the V_3 form. In male castrated ferrets aortic constriction resulting in a 45% increase in LV mass did not alter the volume densities of mitochondria or myofibrils [92]. Since noncastrated controls were not included in the study the influence of testosterone on the findings is speculative. However, the fact the V_{mito}/V_{myo} volume ratio was normal stands in contrast to other studies on pressure overload.

SUMMARY AND CONCLUSIONS

Subcellular adaptations during cardiac hypertrophy are dependent upon factors associated with the stimulus evoking the hypertrophy. While pressure overload causes a greater expansion of myofibrils than mitochondria, anemia or thyroxine-induced hypertrophy facilitate a greater mitochondrial volume density. Exercise training leads to either a proportional growth of these organelles or to enhanced mitochondrial volume density. Thus, exercise-induced hypertrophy is more akin to chronic volume-overload hypertrophy which is characterized by a proportional growth of mitochondria and myofibrils. The signals which enable the cardiocyte to produce mitochondrial and contractile proteins at specified rates, in response to a particular condition evoking hypertrophy, have not been identified. Interestingly, increased afterload of the right ventricle does not lead to the decreased V_{mito}/V_{myo} volume ratio characteristic of the left ventricle, a fact which suggests that different mechanisms may be called into play during pulmonary and systemic hypertension.

The relationship between hemodynamic load and cardiac hypertrophy is not as absolute as one might expect since cardiac hypertrophy may persist even when hypertension is reversed. This conclusion is supported by experiments which have used pharmacological interventions to reduce blood pressure without substantially altering myocardial hypertrophy. That mitochondrial and myofibrillar growth may be independent of the magnitude of hypertrophy is also well documented. Experimental evidence from studies on sympathec-tomy, adrenal demedullation, β_1 blockade, and α-methyldopa implicates the adrenergic system in such a role. Exercise training, at least in young rats, during the period of developing LVH and hypertension, enables normal growth of these organelles, independent of the magnitude of blood pressure and cardiac mass.

It would appear that intracellular growth patterns reflect the major func-tional demand placed on the cardiocyte by the condition evoking hypertrophy. They should therefore be considered as compensatory adaptations aimed at facilitating normal ventricular function at least under the conditions imposed (increased afterload, preload, metabolism and O_2 utilization).

REFERENCES

1. Oparil, S., Bishop, S.P., and Clubb, F.J. Jr. 1984. Myocardial cell hypertrophy or hyperplasia. *Hypertension* 6 (Suppl. III):III-38–III-43.
2. Alpert, N.R., and Mulieri, L.A. 1984. The inhomogeneity and appropriateness of the myocardial response to stress. *Hypertension* 6 (Suppl. III):III-50–III-57.
3. Clubb, F.J. Jr., and Bishop, S.P. 1984. Formation of binucleated myocardial cells in the neonatal rat. An index for growth hypertrophy. *Lab. Invest.* 50:571–577.
4. Sandritter, W., and Scomazzoni, G., 1964. Deoxyribonucleic acid content (Feulgen photometry) and dry weight (interference microscopy) of normal and hypertrophic heart muscle fibers. *Nature* 202:100–101.
5. Smith, H.E. and Page, E. 1977. Ultrastructural changes in rabbit heart mitochondria during the perinatal period. *Develop. Biol.* 57:109–117.
6. Page, E., Early, J., and Power, B. 1974. Normal growth of ultrastructures in rat left ventricle myocardial cells. *Circ. Res.* 34 and 35 (Suppl. II):II-12–II-16.
7. Sheridan, D.J., Cullen, M.J., and Tynan, M.J. 1979. Qualitative and quantitative observations on ultrastructural changes during postnatal development in the cat myocardium. *J. Molec. Cell. Cardiol.* 11:1173–1181.
8. David, H. Rudolph, M., Marx, I., Guski, H., and Wenzelides, K. 1979. Morphometric characterization of left ventricular myocardial cells of male rats during postnatal development. *J. Molec. Cell. Cardiol.* 11:631–638.
9. Ferrans, V.J. 1983. Morphology of the heart in Hypertrophy. *Hosp. Pract. Jul.* 18:67–78.

10. Ferrans, V.J., Buja, L.M., and Maron, B.J. 1976. Sarcolemmal alterations in cardiac hypertrophy and degeneration. *Recent Adv. Stud. Cardiac Struct. Metab.* 9:395–419.
11. Ferrans, V.J., Jones, M., Maron, B.J., and Roberts, W.C. 1975. The nuclear membranes in hypertrophied human cardiac muscle cells. *Am. J. Pathol.* 78:427–60.
12. Goldstein, M.A. 1974. Nuclear pores in ventricular muscle cells from adult hypertrophied hearts. *J. Molec. and Cell. Cardiol.* 6:227–235.
13. Adomian, G.E., Laks, M.M., Morady, F., and Swan, H.J.C. Significance of the multiple intercalated disc in the hypertrophied canine heart. 1974. *J. Molec. Cell. Cardiol.* 6:105–110.
14. Legato, M.J., Mulieri, L.A., and Alpert, N.R. 1984. The ultrastructure of myocardial hypertrophy: why does the compensated heart fail? *Eur. Heart J.* 5 Suppl. F:251–269.
15. Bishop, S.P. 1983. Ultrastructure of the myocardium in physiological and pathological hypertrophy in experimental animals. *Perspectives in Cardiovascular Research* 7:121–147.
16. Legato, M.J., Mulieri, L.A., and Alpert, N.R. 1983. Parallels between normal growth and compensatory hypertrophy in the rabbit. *Perspectives in Cardiovascular Research* 7:111–126.
17. Aguirre, A., and Baba, N. 1969. Electron microscopic observations of experimental left ventricular hypertrophy. *Lab. Invest.* 20:573.
18. Anversa, P., Loud, A.V., and Vitali-Mazza, L. 1976. Morphometry and autoradiography of early hypertrophic changes in the ventricle myocardium of adult rat. An electron microscopic study. *Lab. Invest.* 35:475–483.
19. Albin, R., Dowell, R.T., Zak, R., and Rabinowitz, M. 1973. Synthesis and degradation of mitochondrial components in hypertrophied rat. *Biochem. J.* 136:629–637.
20. Zak, R., Rabinowitz, M., Rajamanickan, C., Merten, S., and Kwiatkonskapatzer, 1980. Mitochondrial proliferation in cardiac hypertrophy. *Basic Res. Cardiol.* 75:171–178.
21. Meerson, FZ. 1964. Structure and mass of mitochondria in the process of compensatory hyperfunction and hypertrophy of the heart. *Exp. Cell. Res.* 36:568–578.
22. Samuel, J.L., and Bertier, B. 1984. Different distributions of microtubules, desmin filaments, and isomyosins during the onset of cardiac hypertrophy in the rat. *Europ. J. Cell Biol.* 34:300–306.
23. Page, E., Polimeni, P.I., Zak, R., Early, J., and Johnson, M. 1972. Myofibrillar mass in rat and rabbit heart muscle. *Circ. Res.* 30:430–439.
24. Anversa, P., Olivetti, G., Melissari, M., and Loud, A.V. 1980. Stereological measurement of cellular and subcellular hypertrophy and hyperplasia in the papillary muscle of adult rat. *J. Molec. Cell. Cardiol.* 12:781–795.
25. Hatt, P.Y. 1977. Cellular changes in the mechanically overloaded heart. *Basic Res. Cardiol.* 72:198–202.
26. Lund, D.D., and Tomanek, R.J. 1978. Myocardial morphology in spontaneously hypertensive and aortic constricted rats. *Am. J. Anat.* 152:141–152.
27. Sung, R., Stephens, M., Blayney, L., and Henderson, A. 1982. Cardiac hypertrophy and its regression in rat: comparison of morphological changes in response to aortic constriction, iron deficiency anaemia, and isopremaline. *J. Molec. Cell. Cardiol.* 14:501–512.
28. Dämmrich, J., and Pfeifer, U. 1983. Cardiac hypertrophy in rats after supravalvular aortic constriction. II. Inhibition of cellular autophagy in hypertrophying cardiomyocytes. *Virchow Arch.* [Cell Pathol.] 43:287–307.
29. Breisch, E.A., White, F.C., Bloor, C.M. 1984. Myocardial characteristics of pressure-overload hypertrophy. A structural and functional study. *Lab. Invest.* 51:333–342.
30. Anversa, P., Olivetti, G., Melissari, M., and Loud, A.V. 1979. Morphometric study of myocardial hypertrophy induced by abdominal aortic stenosis. *Lab. Invest.* 40:341–349.
31. Anversa, P., Vitali-Mazza, L., Visioli, O., and Marahetti, G. 1971. Experimental cardiac hypertrophy: a quantitative ultrastructural study in the compensatory stage. *J. Mol. Cell. Cardiol.* 3:213–227.
32. Goldstein, M.A., Sordahl, L.A., and Schwartz, A. 1974. Ultrastructural analysis of left ventricular hypertrophy in rabbits. *J. Mol. Cell. Cardiol.* 6:265–273.
33. Tomanek, R.J., and Hovanec, J.M. 1981. The effects of long-term pressure overload and aging on the myocardium. *J. Mol. Cell. Cardiol.* 13:471–488.
34. Kawamura, K., Kashii, C., and Imamura, K. 1976. Ultrastuctural changes in hypertrophied myocardium of spontaneously hypertensive rats. *Jap. Circ. J.* 40:1119–1145.
35. Anversa, P., Loud, A.V., Giacomelli, F., and Wiener, J. 1978. Absolute morphometric study of myocardial hypertrophy in experimental hypertension. II Ultrastructure of myocytes and

interstitium. *Lab. Invest.* 38:597–609.

36. Wendt-Gallitelli, M.F., and Jacob, R. 1977. Time course of electron microscopic alterations in the hypertrophied myocardium of Goldblatt rats. *Basic Res. Cardio.* 72:222–227.

37. Wiener, J., Giacomelli, F., Loud, A.V. and Anversa, P. 1979. Morphometry of cardiac hypertrophy induced by experimental renal hypertension. *Am. J. Cardiol.* 44:919–929.

38. Rakusan, K., and Tomanek, R.J., Distribution of mitochondria in normal and hypertrophic myocytes from the rat heart. *J. Mol. Cell. Cardiol.*, in press.

39. Poche, R., De Mello-Mattos, C.M., Rembarz, H.W., and Steopel, K. 1968. Über das Verhältnis Mitochondrien: myofibrillar in den Herzmuskelzellen der Ratte bei Druchhypertrophie des Herzens. *Virchow. arch.* [Path Anat] 344:100–110.

40. Takatsu, T., and Kashii, C. 1972. Cardiac hypertrophy in spontaneously hypertensive rats. In *Spontaneous Hypertension. Its pathogenesis and complications*, ed. Okamoto K. pp. 166–172. Berlin, Heidelberg, New York.

41. Wollenberger, A., and Schulze, W.J. 1961. Mitochondrial alterations in the myocardium of dogs with aortic stenosis. *J. Biophys. Biochem. Cytol.* 10:285–288.

42. Walker, J.G., and Bishop, S.P. 1971. Mitochondrial function and structure in experimental canine congestive heart failure. *Cardiovas. Res.* 5:444–450.

43. Page, E., and McCallister, L.P. 1973. Quantitative electron miscroscopic description of heart muscle cells. Application to normal hypertrophied and thyroxin-stimulated hearts. *Amer. J. Cardiol.* 31:172–181.

44. Anversa, P., Levicky, V., Beghi, C., McDonald, S.L., and Kikkawa, Y. 1983. Morphometry of exercise-induced right ventricular hypertrophy in the rat. *Circ. Res.* 52:57–64.

45. Anversa, P., Olivetti, G., Loud, A.V. 1983. Morphometric studies of left ventricular hypertrophy. Perspectives in Cardiovascular Research Vol. 8, pp. 27–37.

46. Lamers, J.M.J., and Stinis, J.T. 1979. Defective calcium pump in the sarcoplasmic reticulum of the hypertrophied rabbit heart. *Life Sci.* 24:2313–2320.

47. Tomanek, R.J., Trout, J.J., and Lauva, I.K. 1984. Cytochemistry of myocardial structures related to degenerative processes in spontaneously hypertensive and normotensive rats. *J. Mol. Cell. Cardiol.* 16:227–237.

48. Marino, T.A., Houser, S.R., and Cooper, G., IV. 1983. Early morphological alteration of pressure-overloaded cat right ventricular myocardium. *Anat. Rec.* 207:417–426.

49. Marino, T.A., Kent, R.L., Uboh, C.E., Fernandez, E., Thompson, E.W., and Cooper, G., IV. 1985. Structural analysis of pressure-versus volume-overload hypertrophy of cat right ventricle. *Am. J. Physiol.* 249:H371–H379.

50. Anversa, P., Beghi, C., McDonald, S.L., Levicky, V., Kikkawa, Y., and Olivetti, G. 1984. Morphometry of right ventricular hypertrophy induced by myocardial infarction in the rat. *Am. J. Pathol.* 116:504–513.

51. Lauva, I.K., and Tomanek, R.J. 1985. Left ventricular performance in spontaneously hypertensive rats after chronic β_1-adrenoceptor blockade with atenolol. *J. Cardiovas. Pharmacol.* 7:232–237.

52. Pfeffer, M.A., Pfeffer, J.M., and Frohlich, E.D. 1976. Pumping ability of the hypertrophying left ventricle of the spontaneously hypertensive rat. *Circ. Res.* 38:423–429.

53. Lundin, S., Friberg, P., Hallback-Nordlander, M. 1978. Left ventricular hypertrophy improves cardiac function in spontaneously hypertensive rats. *Clin. Sci.* 61:1095–1115.

54. Michael, L.H., and Seidel, C.L. 1981. Hydralazine: Effect on contraction mechanics of WKY and SHR rat heart muscle. *Hypertension* 3:356–361.

55. Heller, L.J. 1978. Cardiac muscle mechanics from Doca- and aging spontaneously hypertensive rats. *Am. J. Physiol.* 235:H82–H86.

56. Nakata, K. 1977. Quantitative analysis of ultrastructural changes in developing rat cardiac muscle during normal growth and during acute volume load. *Jap. Circ. J.* 41:1237–1250.

57. Winkler, B., Schaper, J., and Thiedemann, K-U. 1977. Hypertrophy due to chronic volume overloading in the dog heart. A morphometric study. *Basic Res. Cardiol.* 72:222–227.

58. Fleischer, M., Wippo, O., Themann, H., and Achatzy, R.S. 1980. Ultrastructural morphometric analysis of human myocardial left ventricles with mitral insufficiency. *Virchows Arch* A 389:205–210.

59. Hatt, P.Y., Rakusan, K., Gastineau, P., and Laplace, M. 1979. Morphometry and ultrastructure of heart hypertrophy induced by chronic volume overload (aorto-caval fistula in the rat) *J. Mol. Cell. Cardiol.* 11:989–998.

60. Lund, D.D., and Tomanek, R.J. 1980. The effects of chronic hypoxia on the myocardial cell of normotensive and hypertensive rats. *Anat. Rec.* 196:421–430.
61. Friedman, I., Moravec, J., Reichart, E., and Hatt, P.Y. 1973. Subacute myocardial hypoxia in the rat. An electron microscopic study of the left ventricular myocardium. *J. Mol. Cell Cardiol.* 5:125–132.
62. Guski, H., Meerson, F.Z., and Wassilew, G. 1981. Comparative study of ultrastructure and function of the rat heart hypertrophied by exercise or hypoxia. *Exp. Path.* 20:108–120.
63. Herbener, G.H., Swigart, R.H., and Lang, C.A. 1973. Morphometric comparison of the mitochondrial populations of normal and hypertrophic hearts. *Lab. Invest.* 28:96–103.
64. Kainulainen, H., Pilström, L., and Vihko V. 1979. Morphometry of myocardial apex in endurance-trained mice of different ages. *Acta. Physiol. Scand.* 107:109–114.
65. Anversa, P., Levicky, V., Beghi, C., McDonald, S.L., and Kikkawa, Y. 1983. Morphometry of exercise-induced right ventricular hypertrophy in the rat. *Circ. Res.* 52:57–64.
66. Anversa, P., Beghi, C., Levicky, V., McDonald, S.L., and Kikkawa, Y. 1982. Morphometry of right ventricular hypertrophy induced by strenuous exercise in rat. *Am. J. Physiol.* 243:H856–H861.
67. Anversa, P., Beghi, C., Levicky, V., McDonald, S.L., Kikkawa, Y., and Olivetti, G. 1985. Effects of strenuous exercise on the quantitative morphology of left ventricular myocardium in the rat. *J. Mol. Cell. Cardiol.* 17:587–595.
68. Edington, D.W., and Cosmas, A.C. 1972. Effect of maturation and training on mitochondrial size distributions in rat hearts. *J. Appl. Physiol.* 33:715–718.
69. Craft-Cormney, C., and Hauser, J.T. 1980. Early ultrastructural changes in the myocardium following thyroxine-induced hypertrophy. *Virchows Arch B cell Path* 33:267–273.
70. Reith, A., and Fuchs, S. 1973. The heart muscle of the rat under influence of triiodothyronine and riboflavin deficiency with special reference to mitochondria. A morphological and morphometric study by electron microscopy. *Lab. Invest.* 29:229–235.
71. McCallaster, L.P., and Page, E. 1973. Effects of thyroxin on ultrastructure of rat myocardial cells: A stereological study. *J. Ultrastr. Res.* 42:136–155.
72. Datta, B.N., and Silver, M. 1975. Cardiomegaly in chronic anemia in rats: an experimental study including ultrastructural, histometric, and stereologic observations. *Lab. Invest.* 32:503–514.
73. Schwarz, F., Flameng, W., Schaper, J., and Hehrlein, F. 1978. Correlation between myocardial structure and diastolic properties of the heart in chronic aortic valve disease: effects of corrective surgery. *Am. J. Cardiol.* 42:895–903.
74. Warmuth, H., Fleischer, M., Themann, H., Achatzky, R.S., and Dittrich, H. 1978. Feinstrukturell-morphologische Befunde an der Kammerwond hypertrophierter menschlicker limber Ventricle. *Virchows Arch* [Path Anat], 380:135–147.
75. Schaper, J. 1983. Hypertrophy in the Human Heart: Evaluation by Qualitative and Quantitative Light & Electron Microscopy. *Perspectives in Cardiovascular Research* 7:177–196.
76. Zak, R. 1984. Cardiac growth, maturation and aging. In *Growth of the Heart in Health and Disease*, ed. R. Zak, pp. 131–185. New York: Raven Press.
77. Tomanek, R.J., Davis, J.W., and Anderson, S.C. 1979. The effects of α-methyldopa on cardiac hypertrophy in spontaneously hypertensive rats: ultrastructural stereological and morphometric analysis. *Cardiovas. Res.* 23:173–182.
78. Tomanek, R.J. 1979. The role of prevention or relief of pressure overload on the myocardial cell of the spontaneously hypertensive rat. *Lab. Invest.* 40:83–91.
79. Tomanek, R.J. 1982. Selective effects of α-methyldopa on myocardial cell components independent of cell size in noromtensive and genetically hypertensive rats. *Hypertension* 4:499–506.
80. Laks, M.M., Morady, F., and Swan, H.J.C. 1973. Myocardial hypertrophy produced by chronic infusion of such hypertensive doses of norepinephrine in the dog. *Chest* 64:75–78.
81. Ostman, I., and Sjostrand, N.O. 1971. Effect of heavy physical training on the catecholamine content of the heart and adrenals of the guinea pig. *Experientia* 27:270–271.
82. Womble, J.R., Haddox, M.K., and Russel, D.H. 1978. Epinephrine elevation in plasma parallels of canine cardiac hypertrophy. *Life Sci.* 23:1951–1958.
83. Cutilleta, A.F., Erinoff, L., Heller, A., Low, J., and Oparil, S. 1977. Development of left ventricular hypertrophy in young spontaneously hypertensive rats after peripheral sympathectomy. *Circ. Res.* 40:428–434.

84. Page, E., and Oparil, S. 1978. Effect of peripheral sympathectomy of left ventricular ultrastructure in young spontaneously hypertensive rats. *J. Mol. Cell. Cardiol.* 10:301–305.
85. Tomanek, R.J., Bhatnagar, R.K., Schmid, P.D., and Brody, M.J. 1982. The role of catecholamines in myocardial cell hypertrophy in spontaneously hypertensive rats. *Am. J. Physiol.* 242:H1015–H1021.
86. Lauva, I.K., and Tomanek, R.J. 1983. The effects of adrenoceptor blockade with atenolol on myocardial cellular and subcellular hypertrophy in spontaneously hypertensive rats. *Anat. Rec.* 207:615–622.
87. Blomqvist, C.G. 1983. Cardiovascular adaptations to physical training. *Ann. Rev. Physiol.* 45:169–189.
88. Crisman, R.P., and Tomanek, R.J. 1985. Exercise-training modifies myocardial mitochondria and myofibril growth in spontaneously hypertensive rats. *Am. J. Physiol.* 248:H8–H14.
89. Tomanek, R.J. 1979. Dissociation between blood pressure and cardiac hypertrophy in SHR: Stereological and ultrastructural analysis. *Jap. Heart J.* 20:249–251.
90. Cooper, G. IV, Kent, R.L., Uboh, C.E., Thompson, E.W., and Marino, T.A. 1985. Hemodynamic versus adrenergic control of cat right ventricular hypertrophy. *J. Clin. Invest.* 75:1403–1414.
91. Aschenbrenner, V., Nolan, A.C., and Zak, R. 1984. Study of conditions necessary for the induction of cardiac hypertrophy in hypothyroid rats. *Circulation* 70:(Suppl. II) II-97.
92. Breisch, E.A., Bove, A.A., and Phillips, S.J. 1980. Myocardial morphometrics in pressure overload left ventricular hypertrophy and regression. *Cardiovas. Res.* 14:161–168.

4. CAPILLARITY AND THE DISTRIBUTION OF CAPILLARIES AND MITOCHONDRIA IN CARDIAC GROWTH

NATALIO BANCHERO

The myocardial cell has a high oxygen consumption and is very sensitive to oxygen deprivation. It also requires a constant supply of ATP. These features make it vulnerable to the slightest blood-flow deficit.

The gross anatomy and pathology of the coronary vasculature are well known to the cardiologist and the cardiac surgeon. Less is known, however, about the adaptive changes in cardiac capillarity and myocyte ultrastructure during normal and abnormal hypertrophy. Because it is in the microcirculation that most of the exchange with the myofibers takes place, the numbers and geometrical distribution of capillaries are of great importance in the delivery of oxygen and other substances and in the removal of waste products. Thus, knowledge about the magnitude of changes in cardiac capillarity and in capillary distribution, elicited by physiological factors, is indispensable to evaluate the effect of pathological conditions. It is also important to understand these normal physiological processes in other mammals. Considerable attention has recently been given to the volume density and distribution of the mitochondria within the myocyte. Energy is synthesized in the mitochondria and is then transferred into the myofibrils through the ATP-CP shuttle system [1]. Because ATP is indispensable in cross-bridge cycling, the mitochondria are found in rows between the myofibrils, along the entire length of the fiber [1]. The work of Kayar and Banchero [2] has attempted to determine the exact location of mitochondria within the myocyte, as well as the influence of capillary density and capillary distribution and cell volume on mitochondria.

HEART WEIGHT IN MAMMALIAN SPECIES

In mammals, the weight of the heart (HW) increases linearly with body weight (BW) [3]. The allometric equation relating these two variables in adult mammals of 104 species is as follows: $HW = 0.006 BW^{.98}$ [4]. Thus, the hearts of adult mammals weigh approximately 0.6% of their BW. Extreme examples are the whale's heart, which weighs approximately 500 kg, and the Etruscan shrew's heart, which weighs about 15 mg. Large variations do occur among mammals in the ratio HW/BW. The HW/BW ratio of the Artic weasel is 16.7 g/kg; that of the adult dog is 7, that of the adult guinea pig 3.2, and that of the adult rat approximately 2. However, agreement among laboratories on the HW/BW ratios in a given species is poor. A number of authors have used previously published values that do not conform with more recent observations [3, 5, 6]. For example, the HW/BW ratio in the newborn sheep has been measured by Meier et al. [7] at 6.4 g/kg, which is much lower than the value of 8 g/kg reported by Lee et al. [5]. Our laboratory has consistently found values close to 3.2 g/kg for the adult guinea pig of the Hartley strain; the value reported by Lee et al. [5] is only 1.92 g/kg.

BODY GROWTH SPAN

Body growth in a given animal species affects the spectrum of heart weights. Guinea pigs are born at 100 grams and grow to be about 1.1 kg, for a total elevenfold weight increase. Rats, however, are born at about 6 grams and grow continuously to about 900 grams, for a total 150-fold weight increase. The average human is born weighing 3.5 kg and may reach 70 kg in adulthood: a total twentyfold weight increase. In humans, the total gain varies greatly because of the considerable differences in body weight and composition.

NORMAL CARDIAC GROWTH

In a given animal species the weight of the heart increases with body weight [3, 8–13]. Important variations do occur, however, in the exponential value of the equation $HW = K \times BW^{\alpha}$. The ratio HW/BW is usually greater in the newborn, decreasing rapidly with age [7]. Animals that are born at very immature stages, such as the rat, show cardiac hyperplasia in the early postnatal period, but the increase in cell numbers ceases by weaning time [14, 16]. Animals that are fairly mature at birth, such as the guinea pig, probably have no cardiac hyperplasia. In guinea pigs, the weight of the whole heart, as well as the weights of the right and left ventricular free walls, increase linearly with body weight (figure 4–1) [12, 13]. The guinea pig's left ventricle (LV) weighs about twice as much as its right ventricle (RV). In humans, also, heart weight is linearly related to body weight [8, 9]. Even though humans stop growing by the time they reach their late teens, their hearts continue to increase in weight until the ninth decade, after which heart weight decreases. In centenarians the weight of the heart is about 8 g/kg BW [17].

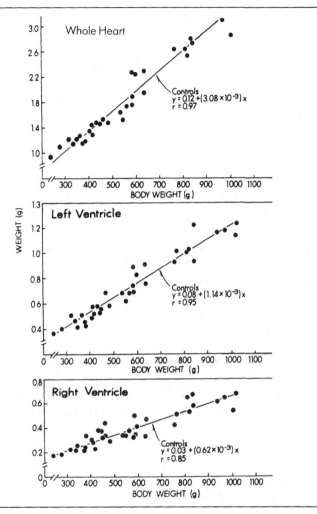

Figure 4–1. Changes in heart weights with body weight in control guinea pigs of the Hartley strain.

To understand the growing process, one must determine the magnitude of the changes—in length and cross-sectional area of the individual myocyte—that accompany normal cardiac growth. Anversa et al. [15, 16], reviewing the absolute and the differential growth of the LV and RV myocytes of the rat in the early postnatal period, found that mean cell volume, cell length, and percent of binucleation were similar in both ventricles during the first 11 days after birth. Korecky and Rakusan [14] isolated cardiac myocytes in growing rats with BWs ranging from 75 to 750 grams. Over this range of BWs, the length and the width of the myocyte increased by 64% and 68%, respectively, while cell volume increased fivefold. In rats of these sizes, cardiac growth occurs solely by hypertrophy of existing fibers [14]. Legato has observed occasional mitotic activity in the hearts of very young dogs [18, 19]. Munnel and Getty [20] measured myocytes in dogs ranging from 2 days to 19 years. Fiber diameter increased from about 13–15 μm, with concomitant length increases, but in the first 100 days postpartum the increases were insignificant. Measuring human myocytes, Ashley [21] found no difference between left and right ventricles in the diameter of the myocytes during the early postnatal period (10.8 and 9.5 μm for the LV and RV, respectively). Subsequently, the LV myocytes grew to 20 μm, but the RV myocytes reached only 16–17 μm. These values were slightly larger than those reported earlier by Roberts and Wearn [8]. The increase in the HW/BW ratio in humans results mainly from hypertrophy of the myofibers. Linzbach [22] believes that moderate hyperplasia does occur in the LV and RV during the early postnatal period, and again with massive hypertrophy. Astorri et al. [23] confirmed this view in a study on RV hypertrophy.

The cross-sectional area of the myofibers (FCSA) can be measured with reasonable accuracy in transverse sections of myocardia, provided they are cut perpendicular to the long axis of the fibers. The linear relationship between HW and the fiber cross-sectional area has been known for many years [8]. Figure 4–2 shows the relationship between FCSA and ventricular weights in the guinea pig [13]. There are significant differences between the right and left ventricles. The myofibers of the LV have larger FCSAs than the myofibers of the RV. This difference, however, is too small to explain the large weight difference between the two ventricles. The difference in weight is because the LV has considerably more fibers than the RV. Using FCSA and cardiac weight to calculate changes in fiber length, Kayar and Banchero [13] analyzed the magnitude of changes in the size of the myofiber during normal growth in guinea pigs weighing between 225 and 1100 grams. The weight of the myocardium was assumed to be proportional to its volume, i.e., tissue density was constant and equal to 1. The changes in weight had to be proportional to the changes in FCSA, or the difference would provide an index of length changes.

$$\Delta L = (\Delta W)^{1/3} \text{ and}$$

$$\Delta FCSA = (\Delta L)^2 + (\Delta W)^{2/3}$$

The LV of the normal guinea pigs increased in weight from approximately 0.4 to 1.2 grams, or by a factor of 3. Theoretically then, the increase in FCSA should be $3^{2/3} = 2.1$. The actual change in FCSA, measured in the LV, was from 157 to 294 μm², or 1.9x, which agrees with the predicted values. The fiber length change should then be $3^{1/3} = 1.44$x. The RV weight increased from 0.2 to 0.7 grams (3.5x). The expected changes should then be $3.5^{2/3} = 2.31$, but the actual change was from 131 to 235 μm² (1.79x). This discrepancy suggests that length showed a disproportionate increase which was calculated as 1.96x. Thus, the RV myofibers of the normal guinea pig grew less than the

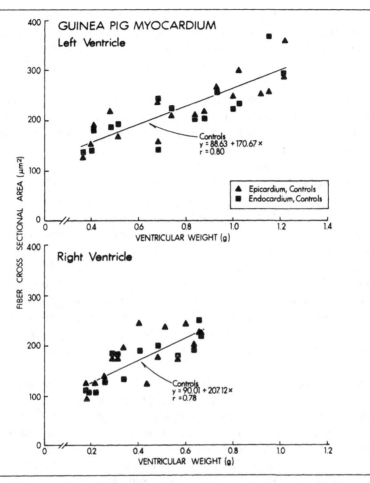

Figure 4-2. Changes in myofiber cross-sectional area with ventricular weight in normal guinea pig hearts.

LV myofibers. The estimate of hyperplasia carried out by Pietschmann and Bartels [24] assumes the constant length/width ratio that was reported by Koreczy and Rakusan [14], but there is no reason to believe that these ratios are constant in situations other than normal growth.

CAPILLARITY IN THE NORMAL HEART

Before analyzing the effects on capillarity of physiological conditions, such as exercise or by pathological alterations, it is necessary to know how much cardiac capillarity changes with normal body growth [10, 13, 25–27]. This is particularly important if changes in the size of the myofibers occur. The changes in capillarity with growth are species-specific and are influenced by biological and technical factors. For example, the Etruscan shrew, the smallest of the mammals, has 7287 cap/mm^2 and a C/F of 1.71, with fiber cross section of 240 μm^2 [28]. Cardiac capillarity in the guinea pig is less than half what it is in the shrew. Investigators should be aware that data available in the literature are not necessarily suitable for comparisons. In fact, investigators should study their own control animals to determine the relationship between fiber size and capillarity.

Measurement of capillary density (CD) is not necessarily accurate as different technical artifacts can affect CD. Shrinkage of the tissue during fixation can be considerable, and was particularly important in early studies, in which formalin fixation shrank cross sections by up to 50%. Large differences have been measured between cardiac muscle fixed by arterial perfusion at about 100 cm H_2O pressure and that fixed by immersion [26]. In guinea pig hearts that were immersion-fixed in glutaraldehyde the average FCSA was 40–60% larger, and the CD accordingly lower, than in those fixed by arterial perfusion. The state of contraction of the myofibers also affects FCSA and CD, but a systematic comparison to assess these effects has not yet been made. It is, therefore, important that all hearts be contracted similarly at the time of sampling and that the fixation procedure be the same [25]. The method used to kill the animal may be important in this respect. Because capillaries do not necessarily run as straight tubes parallel to the myofibers, and their orientation is not always perpendicular to the plane of section, corrections should be introduced in the measurement of CD [29]. The correction factor is generally not large (5–10%) but it should not be disregarded.

It has been known for a long time that cardiac CD is related to fiber cross sectional area and hence to ventricular weight [10, 13, 26]. As normal growth occurs mainly through hypertrophy of the myofibers, the surrounding capillaries are pushed farther apart and CD decreases as the girth of the fibers increases. In guinea pigs, the decrease in CD with increasing FCSA has been shown to be hyperbolic with no gender difference (figure 4–3) [13, 26]. The transmural distribution of capillaries was homogenous, but the scatter of the data was considerable. The same homogeneity in transmural capillarity was observed by Wright and Hudlicka [25]. As CD decreases with increasing FCSA, there is an increase in the ratio of capillary density to fiber density (C/F) (figure 4–4), and in the number of capillaries around the myofiber (CAF) (figure 4–5). This means that new capillaries develop as the myofibers increase in girth, but they are insufficient to maintain a constant CD. Some investigators have found it difficult to trace the fiber profiles in the cross section, and have used instead, as their control relationship, the changes in capillary density with ventricular weight [25, 27]. As would be expected, this relationship is not hyperbolic; CD decreases with HW, but remains fairly constant after the heart and body have stopped growing [25, 27]. Furthermore, not all increases in HWs are accompanied by proportional increases in the girth of the fibers. There is no reason to believe that fiber elongation should increase CD, but it would, of course, increase the total length of the capillary network.

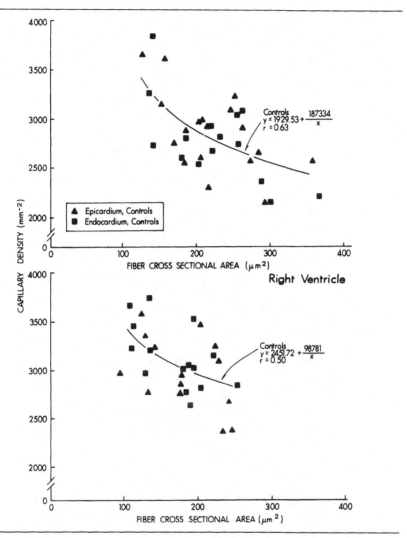

Figure 4–3. Changes in capillary density with changes in fiber cross-sectional area in guinea pig myocardium.

Capillary Distribution

Oxygen gradients within tissues are related not only to capillary density but also to geometrical arrays. Yet quantitative analyses of capillary distribution and measurement of diffusion distances in myocardium have been difficult. Without data on capillary geometrical arrangement, the estimates of capillary distances have relied on assumptions. First approximations assumed that capillaries were distributed uniformly on the cross section, and thus, calculated only the mean value for intercapillary distance. This value does not provide

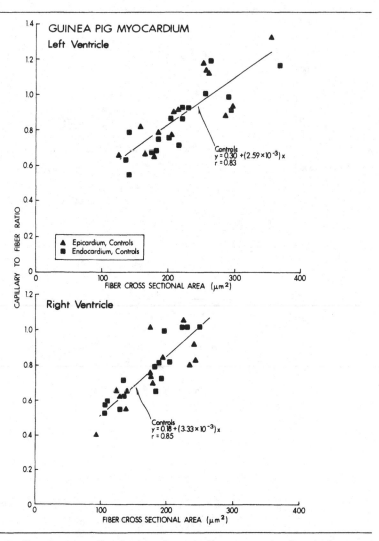

Figure 4–4. Capillary density-to-fiber density ratio versus fiber cross-sectional area in the myocardium of normal guinea pigs. From Kayar and Banchero [13].

adequate information to judge tissue oxygenation. Loats et al. [30] published a method, using concentric circles of known radii for calculating diffusion distances on transverse sections of skeletal muscle, and Rakusan et al. [31] used this method to calculate diffusion distances in rat myocardium. Later, Turek and Rakusan [32] measured the distribution of capillaries, using lognormal distributions from data obtained by the method of concentric circles. Turek and Rakusan [32], as well as Vetterlein et al. [33], found that the distribution of distances to the nearest capillary was asymmetric, with larger numbers for the long distances, and concluded that the distribution of capillaries in cardiac

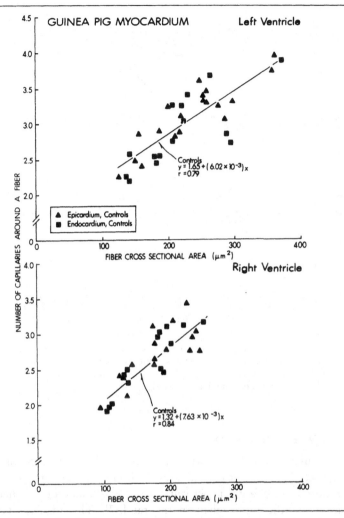

Figure 4–5. Number of capillaries around the fiber versus fiber cross-sectional area in guinea pig myocardium. From Kayar and Banchero [13].

muscle was inhomogeneous. However, mathematical skewness and inhomogeneity of capillary distribution are not necessarily the same. Kayar et al. [34] have recently reported an improved method for analyzing capillary distribution and diffusion distances in tissues. To calculate median and maximal diffusion distances, these investigators used the closest-individual method, which also permits the identification of the capillary array. As figure 4–6 shows, the array of capillaries in guinea pig myocardium is ordered and square, not random. The diffusion distances calculated by Kayar and Banchero [35], using this method for the LV and RV of growing guinea pigs, are shown in table 4–1.

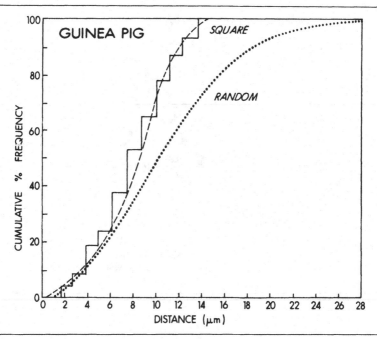

Figure 4–6. Cumulative frequency distribution of distances, to the nearest capillary, in the left ventricle of a 486 g guinea pig (10 fields, 250 measurements). Data are compared to expected distributions if the same density of capillaries (2308 capillaries/mm^2) were in a random or square-ordered array. From Kayar and Banchero [35].

Mitochondria in the Normal Heart

The myofibrillar and mitochondrial fractions of cell volume remain constant during myocardial cell growth in rats weighing 36–270 grams [36]. The concentration of mitochondria per cell volume is a function of cardiac activity and is lower in the rabbit than in the rat [37]. The absolute volume of mitochondria and myofibrils increases with cell volume. The size distribution of mitochondrial profiles also remains constant [38]. The ratio of mitochondria to myofibrils remains intact in physiologic hypertrophy and in exercise training [39]. This normal growth of the myofiber is different in cardiac hypertrophy, elicited by pressure overload, such as aortic constriction. In that case, the mitochondria/myofibril ratio decreases [40]. However, although there were no changes when spontaneously hypertensive rats were trained to run on a treadmill, this ratio was maintained at normal values without changes in the magnitude of the hypertension and cardiac hypertrophy [41].

The location of mitochondria, relative to capillaries, as well as their distribution within the myofiber, has been the subject of intense research. However, it has been difficult to obtain and interpret data. Mainwood and Rakusan [42] proposed a method for the indirect assessment of these distances

Table 4–1. Capillary densities (CD), mean (R) and maximal (R95) diffusion distances in LV and RV.

Body Wt. (g)		CD ± 1 SE (caps/mm²)	R ± 1 SE (μm)	Measured R95 (μm)	Predicted R95 (μm)	n
452	LV	2441 ± 220	7.7 ± 0.2	12.3	12.1	9
	RV	2456 ± 156	7.7 ± 0.2	13.5	12.1	9
486	LV	2308 ± 115	7.1 ± 0.2	12.3	12.5	10
	RV	2284 ± 279	7.8 ± 0.3	13.5	12.6	4
501	LV	2273 ± 205	8.0 ± 0.2	13.5	12.6	10
	RV	2432 ± 119	7.8 ± 0.2	13.5	12.2	10
668	LV	1962 ± 253	7.1 ± 0.2	12.3	13.5	5
	RV	2539 ± 160	6.6 ± 0.2	11.0	11.9	10
690	LV	1695 ± 47	7.8 ± 0.2	12.3	14.6	10
	RV	2059 ± 157	7.9 ± 0.2	12.3	13.2	10
723	LV	1745 ± 93	8.1 ± 0.2	12.3	14.4	10
	RV	1861 ± 128	7.8 ± 0.2	12.3	13.9	10
960	LV	2052 ± 160	8.7 ± 0.3	18.4	13.2	10
	RV★					

★ Sample lost
Note: In a cumulative frequency distribution of measurements, any heterogeneity would be most evident at the higher frequencies. Predictions of R95 assuming a square array $(0.60 \sqrt{D^{-1}})$ of capillaries at these densities. Number of fields analyzed in n. From Kayar and Banchero [35]

by assuming that the mitochondria were either distributed around capillaries or distributed homogeneously throughout the myofiber. Kayar and Banchero [2] used a template of concentric rings of equal areas and a lattice of points distributed evenly to measure, by stereology, the relative volume density of mitochondria as a function of diffusion distances from the center of a cardiac capillary (figure 4–7). The point-counting technique for measuring relative volume densities was applied to each ring, at increasing distances from the center of a capillary. Volume density of mitochondria was greatest close to the capillary at 29–35% (mean = 31.6%) and decreased significantly (p < 0.001) to 22–29% (mean = 25.2%) at the greatest distance from the capillary [2]. Both in normal guinea pigs and in those with cardiac hypertrophy, the highest volume density of mitochondria occurred at a distance of approximately 15% of the maximal diffusion distance, measured by the closest-individual method [34]. The particular distribution of mitochondria in relation to the capillary did not differ between controls and guinea pigs with pressure overload hypertrophy, induced by hypobaria [2]. These results indicate that the mitochondria increase with fiber girth, and that as capillary density decreases with normal growth, the consequent increases in diffusion distances are counterbalanced by a continuous change in the relative position of the mitochondria. Mitochondrial positions change so that the mitochondria are always more dense at about 15% of the maximal diffusion distance from the center of the capillary [2]. Because the distributions of capillaries in guinea pig myocardium can be

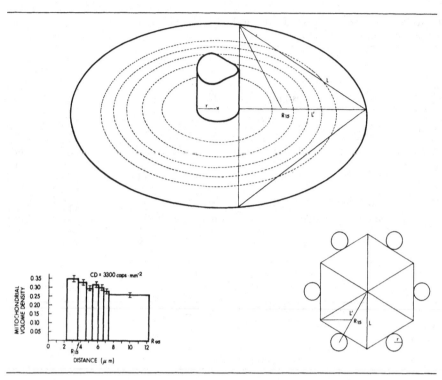

Figure 4–7. The volume density of mitochondria is measured by the point-counting technique, the distances from the center of the capillary is measured by the concentric rings technique [30]. These distances are plotted as shown on the inset at the left-hand side of the illustration. A hexagonal array of capillaries is depicted on the right-hand side. Modified from Kayar and Banchero [2].

hexagonal or square, a hexagonal arrangement was used to model the system (figure 4–7). The model has obvious oversimplifications; for instance, it ignores the fact that not all capillaries contribute the same amount of oxygen to the tissue.

NORMAL GROWTH VERSUS PHYSIOLOGIC CARDIAC HYPERTROPHY

It has been firmly established that the growth of the heart occurs first by hyperplasia and later by myofiber hypertrophy. The number of cell replications appears to be fixed for a given species. These replications occur mostly in utero, but some may occur early in the postnatal period [4, 43]. When a hyperplastic development occurs after birth, it is often related to the state of maturation at birth. Prothero [4] has indicated that cardiac muscle fibers may be able to divide up to, but not beyond, a fixed, species-specific number of cell replications. Yet unknown are both the mechanism that stops hyperplastic growth and the mechanism responsible for normal hypertrophic growth. Hypertrophy is known to occur within well-defined limits. Some investigators believe that the changes in ventricular size may be related to hemo-dynamic factors. Others say that they cannot fully explain the changes in ventricular volumes that occur in normal life.

One common type of physiological hypertrophy of the myofiber, which is not connected to body growth, has been observed in the hearts of athletes whose ventricles are larger and heavier than normal. During exercise, the athlete's stroke volume increases due mainly to a decrease in end-systolic volume. At the same time, the end-diastolic volume of an athlete is larger, and the size and weight of the ventricles increase. This type of cardiac hypertrophy is thus accompanied by increases in cardiac performance: the ejection fraction (SV/EDV) is increased. Clearly, the contractile machinery of the myofiber must function optimally in these athletes.

The increases in cardiac output occur only while the subject is exercising. Changes in mean systemic arterial blood pressure and mean pulmonary arterial pressure during intense endurance exercise are moderate, whereas changes in systolic arterial pressure reflect changes in stroke volume. Hence, the load increase applies equally to both ventricles. Anversa et al. [40] found data suggesting that this may not be the case in the rat.

Anversa and co-workers [40] have found the hypertrophy of the RV (31%) to be larger than that of the LV (13%) in rats after a seven-week period of treadmill running. The hypertrophy of the LV was not statistically significant. Interestingly, cardiac hypertrophy was not the result of a larger FCSA in either ventricle. This observation was corroborated by the measurement of wall thickness in both ventricles, which remained the same. It seems logical to conclude that an elongation of the fibers had occurred (26% for the RV). This elongation may be explained by replication of sarcomeres in the longitudinal direction of the myocyte. The capillary numerical density increased by 16% for the RV and by 4% for the LV. The increase in the total length of the capillary network (41%) reflected, in addition, the change in the length of the RV fibers. If these changes had been analyzed as changes in CD as a function of HW, the very significant differences in capillarity might have gone unnoticed. Kayar et al. [44] have measured a decrease in CD, with no change in either C/F or total capillary length, in rats exercised for six weeks on a laddermill. The peak density of mitochondrial volume, 42%, occurred 4–5 μm from the center of the capillary.

It is known that athletes have markedly slow resting-heart rates. Wright and Hudlicka [25] have reported an increase of up to 70% in the capillary density of rabbits whose hearts were made bradycardic (55% of normal heart rates) by chronic electrical pacing for more than three weeks. The hearts of these animals did not exhibit hypertrophy as judged by the weights of the ventricles. Thus, the authors claim, the increase in cardiac capillarity represents an additional advantage to oxygen delivery [25]. Wright's and Hudlicka's data could, however, have resulted from a reduction in FCSA, with a proportional lengthening of the myofibers. The authors found a reduction in FCSA in the

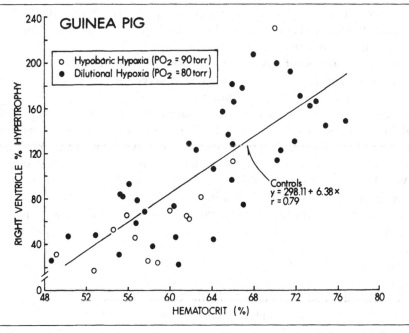

Figure 4–8. Variation in the degree of hypertrophy of the right ventricle with hematocrit in guinea pigs reared in hypoxic environments. Percent of hypertrophy was calculated as the weight of the RV of the hypoxic guinea pig minus the calculated average weight of the RV of a control animal of the same body weight, divided by the control RV weight.

myofibers of the bradycardic rabbits, but they did not quantitate it. This observation simply emphasizes the importance of FCSA on CD.

Right ventricular hypertrophy occurs in normal human high altitude residents, and is tolerated well [45–47]. Most mammals exposed to chronic hypoxia also show significant RV hypertrophy. These changes in RV weight, in chronically hypoxic animals, were linearly related to BW [11–13]. Bartels et al. [48] have reported considerable differences in RV hypertrophy between rats and guinea pigs exposed to the same degree of hypoxia. Large differences in the degree of RV hypertrophy also occur within one species. Guinea pigs exposed to laboratory hypoxia had a 20% incidence of right heart failure and these animals had heavier right ventricles [49]. Figure 4–8 shows the correlation between the degree of right ventricular hypertrophy and hematocrit values, and suggests that increased blood viscosity plays an important role in the development of right heart failure [50]. The mortality rate was not as high in guinea pigs exposed to the same degree of hypoxia plus 6°C cold [51]. The rate of development of right ventricular hypertrophy was different in these two groups (figure 4–9). In the guinea pigs, exposed to the combined effects of cold and hypoxia, the levels of hemoglobin concentration and hematocrit were not as high, and the degree of right ventricular hypertrophy

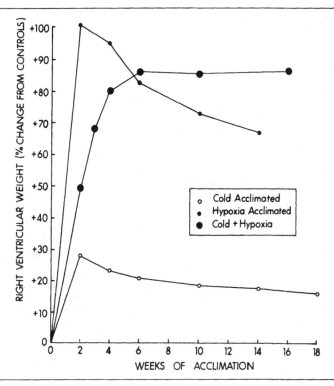

Figure 4–9. Changes in RV weight, expressed as percent change from RV weights in control animals. Guinea pigs acclimated to 5°C cold are represented by open circles; guinea pigs acclimated to an altitude of 5100 m are represented by small closed circles; and, guinea pigs acclimated to the combined stresses of cold plus hypoxia are represented by large closed circles.

was not as marked, as in those animals in simple normothermic hypoxia (figure 4–10).

An increase in cardiac capillarity has been reported in animals born at high altitudes. The early observations made by Becker et al. [52] and Valdivia [53] on a small number of animals, utilizing inadequate fixing and sampling techniques, are questionable. Becker et al. [52] reported a larger relative volume of cardiac capillaries in puppies born at simulated altitude, while Valdivia [53] found an increase in the C/F ratio in Andean guinea pigs. These findings alone do not necessarily indicate increased cardiac capillarity. In rats adapted to a simulated altitude of 3500 m, Turek et al. [11] found an increase in fiber diameter and a significant increase in CD and in C/F, which resulted in decreased diffusion distances. As Pietschmann and Bartels [24] have indicated, the values for C/F in hypoxic animals, reported by Turek et al. [11], were higher than any other value for C/F recorded in the literature. Grandtner et al. [54] reported increased capillarity in rats born at simulated altitude. In contrast, Turek et al. [55] reported a decrease in CD, with constant values for C/F in the RV of rats with RV hypertrophy induced by ligation of a coronary

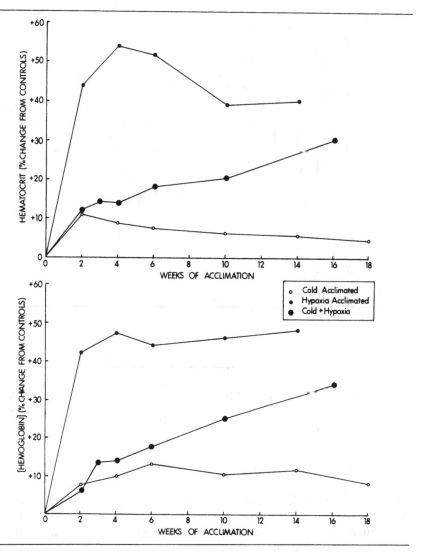

Figure 4–10. Changes in hemoglobin and hematocrit in guinea pigs acclimated to three different environments. Symbols are the same as indicated in figure 4–9.

artery followed by myocardial infarction of the LV. These results imply that the large hypertrophy of the RV in the hearts with myocardial infarction was different from the hypertrophy associated with chronic hypoxia, and that this difference was related to an inability of the noninfarcted myocardium to develop more capillaries. Kayar and Banchero [26] reported increased CD, C/F, and CAF in the RV of chronically hypoxic guinea pigs, without evidence of cardiac failure. The median and maximal diffusion distances measured by the closest-individual method were shorter than in controls. In hypoxic animals with signs of RV failure, CD, C/F, and oxygen diffusion distances, did not differ from those of normoxic controls. These guinea pigs with right heart failure had larger FCSA's than the controls. Pietschmann and Bartels [24] have recently reported an increased C/F in rats exposed to a simulated altitude of 5000 m, but the increases were related to an increase in FCSA, as CD remained unchanged. Rakusan et al. [56] found no differences in number and distribution of capillaries between guinea pigs native to the Andes and control guinea pigs born in the Netherlands. This summary of studies on capillarity in chronic hypoxia indicates that some of the discrepancies in the literature may reflect differences in the size of RV myofibers, and in the magnitude of the hypertrophy.

Many small mammals are exposed either seasonally or nocturnally to low temperatures. On occasion, this exposure to low temperatures occurs at high elevations. Hence the animals are exposed naturally to cold plus hypoxia. Exposing small mammals to low temperatures produces a rapid increase in oxygen consumption. Guinea pigs exposed to 5°C doubled their cardiac output and oxygen consumption [57]. Simple calculations made by Kayar and Banchero [13] on guinea pigs exposed to cold show modest volume-overload hypertrophy in both ventricles. In the LV this was due mainly to fiber elongation whereas in the RV it was due to FCSA. Because of mechanical considerations related to the volume of a sphere and its radius ($Vs = \frac{4}{3}\pi r^3$), an enlarged ventricle can pump a larger stroke volume than a smaller ventricle with the same degree of fiber shortening. As the LV enlarges, the end-diastolic pressure and volume increase. In turn, the oxygen consumption of the myocardium is increased considerably, because the tension required to pump at a given blood pressure increases as the radius increases. This is stated in the Laplace equation:

$$T = P \times \frac{R}{2}; \text{ where } T = \text{tension}, P = \text{pressure and } R = \text{radius}.$$

Cardiac capillarity does seem to change in response to volume-overload hypertrophy. Heroux and St. Pierre [58] measured cardiac capillarity in rats exposed to 6°C and found no change in CD, but they failed to report changes in fiber size or heart weights. Thus, the interpretation of their results is equivocal. Kayar and Banchero [13] found no change in the capillarity of the LV and RV of guinea pigs exposed to 5°C. Hence, diffusion distances were the same in the hearts of cold-acclimated guinea pigs and in the hearts of animals at normal laboratory temperature.

Abnormal Cardiac Growth

Chronic increases in the work of the heart result in myocardial hypertrophy. Massive hypertrophy is the result of severe pathological alteration. In physical terms, work is the product of pressure times flow. For the ventricles, work is calculated as the product of the mean blood pressure, against which the ventricle pumps, and the blood flow through that chamber. When the resistance to flow increases, the intracavitary pressure generated by the ventricle increases, and a pressure overload occurs. When blood flow increases with no alteration in the blood pressure generated by the ventricle, a volume overload occurs. Cardiac hypertrophy may result from both mechanisms acting together. Despite the tremendous growth potential of the myofibers, large and sustained increases in their work often result in diminished contractile force and eventual failure. The rapidity of the change in cardiac work may affect the performance of the myofibers. Right heart failure is more common in those animals with sudden increases in RV weights. The mechanisms responsible for myofiber failure remain elusive. There is reason to believe that these two forms of cardiac hypertrophy, pressure and volume overload, differ not only in their pathogenesis but also in their implications for cardiac function.

ACKNOWLEDGMENTS

The author wishes to thank Drs. José Faura, Catherine R. Jackson, and Cynthea I. Blake for their assistance in the preparation of the manuscript. The experimental work was supported by NIH grants HL-18145, HL-28849, and HL-32180.

REFERENCES

1. Mela-Riker, L.M., and Bukoski, R.D. 1985. Regulation of mitochondrial activity in cardiac cells. Ann. Rev. Physiol. 47:645–663.
2. Kayar, S.R., and Banchero, N. 1986. Volume density and distribution of mitochondria in myocardial growth and hypertrophy. Resp. Physiol.
3. Grande, F., and Taylor, H.L. 1965. Adaptative changes in the heart, vessels, and patterns of control under chronically high loads. In Handbook of Physiology: Circulation. Hamilton, W.F., and Dow, P., eds. Washington, DC: Am. Physiol. Soc. III:2615–2677.
4. Prothero, J. 1979. Heart weight as a function of body weight in mammals. Growth 43:139–150.
5. Lee, J.C., Taylor, J.F.N., and Downing, S.E. 1975. A comparison of ventricular weights and geometry in newborn, young, and adult mammals. J. Appl. Physiol. 38:147–150.
6. Holt, J.P., Rhode, E.A., and Kines, H. 1968. Ventricular volumes and body weight in mammals. Am. J. Physiol. 215:704–715.
7. Meier, P.R., Manchester, D.K., Battaglia, F.C., and Meschia, G. 1983. Fetal heart rate in relation to body mass. Proc. Soc. Exp. Biol. Med. 172:107–110.
8. Roberts, J.T., and Wearn, J.T. 1941. Quantitative changes in the capillary-muscle relationship in human hearts during normal growth and hypertrophy. Am. Heart. J. 21:617–633.
9. Rosahn, P.D. 1941. The weight of normal heart in adult males. Yale J. Biol. Med. 14:209–223.
10. Shipley, B.R., Shipley, L.J., and Wearn, J.T. 1937. The capillary supply in normal and hypertrophied hearts of rabbits. J. Exp. Med. 65:29–42.
11. Turek, Z., Grandtner, M., and Kreuzer, F. 1972. Cardiac hypertrophy, capillary and muscle fiber density, muscle fiber diameter, capillary radius and diffusion distance in the myocardium of growing rats adapted to a simulated altitude of 3,500 m. Pflügers Arch 335:19–28.
12. Bui, M.V., and Banchero, N. 1980. Effects of chronic exposure to cold or hypoxia on ventricular weights and ventricular myoglobin concentrations in guinea pigs during growth. Pflügers Arch 385:155–160.
13. Kayar, S.R., and Banchero, N. 1985. Volume overload hypertrophy elicited by cold and its

effects on myocardial capillarity. *Respir. Physiol.* 59:1–14.

14. Korecky, B., and Rakusan, K. 1978. Normal and hypertrophic growth of the rat heart; changes in cell dimensions and number. *Am. J. Physiol.* 234:123–128.

15. Anversa, P., Olivetti, G., and Loud, A.V. 1980. Morphometric study of early postnatal development in the left and right ventricular myocardium of the rat. I. Hypertrophy, hyperplasia, and binucleation of myocytes. *Circ. Res.* 46:495–502.

16. Olivetti, G., Anversa, P., and Loud, A.V. 1980. Morphometric study of early postnatal development in the left and right ventricular myocardium of the rat. II. Tissue composition capillary growth, and sarcoplasmic alterations. *Circ. Res.* 46:503–512.

17. Linzbach, A.J., and Akuamoa-Boateng, E. 1973. Die Alternsveranderungen des menschlichen herzens. I. Das herzgewicht im *Alter Klin Wochenschr* 51:156–163.

18. Legato, M.J. 1979. Cellular mechanisms of normal growth in the mammalian heart. I. Qualitative and quantitative features of ventricular architecture in the dog from birth to five months of age. *Circ. Res.* 44:250–262.

19. Legato, M.J. 1979. Cellular mechanisms of normal growth in the mammalian heart. II. A quantitative and qualitative comparison between the right and left ventricular myocytes in the dog from birth to five months of age. *Circ. Res.* 44:263–279.

20. Munnell, J.F., and Getty, R. 1968. Nuclear lobulation and amitotic division associated with increasing cell size in the aging canine myocardium. *J. Gerontol.* 23:363–369.

21. Ashley, L.M. 1945. A determination of the diameters of myocardial fibers in man and other mammals. *J. Anat.* 77:325–347.

22. Linzbach, A.J. 1960. Heart failure from the point of view of quantitative anatomy. *Am. J. Cardiol.* 5:370–382.

23. Astorri, E., Chizzola, A., Visioli, O., Anversa, P., Olivetti, G., and Vitali-Mazza, L. 1971. Right ventricular hypertrophy—a cytometric study on 55 human hearts. *J. Mol. Cell. Cardiol.* 2:99–110.

24. Pietschmann, M., and Bartels, H. 1985. Cellular hyperplasia and hypertrophy, capillary proliferation and myoglobin concentration in the heart of newborn and adult rats at high altitude. *Resp. Physiol.* 59:347–360.

25. Wright, A.J.A., and Hudlicka, O. 1981. Capillary growth and changes in heart performance induced by chronic bradycardial pacing in the rabbit. *Circ. Res.* 49:460–478.

26. Kayar, S.R., and Banchero, N. 1985. Myocardial capillarity in acclimation to hypoxia. *Pflügers Arch* 404:319–325.

27. Hudlicka, O. 1984. Development of microcirculation: capillary growth and adaptation. In *Handbook of Physiology*. The cardiovascular system IV. Capillary growth, Renkin, E.M., and Michel, C.C., eds., Washington, DC, *Am. Physiol. Soc.* 165–216.

28. Pietschmann, M., Bartels, H., and Fons, R. 1982. Capillary supply of heart and skeletal muscle of small bats and nonflying mammals. *Resp. Physiol.* 50:267–282.

29. Mathieu, O., Cruz-Orive, L.M., Hoppeler, H., and Weibel, E.R. 1983. Estimating length density and quantifying anisotropy in skeletal muscle capillaries. *J. Microscopy* 131:131–146.

30. Loats, J.T., Sillau, A.H., and Banchero, N. 1978. How to quantify skeletal muscle capillarity. In *Oxygen Transport to Tissue—III*, Silver, I.A., Erecinska, M., and Bicher, H.I., eds., pp. 41–48. New York: Plenum Press.

31. Rakusan, K., Moranec, J. and Hatt, P.Y. 1980. Regional capillary supply in the normal and hypertrophied rat heart. *Microvasc. Res.* 20:319–326.

32. Turek, Z., and Rakusan, K. 1981. Lognormal distribution of intercapillary distance in normal and hypertrophic rat heart as estimated by the method of concentric circles: its effect on tissue oxygenation. *Pflügers Arch* 391:17–21.

33. Vetterlein, F., dal Ri, H., and Schmidt, G. 1982. Capillary density in rat myocardium during timed plasma staining. *Am. J. Physiol.* 242:H133–141.

34. Kayar, S.R., Archer, P.G., Lechner, A.J., and Banchero, N. 1982. The closest-individual method in the analysis of the distribution of capillaries. *Microvasc. Res.* 24:326–341.

35. Kayar, S.R., and Banchero, N. 1983. Distribution of capillaries and diffusion distances in guinea pig myocardium. *Pflügers Arch* 396:350–352.

36. Page, E., Earley, J., and Power, B. 1974. Normal growth of ultrastructures in rat left ventricular myocardial cells. *Circ. Res.* 34–35:(Suppl. II) 12–16.

37. Page, E., Polimeni, P.I., Zak, R., Earley, J., and Johnson, M. 1972. Myofibrillar mass in rat and rabbit heart muscle: correlation of microchemical and stereological measurements in

normal and hypertrophic hearts. *Circ. Res.* 30:430–439.
38. Smith, H.E., and Page, E. 1976. Morphometry of rat heart mitochondrial subcompartments and membranes: application to myocardial cell atrophy after hypophysectomy. *J. Ultrastruc. Res.* 55:31–41.
39. Guski, H., Meerson, F.Z., and Wassilew, G. 1981. Comparative study of ultrastructure and function of the rat heart hypertrophied by exercise or hypoxia. *Exp. Pathol.* 20:108–120.
40. Anversa, P. Levicky, V., Beghi, C. McDonald, S.L., and Kikkawa, Y. 1983. Morphometry of exercise-induced right ventricular hypertrophy in the rat. *Circ. Res.* 52:57–64.
41. Crisman, R.P., and Tomanek, R.J. 1985. Exercise training modifies myocardial mitochondria and myofibril growth in spontaneously hypertensive rats. *Am. J. Physiol.* 248:H8–14.
42. Mainwood, G.W., and Rakusan, K. 1982. A model for intracellular energy transport. *Can. J. Physiol. Pharmacol.* 60:98–102.
43. Winick, M., and Noble, A. 1965. Quantitative changes in DNA, RNA, and protein during prenatal and postnatal growth in the rat. *Development. Biology.* 12:451–466.
44. Kayar, S.R., Conley, K.E., Claassen, H., and Hoppeler, H. 1986. Capillarity and mitochondrial distribution in rat myocardium following exercise training. *J. Exp. Biol.* 120:189–199.
45. Arias-Stella, J., and Recavarren, S. 1962. Right ventricular hypertrophy in native children living at high altitude. *Am. J. Pathol.* 41:55–64.
46. Recavarren, S., and Arias-Stella, J. 1964. Growth and development of the ventricular myocardium from birth to adult life. *Brit. Heart J.* 26:187–192.
47. Banchero, N., Sime, F., Penaloza, D., Cruz, J., Gamboa, R., and Marticorena, E. 1966. Pulmonary pressure, cardiac output, and arterial oxygen saturation during exercise at high altitude and at sea level. *Circulation* 33:249–262.
48. Bartels, H., Bartels, R., Rathschlage-Schaefer, A.M., Robbel, H., and Ludders, S. 1979. Acclimatization of newborn rats and guinea pigs to 3000 to 5000 m simulated altitudes. *Resp. Physiol.* 36:375–389.
49. Banchero, N., Kayar, S.R., and Lechner, A.J. 1985. Increased capillarity in skeletal muscle of growing guinea pigs acclimated to cold plus hypoxia. *Respiration Physiology* 62:245–255.
50. Banchero, N., Kayar, S.R., and Blake, C.I. 1983. Factors influencing right ventricular hypertrophy and survival of guinea pigs in hypoxia. *The Physiologist* (26):A-33.
51. Banchero, N. Bui, M.V., and Kayar, S.R. Effect of cold plus hypoxia on ventricular weights. Submitted.
52. Becker, L.E., Cooper, R.G., Hataway, G.D. 1955–1956. Capillary vascularization in puppies born at a simulated altitude of 20,000 feet. *J. Appl. Physiol.* 8:166–168.
53. Valdivia, E. 1957. Right ventricular hypertrophy in guinea pigs exposed to simulated high altitude. *Circ. Res.* 5:612–616.
54. Grandtner, M., Turek, Z., and Kreuzer, F. 1974. Cardiac hypertrophy in the first generation of rats native to simulated high altitude. *Pflügers Arch* 350:241–248.
55. Turek, Z., Grandtner, M., Kubat, K., Ringnalda, B.E.M., and Kreuzer, F. 1978. Arterial blood gases, muscle fiber diameter and intercapillary distance in cardiac hypertrophy of rats with an old myocardial infarction. *Pflüger Arch* 376:209–215.
56. Rakusan, K., Turek, Z., and Kreuzer, F. 1981. Myocardial capillaries in guinea pigs native to high altitude (Junin, Peru, 4,105m). *Pflügers Arch* 391:22–24.
57. Blake, C.I., and Banchero, N. 1985. Effects of cold and hypoxia on ventilation and oxygen consumption in awake guinea pigs. *Respir. Physiol.* 61:357–368.
58. Heroux, O., and St. Pierre, J. 1957. Effect of cold acclimation on vascularization of ears, heart, liver, and muscles of white rats. *Am. J. Physiol.* 188:163–168.

5. THE CORONARY VASCULATURE DURING MYOCARDIAL HYPERTROPHY

WILLIAM M. CHILIAN, ROBERT J. TOMANEK, AND MELVIN L. MARCUS

CHARACTERISTICS OF LEFT VENTRICULAR HYPERTROPHY

Left ventricular hypertrophy is generally viewed as a compensatory response to pressure or volume overload that results in normalization of left ventricular wall stress. For example, during systemic hypertension, the increase in arterial pressure causes an initiation of ventricular hypertrophy that stabilizes after some period. During the period of stable hypertrophy, there is no change in ventricular volume or the total mass of the myocardium [1, 2]. During this period of stable hypertrophy, resting ventricular systolic wall stress is normal because the increased wall thickness compensates for increased ventricular pressure [3, 4, 5]. With the normalized systolic wall stress, resting left ventricular oxygen consumption per unit mass of myocardium, is reported as normal. [6, 7] Since myocardial perfusion is primarily regulated by myocardial oxygen consumption, during stable left ventricular hypertrophy, myocardial perfusion, per unit mass of myocardium, is usually found to be normal with respect to that in normal, unhypertrophied hearts [7, 8, 9, 10, 11, 12, 13]. Despite normalized wall stress and normalized blood flow at rest there are many pathological manifestations of cardiac hypertrophy.

Pressure-overload-induced left ventricular hypertrophy is usually associated with abnormalities of cardiac muscle and of the coronary vascular system. Cardiac muscle is characterized by decreased contractility [14], increased

The original work upon which this review was based was supported by the following U.S. Public Health Service Grants:

Program Project Grant HL-14388, National Heart, Lung and Blood Institute Grants HL-20827, HL-06496, HL-01570, HL-29271, and HL-18629 collagen content [15] decreased mitochondrial volume density [16] decreased surface area of the external sarcolemma (excluding the T-tubules) per cell volume [16], abnormal electrophysiological properties [17] and altered diastolic function [18].

Abnormalities associated with alterations of the coronary vascular system, however, appear to be the dominant mechanism associated with pathophysiological manifestations of hypertrophy [19]. Within this context, cardiac hypertrophy is associated with a decrease in coronary vasodilator reserve [11, 13, 20, 21, 22] and an increase in minimal coronary resistance per unit weight of myocardium [8, 10, 20, 23, 24]. Although there are several mechanisms by which cardiac hypertrophy can adversely influence the coronary vasculature and damage the heart, there are several explanations which can account for the decrease in coronary reserve and the increase in minimal coronary vascular resistance. Such mechanisms can include inadequate growth of extramural coronary arteries, arteriolar rarefaction, increased arteriolar wall-to-lumen ratios, increased diffusion distance from capillaries to the myocardial cells, increased heterogeneous spacing of capillaries, augmented extravascular compressive forces, and alterations in coronary vascular reactivity in the hypertophied heart.

CORONARY ANATOMY DURING PATHOLOGICAL CARDIAC HYPERTROPHY

Many laboratories report that the size of epicardial coronary arteries increases appropriately during myocardial hypertrophy [25, 26] but Stack et al. [27] found that epicardial coronaries did not enlarge appropriately during pressure-overload-induced hypertrophy. Thus, either resistance of the epicardial coronary vascular system remains normalized per unit mass of the myocardium or it may slightly increase during cardiac hypertrophy. However, this would alter total coronary resistance only to a very minor extent, since the epicardial coronary conduit arteries only constitute a very minor fraction of total coronary resistance [28].

The effects of cardiac hypertrophy on coronary resistance vessels are less well-documented. Recently Tomanek et al. [29] reported no consistent morphological abnormalities in coronary resistance vessels obtained from dogs with six weeks of pressure-induced left ventricular hypertrophy secondary to renal vascular hypertension. Specifically, the wall-to-lumen ratios of coronary arteries and arterioles, ranging from the epicardial conduit arteries to arterioles approximately 10–30 microns in diameter, were not significantly different from the wall-to-lumen ratios in similarly sized coronary arteries and arterioles from control animals (figure 5–1). However, in the larger coronary arteries from hypertensive animals there was a significant increase in the thickness of the tunica media and diffuse fibrosis of coronary arteries (figure 5–2). These results contrast with the reports of anatomical abnormalities associated with systemic hypertension in other vascular organ systems [30]. In addition, arteriolar rarefaction has been

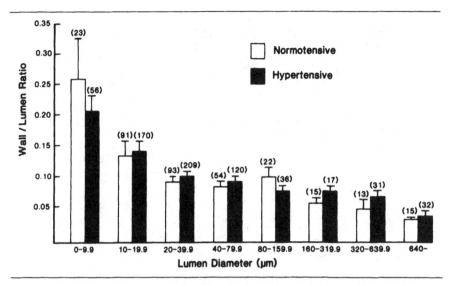

Figure 5–1. Wall-to-lumen ratios for arteries and arterioles in control dogs and dogs with left ventricular hypertrophy. Values for the various lumen diameter classes are shown as means ± SEM. The total number of vessels in each class for the control and hypertrophy groups is indicated in parenthesis. None of the intergroup differences are statistically significant at p < 0.05. The data in this figure were originally published by Tomanek et al. [29].

observed in other vascular beds during systemic hypertension, e.g., skeletal muscles [31, 32], mesentery [33], and cutaneous [34]. Rarefaction of arterioles in the myocardium during hypertrophy has not received extensive evaluation. In this regard, recently Breisch et al. [35] reported a decrease in arteriolar density (less than 100 microns in diameter) in the hypertrophied myocardium. This, however, may not represent true rarefaction, but a relative dilution in the numbers of vessels per unit mass, due to the hypertrophying myocardium.

Coronary vascular abnormalities of the capillary circulation are also associated with myocardial hypertrophy. Generally, most investigators report a decrease in capillary density [36, 37, 38, 39, 40, 41]. Furthermore, some studies have found that the decrease in capillary density occurs mostly to the largest extent in the subendocardial layers of the hypertrophied ventricle [42]. A decrease in capillary density will increase in diffusion distance for oxygen, from the capillary lumen to the myocyte, and this may lead to problems in oxygen supply to the myocytes. Within this context, Henquell et al. [43] reported that intercapillary distances were increased from 12.9 µm in controls to 15.3 µm in pressure-overloaded, hypertrophied hearts. Although this represents a small increase in intercapillary distance, these investigators postulated that such an increase could decreased tissue PO_2 and produce anoxic foci. Furthermore, the amount of anoxic tissue produced by such an increase in intercapillary distance may cause the fibrosis and necrosis observed in left ventricular hypertrophy. Also, if the capillaries are not evenly spaced (arranged in a heterogenous array) this could potentially lead to focal areas of

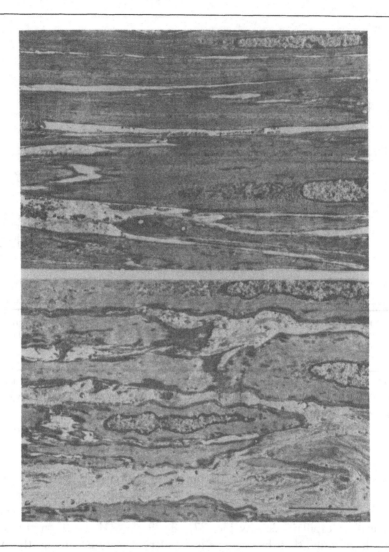

Figure 5–2. Electron micrographs of the tunica media of a large epicardial artery. The upper panel is from a normotensive dog and the lower panel is from a hypertensive dog. Note the larger extracellular compartment relative to the myocytes in the vessel from the hypertensive animal. Bar = 5 μm. These figures were originally published by Tomanek et al. [29].

inadequate oxygen supply. In our opinion, it is not unreasonable to speculate that the heterogeneity of capillary spacing may be an important lesion, which increases the susceptibility of the hypertrophied myocardium to ischemic damage. We must emphasize that the physiological effects of increased diffusion distance, due to a decrease in capillary density, are uncertain because there can be compensatory changes in capillary permeability [44] which may enhance nutritional support of the hypertrophied myocardium and partially offset the increase in diffusion distance.

It is plausible that augmented extravascular compressive forces in the hyper-trophied ventricle, e.g., impaired diastolic relaxation and decreased ventricular compliance, could also compromise myocardial perfusion. Harrison et al [45] found that minimal coronary resistance in the isolated canine heart, following pressure-overload hypertrophy, was equivalent to that of control, normo-tensive animals. This implies that the increase in minimal coronary resistance in pressure overload hypertrophy [8, 24, 46] may be due to augmented mechanical compression of the coronary microvasculature, rather than a direct abnormality of the vasculature. This issue, however, remains unsettled, because Scheel et al. [47] have reported an increase in minimal coronary resistance in an isolated heart preparation with pressure-overload left ventri-cular hypertrophy.

Although pathological cardiac hypertrophy is associated with a decrease in coronary reserve and an increase in minimal coronary resistance, the anatomical abnormalities documented to date are not severe enough to fully account for the physiological dysfunction of the coronary vascular system during pathological hypertrophy. Clearly, more extensive anatomical, physio-logical, and biochemical studies regarding quantification of arteriolar rarefac-tion, heterogeneous spacing of capillaries, altered properties and membrane transport, factors which influence microvascular reactivity, etc., are needed to fully understand these pathological manifestations of cardiac hypertrophy.

FACTORS THAT INFLUENCE THE RELATIONSHIP BETWEEN CARDIAC HYPERTROPHY AND THE CORONARY VASCULAR SYSTEM

There are several more factors that must be considered when assessing the influence of cardiac hypertrophy on the function of the coronary vascular system, such as:

1. different types of species used as the experimental model, e.g., dogs, rats, cattle, ponies [8, 20, 22, 46, 48];
2. different stimuli used to provoke the cardiac hypertrophy, e.g., pressure overload, volume overload, exercise, thyroxine [23, 49, 50, 51];
3. age when the hypertrophy is induced, e.g., fetus, neonate, adult [48, 50, 52, 53];
4. the duration of hypertrophy relating to the stabilization of wall stress [20, 41]; and
5. right versus left ventricular hypertrophy [21, 22, 48, 54].

Animal Species

It is important to consider the animal species employed in any evaluation of the effects of cardiac hypertrophy on the coronary circulation. Pressure-induced left ventricular hypertrophy is associated with a decrease in coronary reserve in animals [11, 13, 20, 21, 55] and man [46, 56, 57]. Volume-overload-induced hypertrophy, however, produces disparate results on coronary vascular reserve in animals versus man. Hiratzka et al. [58] found that volume-overload-induced hypertrophy was associated with a substantial decrease in coronary reserve in man, whereas coronary resistance per unit weight of myocardium and coronary reserve is reported to be normal in animals with volume-overload hypertrophy [49]. However, Hultgren and Bove [59] found that volume-overload induced hypertrophy in the canine produced a decrease in capillary density. The reasons for these different results regarding volume-overload-induced hypertrophy may be related to the duration and intensity of the hypertrophy.

Initiating Stimulus

The stimulus that initiates cardiac hypertrophy also influences the response of the coronary vascular system. Although, as previously discussed, pressure-overload-induced hypertrophy and volume-overload-induced hypertrophy may decrease coronary vasodilator reserve, we have recently shown that left ventricular hypertrophy, secondary to thyrotoxicosis, is associated with a decrease in minimal coronary vascular resistance of the entire left ventricle [50]. We also found that capillary density during thyroxine-induced left-ventricular hypertrophy was actually increased and that coronary vasodilator reserve was normal. Despite elevations in mean arterial pressure thyroxine-induced hypertrophy is characterized by several hemodynamic and biochemical alterations that distinguish it from pressure-overload-induced hypertrophy; namely, resting perfusion is augmented, cardiac output and heart rate are increased, myosin adenosine triphosphatase activity is elevated, and there is an increased mitochondrial volume density [16, 50, 60].

Left ventricular hypertrophy, of the same of lesser magnitude secondary to systemic hypertension, is associated with an increased minimal coronary resistance, decreased coronary vasodilator reserve, and increased capillary density [20, 42, 55]. Recently, Tomanek et al. [61] reported that increased minimal coronary resistance in the spontaneously hypertensive rat was returned to control values when arterial pressure was chronically reduced with hydralazine. This suggests that the mechanism responsible for adverse changes in the coronary vasculature is hypertension, rather than hypertrophy.

A comparison of two different models of hypertrophy (pressure-overload vs. thyroxine) on the anatomical and physiological responses of the coronary vascular systems is shown in figure 5–3. This figure summarizes comparisons between seven-month-old spontaneously hypertensive rats (SHR), the normotensive parent strain, Wistar-Kyoto (WKY), and thyroxine-treated WKY rats (TH-WKY). The left-ventricular weight-to-body-weight ratio (LV/BW) was comparable in the SHR and TH-WKY animal, indicating a similar degree of left ventricular hypertrophy. The capillary density in the SHR was approximately 20% lower than that in the WKY rats, whereas in the TH-WKY rats, the capillary density was about 20% higher than that in the WKY animals. The

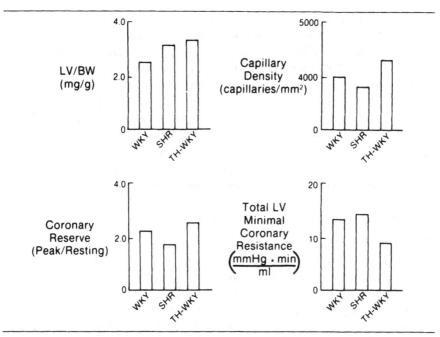

Figure 5–3. Left ventricular weight-to-body weight ratio (LV/BW), capillary density, coronary reserve (maximal peak-to-resting blood flow velocity ratio), and minimal coronary resistance of the entire left ventricle are shown for Wistar-Kyoto (WKY), spontaneously hypertensive rats (SHR), and thyroxine-treated WKY (TH-WKY). This figure was originally presented by Chilian et al. [50] and was adapted from Wangler et al. [20], Tomanek et al. [42], and Peters et al. [55]. Note that, despite similar changes in the LV/BW ratio in SHR and TH-WKY animals, the responses of the coronary vascular system are markedly different.

different stimuli (pressure-overload versus thyroxine) also had markedly disparate effects on coronary reserve. In the SHR rats, coronary reserve was signficantly depressed from that of controls. In contrast, coronary reserve in the TH-WKY rats tended to be higher than that of controls. Minimal coronary resistance for the entire left ventricle was lower in rats with thyroxine-induced left ventricular hypertrophy than that in the control animals or in the spontaneously hypertensive rats. This indicates an enlargement of the coronary cross-sectional area in thyroxine-induced cardiac hypertrophy which was not evident in hypertrophy in the spontaneously hypertensive rat.

These data (figure 5–3) demonstrate that despite a similar degree of left ventricular hypertrophy in two different models (pressure-overload versus thyroxine-induced), the interaction between the coronary vascular system and the cardiac mass is very different: namely, during pressure-overload hypertrophy the effect on the coronary system is adverse (decreased capillary density, decreased coronary reserve), whereas during thyroxine-induced hypertrophy, the response of the coronary vascular system is adequate or more than adequate (increased capillary density, normal coronary reserve). Also,

Scheel and Williams [62] have recently reported that left ventricular hypertrophy in the canine, produced by chronic anemia, is associated with a decrease in minimal coronary resistance and a decrease in collateral resistance. Thus, thyroxine-induced cardiac hypertrophy and anemia-induced cardiac hypertrophy are characterized by adequate growth of the coronary vascular system to match the increase in left ventricular mass. Furthermore, exercise-induced left ventricular hypertrophy is associated with neoformation of capillaries [51], which results in a normal capillary density [63]. Moreover, the volume of the coronary arterial tree is reported to increase during exercise-induced hypertrophy [64]. *Thus, the stimulus (or stimuli) that provokes hypertrophy influences the functional and anatomical responses of the coronary vasculature.*

Age of the Animal when Hypertrophy is Initiated

The age of the animal, when the hypertrophying stimulus is applied to the myocardium, strongly influences the response of the coronary vascular system. For instance, when right ventricular hypertrophy is produced by banding the pulmonary artery in fetal lambs [53], new born lambs [52], or young calves [48], coronary reserve is not decreased, and total right ventricular minimal resistance decreases. This indicates that growth of the coronary vascular bed occurs appropriately with the increase in right ventricular muscle mass. The influence of age on the coronary vascular system response during cardiac hypertrophy is also observed in the left ventricle. We have found a greater increase in capillary proliferation during thyroxine induced hypertrophy in younger (prepubescent) versus older (young adult) animals [50]. Thus, despite many divergent attributes of pressure-overload hypertrophy and thyroxine-induced hypertrophy, a similar characteristic of both models is that the response of the coronary vascular system is dependent on the age of the animal when the hypertrophy is initiated.

Duration of Left Ventricular Hypertrophy

The duration of left ventricular hypertrophy also influences the anatomical and physiological responses of the coronary vascular system. Tomanek et al. [42] found in the spontaneously hypertensive rat a decrease in capillary density during development of left ventricular hypertrophy. During stabilization of the hypertrophy there was normalization of capillary density and capillary surface area due to proliferation of these vessels. Furthermore, Wangler et al. [20] reported an increase in minimal coronary vascular resistance of the left ventricle in spontaneously hypertensive rats during developing left ventricular hypertrophy, but during stabilization of hypertrophy, coronary vascular resistance became normal with respect to control rats. These results, summarized in figure 5-4, imply that during development of cardiac hypertrophy the coronary vessels cannot keep pace with the growing muscle mass, but as the hypertrophy stabilizes and the myocardial mass remains

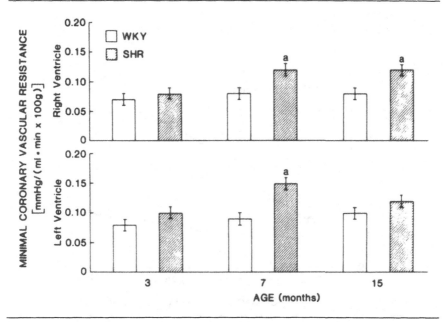

Figure 5–4. Minimal coronary resistance is shown in the left and right ventricles of both Wistar-Kyoto rats (WKY) and spontaneously hypertensive rats (SHR). The statistical significance between the two different strains of rats for a given age is shown by an asterisk. Note that, in the left ventricle of the spontaneously hypertensive rat, there is a normalization of the increase in minimal coronary resistance at seven months, and, of the minimal coronary resistance at fifteen months. Also note the increase in minimal coronary resistance in the right ventricle in the spontaneously hypertensive rat. The data in this figure were adapted from Wangler et al. [20].

relatively constant, the coronary vasculature eventually matches the increased muscle mass. Whether this occurs in other forms of pressure-overload-induced left ventricular hypertrophy is unknown.

Right Versus Left Ventricular Hypertrophy

Right and left ventricular hypertrophy are both reported to decrease coronary vasodilator reserve and increase minimal coronary vascular resistance [8, 20, 48, 54, 55]. However, there is one important difference between the response of the coronary vascular system at rest. Right ventricular hypertrophy is associated with an elevated myocardial perfusion per unit mass of myocardium at rest, which has been attributed to elevated wall stress that does not appear to normalize [54], whereas wall stress in the left ventricle is normalized with time, and myocardial perfusion at rest is normal per unit mass of myocardium [8]. There have been recent reports of two models of left ventricular hypertrophy in which left ventricular perfusion is elevated per unit mass of myocardium [65, 66]. Investigators found pressure-induced left ventricular hypertrophy associated with heart failure or, as a consequence of aortic vascular stenosis, it is characterized by increased resting myocardial perfusion.

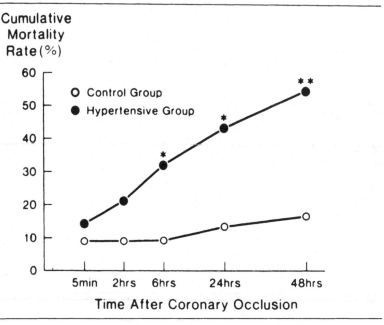

Figure 5–5. The incidence in sudden death, following coronary occlusion in normotensive control dogs and those with hypertrophy as a consequence of renovascular hypertension. Mortality was significantly higher in the hypertensive group and the primary cause of death was ventricular fibrillation. These data suggest that chronic hypertension and left ventricular hypertrophy adversely influence the outcome of sudden coronary occlusion. Statistical significance between groups is represented by * ($p < 0.05$), ** ($p < 0.01$). These data were originally presented by Koyanagi et al. [71].

PATHOPHYSIOLOGICAL CONSEQUENCES OF LEFT VENTRICULAR HYPERTROPHY

One of the important characteristics of the constellation of effects of left ventricular hypertrophy on the coronary circulation relates to interaction between left ventricular hypertrophy and hypertension on effects of myocardial ischemia and coronary artery disease. Systemic hypertension is the dominant cause of left ventricular hypertrophy in humans. Hypertension increases the risk of development of atherosclerotic coronary artery disease [67]. Epidemiological studies have found that the manifestations of coronary artery disease (sudden death, myocardial infarction, cardiovascular morbidity) are more severe in patients with left ventricular hypertrophy as a consequence of systemic hypertension [67, 68, 69]. Specifically, these investigators found that patients with left ventricular hypertrophy had a three-fold increase in sudden death and an increased incidence of cardiac rupture. Pathophysiological mechanisms from clinical epidemiological studies regarding the interaction between coronary vasculature (during myocardial ischemia) and the hypertrophied ventricle can be explained from basic, experimental literature.

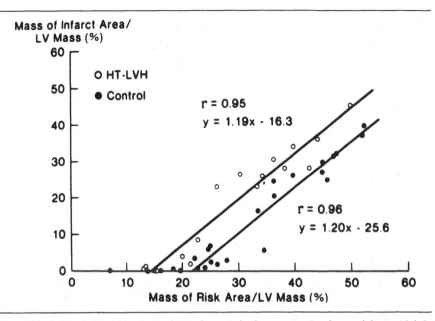

Figure 5-6. The infarct/risk relationship is shown in both normotensive dogs and dogs with left ventricular hypertrophy secondary to chronic hypertension (Ht-LVH). Conscious animals were subjected to coronary occlusion, and 48 hours later infarct size was determined by pathological techniques and the risk area was defined by postmortem coronary arteriography. Dogs with chronic hypertension and left ventricular hypertrophy had larger infarcts per risk area than control animals. These data were originally presented by Koyanagi et al. [70].

Animal Studies

Koyanagi et al. [70, 71] found that dogs with left ventricular hypertrophy, as a consequence of renal vascular hypertension, had a 300% increase in sudden death following coronary artery occlusion (figure 5–5). Also, these investigators reported a substantial increase in the infarct/risk area relationship following coronary occlusion (figure 5–6). Preliminary studies by Inou et al. [72, 73] have shown that the critical factor responsible for the increase in sudden death and the increase in infarct size is hypertension per se. Within this context, these investigators found that acute reduction of arterial pressure in the renovascular hypertensive dog with cardiac hypertrophy prevented the increase in infarct size and sudden death associated with coronary artery occlusion.

Patient Studies

Another clinical observation which is compatible with adverse effects of left ventricular hypertrophy on the coronary circulation has been reported by Marcus et al. [56, 57]. These investigators found that in patients with aortic stenosis there was a substantial decrease in coronary reserve (the ratio of

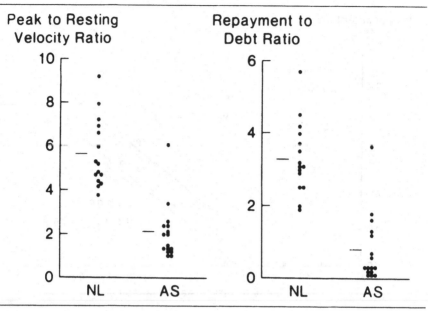

Figure 5-7. Reactive hyperemic response following coronary occlusion (20 seconds) in the left anterior descending artery in patients with aortic stenosis (AS) and controls (NL). Studies were performed at the time of open-heart surgery prior to cardiopulmonary bypass. Coronary vessels in both patient groups were angiographically normal. The left ventricles in the normal group of patients were not enlarged whereas the left ventricles in patients with aortic stenosis were severely hypertrophied. Following release of a 20 second occlusion of the left anterior descending coronary artery, the peak-to-resting blood flow velocity ratio was measured in both groups of patients (individual responses for a given patient are represented by the dots, and the mean responses for each group are represented by the line to the left of the dots). These studies suggest that coronary reserve—the ability to increase blood flow above resting levels—is markedly diminished in patients with aortic stenosis. This figure is adapted from data originally presented by Marcus et al. [57].

maximal coronary blood flow velocity to resting coronary blood flow velocity) (figure 5-7). This decrease in coronary reserve was observed despite angiographically normal coronary blood vessels. Furthermore, coronary vasodilator reserve was so compromised that these patients usually had symptoms of angina pectoris. Coronary reserve was also reported to be compromised in patients with volume-overload-induced right ventricular hypertrophy, but with normal coronary blood vessels [74]. The decrement in coronary reserve in patients is usually much greater than that reported in animal studies of cardiac hypertrophy. Although there are no unequivocal explanations of these differences, they could be related to the severity of hypertrophy and/or the duration of hypertrophy in the animal studies versus that in patients.

SUMMARY AND CONCLUSIONS

In summary, the myriad effects of left ventricular hypertrophy on the coronary circulation depend on several important factors, e.g., age when the

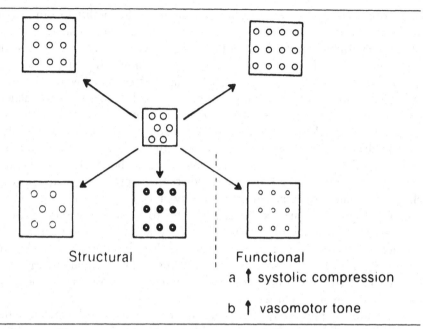

Structural ┊ Functional

a ⬆ systolic compression

b ⬆ vasomotor tone

Figure 5-8. Conceptual representation of the left ventricular mass to the cross-sectional area of coronary resistance vessels. The ventricular mass is represented by the size of the box, and the size of the vascular bed is represented by the total area of the circles within a box. The center box represents the normal relationship between the cross-sectional area of the cardiac mass to that of the coronary vasculature. The arrows point to different relationships between the coronary vasculature and hypertrophied myocardium. See text for details. This figure was originally published by Marcus [75] in *The Coronary Circulation In Health And Disease*.

hypertrophing stimulus is applied, stimulus that provokes hypertrophy, animal species etc. It is our intent to provide a framework from which the effects of hypertrophy on the coronary vascular system can be assessed. A schematic representation of the interaction between left ventricular hyper-trophy and the coronary vascular system is shown in figure 5-8, where the size of the boxes represents the left ventricular mass and the circles within the boxes represent the cross-sectional area of coronary resistance vessels. As can be seen, there is a complex mosaic that represents a different outcome between the coronary vasculature and the hypertrophying cardiac mass. The middle box represents the normal relationship between the cross-sectional area of the vascular system and that of the myocardium. The upper right-hand box represents an example of excess vascular growth in proportion to the magnitude of left ventricular hypertrophy. Physiologically, this would mean a decrease in left ventricular minimal coronary resistance per unit mass of myocardium and/or increased capillary density. The box on the top left represents the situation in which cardiac enlargement is accompanied by adequate vascular growth to match the hypertrophying myocardium. The physiological correlates of this example would be that minimal coronary vascular resistance per unit mass of myocardium would not differ from that in the control situation, and that minimal coronary vascular resistance for the entire hypertrophied ventricle would decrease in proportion to the increase in mass of the myocardium. The bottom three boxes show different mechanisms by which the cross-sectional area of the coronary vascular bed would decrease during left ventricular hypertrophy. Decreased vascular growth, or rarefaction (left bottom box) would increase minimal resistance of the left ventricle. An increase in the wall-to-lumen ratio of the coronary vasculature would also serve to decrease the cross-sectional area of the bed and increase minimal coronary resistance as shown in the center bottom box. Also, augmented extravascular compressive forces (systolic compression, incomplete diastolic relaxation) could also impair dilator capacity and increase minimal coronary resistance (right bottom box). It is unknown to what extent these various mechanisms contribute to impaired coronary vascular reserve in hypertrophied ventricles. However, it is plausible that under various models of hypertrophy, each of these three mechanisms, which would increase the minimal coronary resistance, contribute to impaired coronary vasodilator reserve in the hypertrophied heart.

As mentioned previously, there are several factors which influence the relationship between the hypertrophied myocardium and the coronary vascular system. For instance, left ventricular hypertrophy as a consequence of thyroxine administration or anemia results in a decrease in minimal coronary vascular resistance indicating an adequate response of the coronary vascular system to match the increased myocardial mass. Thus, the upper boxes of figure 5–8 represent the relationship between the coronary system and the cardiac muscle during thyroxine-induced and anemia-induced left ventricular hypertrophy. In contrast, when the stimulus that provokes hypertrophy is pressure overload, the relationship of the interaction between the coronary vascular system and the myocardium can be seen in one or more of the bottom three boxes. In this situation, the response of the coronary vascular system is clearly inadequate to match the growing myocardium. The age of the animal when the hypertrophy is induced would also influence the relationships shown in figure 5–8. Younger animals, especially neonates and fetuses, appear to have better responses of the coronary vascular system to cardiac hypertrophy (upper boxes), whereas adult animals appear to have adverse effects of hypertrophy on the coronary vascular system (lower boxes). Another factor which alters the relationships shown in figure 5–8 is the duration of left ventricular hypertrophy. During the development of left ventricular hypertrophy, the growth of the cardiac muscle exceeds that of the coronary vascular system. This impairs coronary vasodilator reserve, increases coronary minimal resistance, and decreases capillary density of the myocardium (bottom boxes). However, during stabilization of hypertrophy, the coronary vascular system eventually matches the increase in cardiac mass, leading to normalized coronary vasodilator reserve, capillary density, and minimal coronary resistance (upper boxes). There are other factors such as right versus left ventricular hypertrophy and what animal species is used as the experimental model which also influence the relationships between the coronary vasculature and the hypertrophying myocardium shown in figure 5–8.

Despite substantial knowledge about the interaction between the coronary vascular system and cardiac hypertrophy that has been gained in recent years, many important questions remain unanswered. In our opinion, some of the more important ones are:

1. What is the biochemical messenger that stimulates angiogenesis in thyroxine-induced and anemia-induced cardiac hypertrophy, and what is the deficiency of the expression of this messenger in models of pathological cardiac hypertrophy?

2. Is the distribution of coronary microvascular resistance altered in hearts that develop cardiac hypertrophy secondary to systemic hypertension? In organ systems other than the heart (e.g., mesentery, skeletal muscle, cheek pouch) the distribution of microvascular resistance shifts towards larger vessels that bear a greater proportion of the total vascular resistance.

3. What are the anatomical characteristics of the coronary vasculature in different types of hypertrophy? There is surprisingly little information regarding the anatomical features of coronary resistance vessels during different types of cardiac hypertrophy. It is of great importance to understand if wall-to-lumen ratios change significantly in certain types of hypertrophy or in certain groups of resistance vessels. Also, can arteriolar rarefaction be observed in different types of hypertrophy or in different portions of the coronary microvasculature?

4. Is the rate at which tissue necrosis occurs accelerated following coronary occlusion in the hypertrophied heart? Since it is already known that the infarct/risk relationship is altered in the hypertrophied heart it is also important to understand if the rate at which tissue necrosis occurs is also altered. Such information could help in the use of thrombolytic therapy in that such therapy may be of lesser value in patients with left ventricular hypertrophy due to hypertension than in those without such problems.

5. What is the relationship between the coronary vasculature and the myocardium during the regression of cardiac hypertrophy? And, within this context, does coronary reserve return to normal following regression of cardiac hypertrophy and does the rate at which the myocardium regresses exceed that of the coronary vasculature (in hypertrophy as a consequence of thyroxine administration or that due to anemia)?

The answers to these basic questions should help us understand the effects of ventricular hypertrophy on the coronary vascular system and the cardiac mass.

REFERENCES

1. Burger, S.B., and Strauer, B.E. 1981. Left ventricular hypertrophy in chronic pressure load due to spontaneous essential hypertension. I. Left ventricular function, left ventricular geometry, and wall stress. In *The Heart In Hypertension*, Strauer B.E., ed., pp. 13–36. Berlin. Springer Verlag.
2. Meerson, F.Z. 1969. The myocardium in hyperfunction, hypertrophy and heart failure. *Circ. Res.* 25 (Supp. II):1–163.
3. Hood, W.P. Jr., Rackley, C.E., and Rolett, E.L. 1968. Wall stress in the normal and hypertrophied left ventricle. *Am. J. Cardiol.* 22:550–558.
4. Falsetti, H.L., Mates, R.E., Grant, C., Greene, D.G., and Bunnell, I.L. 1970. Left ventricular wall stress calculated from one-plane cineangiography. *Circ. Res.* 26:71–83.
5. Grossman, W., Jones, D., and McLaurin, L.P. 1975. Wall stress and patterns of hypertrophy in human left ventricle. *J. Clin. Invest.* 56:56–64.
6. Strauer, B.E. 1979. Ventricular function and coronary hemodynamics in hypertensive heart disease. *Am. J. Cardiol.* 44:999–1007.
7. Malik, A.B., Abe, T., O'Kane, H., and Geha, A.S. 1973. Cardiac function, coronary flow, and oxygen consumption in stable left ventricular hypertrophy. *Am. J. Physiol.* 225:186–191.
8. Mueller, T.M., Marcus, M.L. Kerber, R.E., Young, J.A., Barnes, R.W., and Abboud, F.M. 1978. Effect of renal hypertension and left ventricular hypertrophy on the coronary circulation in dogs. *Circ. Res.* 42:543–549.
9. O'Keefe, D.D., Hoffman, J.I.F., Cheitlin, R., O'Neill, M.J., Allard, J.R., and Shapkin, E. 1978. Coronary blood flow in experimental canine left ventricular hypertrophy. *Circ. Res.* 43: 43–51.
10. Holtz, J., Restorff, W.V., Bard, P., and Bassenge, E. 1977. Transmural distribution of myocardial blood flow and coronary vascular reserve in canine left ventricular hypertrophy. *Basic Res. Cardiol.* 72:286–292.
11. Rembert, J.C., Kleinman, L.H., Fedor, J.J., Wechsler, A.S., and Greenfield, J.C. Jr. 1978. Myocardial blood flow distribution in concentric left ventricular hypertrophy. *J. Clin. Invest.* 62:379–386.
12. Bache, R.J., and Vrobel, T.R. 1979. Effects of exercise on blood flow in the hypertrophied heart. *Am. J. Cardiol.* 44:1029.
13. Bache, R.J., Vrobel, T.R., Ring, W.S., Emergy, R.W., and Anderson, R.W. 1981. Regional myocardial blood flow during exercise in dogs with chronic left ventricular hypertrophy. *Circ. Res.* 48:78–87.
14. Spann, J.F. Jr. 1969. Heart failure and ventricular hypertrophy: altered cardiac contractility and compensatory mechanisms. *Am. J. Cardiol.* 23:504–509.
15. Tarazi, R.C. 1985. The heart in hypertension. *N. Eng. J. Med.* 312:308–390.
16. Page, E., and McCallister, L.P. 1973. Quantitative description of heart muscle cells. Application to normal, hypertrophied, and thyroxin-stimulated hearts. *Am. J. Cardiol.*: 31:172–181.
17. Aronson, R.S. 1980. Characteristics of action potentials of hypertrophied myocardium from rats with renal hypertension. *Circ. Res.* 47:443.
18. Fouad, F.M., Slominski, J.M., and Tarazi, R.C. 1984. Left ventricular diastolic function in hypertension: Relation to left ventricular mass and systolic function. *Am. Coll. Cardiol.* 3:1500–1506.
19. Paulsen, S., Vatner, M., and Hagerup, L.M. 1975. Relationship between heart weight and the cross-sectional area of the coronary ostia. *Acta. Pathol. Microbiol. Scand.* 83:429–432.
20. Wangler, R.D., Peters, K.G., Marcus, M.L., and Tomanek, R.J. 1982. Effects of duration and severity of arterial hypertension and cardiac hypertrophy on coronary vasodilator reserve. *Circ. Res.* 51:10–18.
21. Murray, P.A., and Vatner, S.F. 1981. Reduction of maximal coronary vasodilator capacity in conscious dogs with severe right ventricular hypertrophy. *Circ. Res.* 48:27–33.
22. Manohar, M., Bisgard, G.E., Bullard, V., Rankin, J.H.G. 1981. Blood flow in the hypertrophied right ventricular myocardium of unanesthetized ponies. *Am. J. Physiol.* 240:H881–H888.
23. Wicker, P., Tarazi, R.C., and Kobayashi, K. 1983. Coronary blood flow during the development and regression of left ventricular hypertrophy in renovascular hypertensive rats. *Am. J. Cardiol.* 51:1744–1749.

24. Einzig, S., Leonard, J.J., Trip, M.R., Lucas, R.V., Swayze, C.R., and Fox, I. 1981. Changes in regional myocardial blood flow and variable development of hypertrophy after aortic banding in puppies. *Cardiovasc. Res.* 15:711–718.
25. Hort, W. 1981. Microscopic pathology of heart muscle and of coronary arterial hypertension. In *The Heart in Hypertension*, B.E. Strauer, ed. pp. 183–191. Berlin: Springer-Verlag.
26. Hutchins, G.M., Bulkley, B.H., Miner, M.M., and Bortnott, J.K. 1977. Correlation of age and heart weight with tortuosity and caliber of normal human coronary arteries. *Am. Heart J.* 94:196–202.
27. Stack, R.S., Rembert, J.C., Shrimer, B., Greenfield, J.C. Jr. 1983. Relation of left ventricular mass to geometry of the proximal coronary arteries in the dog. *Am. J. Cardiol.* 51:1728–1731.
28. Kelley, K.O., and Feigl, E.O. 1978. Segmental alpha-receptor-mediated vasoconstriction in the canine coronary circulation. *Circ. Res.* 43:908–917.
29. Tomanek, R.J., Palmer, P.J., Pieffer, G.W., Schrieber, K., Eastham, C.L., and Marcus, M.L. 1986. Morphometry of canine coronary arteries, arterioles, and capillaries during hypertension and left ventricular hypertrophy. *Circ. Res.* 58:38–46.
30. Folkow, B., Hallback, M., Lundgren, Y., Sivertsson, R., and Weiss, L. 1973. Importance of adaptive changes in vascular design for establishment of primary hypertension, studied in man and in spontaneously hypertensive rats. *Circ. Res.* 32/33 (Supp. I):2–10.
31. Hutchins, P.M., and Darneel, A.E. 1974. Observation of a decreased number of small arterioles in spontaneously hypertensive rats. *Circ. Res.* 34/35 (Supp. I):150–161.
32. Prewitt, R.L., Chen, I.I.H., and Dowell, R. 1982. Development of microvascular refraction in the spontaneously hypertensive rat. *Am. J. Physiol.* 243 (Heart Circ. Physiol. 12): H243–251.
33. Henrich, H., Hertel, R. and Assmann, R. 1978. Structural differences in the mesentery microcirculation between normotensive and spontaneously hypertensive rats. *Pfuegers Arch* 375:153–159.
34. Haack, D.W., Schaffer, J.J., and Simpson, J.G. 1980. Comparisons of cutaneous microvessels from spontaneously hypertensive, normotensive Wistar-Kyoto and normal Wistar rats. *Proc. Soc. Exp. Biol. Med,* 164:453–458.
35. Breisch, E.A., White, F.C., Nimmo, L., and Bloor, C.M. 1985. The interrelationship of coronary vascular structure and flow during pressure overload hypertrophy. *Circulation* 72 (Supp. III):76.
36. Rakusan, K., and Poupa, O. 1966. Differences in capillary supply of hypertrophic and hyperplastic hearts. *Cardiologica* 49:293–298.
37. Rakusan, K. 1971. Quantitative morphology of capillaries of the heart. Number of capillaries in animal and human hearts under normal and pathologic conditions. *Methods Arch. Exp. Pathol.* 5:272–286.
38. Lund, D.D., and Tomanek, R.J. 1978. Myocardial morphology in spontaneously hypertensive and aortic-constricted rats. *Am. J. Anat.* 152:141–151.
39. Anversa, P., Olivetti, G., Melissari, M., and Lored, A.U. 1979. Morphometric study of myocardial hypertrophy induced by abdominal aortic stenosis. *Lab. Invest.* 40:341–349.
40. Breisch, E.A., Houser, S.R., Carey, R.A., Spaan J.F., and Bove, A.A. 1980. Myocardial blood flow and capillary density in chronic pressure overload of the feline left ventricle. *Cardiovasc. Res.* 14:469–475.
41. Tomanek, R.J., and Hovanec, J.M. 1981. The effects of long-term pressure overload and aging on the myocardium. *J. Mol. Cell. Cardiol.* 13:471–488.
42. Tomanek, R.J., Searls, J.C., and Lachenbruch, P.A. 1982. Quantitative changes in the capillary bed during developing, peak, and stabilized cardiac hypertrophy in the spontaneously hypertensive rat. *Circ. Res.* 51:295–304.
43. Henquell, L., Odoroff, C.L., and Honig, C.R. 1977. Intercapillary distance and capillary reserve in hypertrophied rat hearts beating in situ. *Circ. Res.* 41:400–408.
44. Laughlin, M.H., and Diana, J.N. 1975. Myocardial transcapillary exchange in the hypertrophied heart of the dog. *Am. J. Physiol.* 229:838–846.
45. Harrison, D.G., Barnes, D.H., Hiratzka, L.F., Eastham, C.L., Kerber, R.E., and Marcus, M.L. 1985. The effect of cardiac hypertrophy on the coronary collateral circulation. *Circulation* 71:1135–1142.
46. Wusten, B., Buss, D.D., Heist, H., and Schaper, W. 1977. Dilatory capacity of the coronary circulation and its correlation to the arterial vasculature in the canine left ventricle. *Basic Res.*

Cardiol. 72:636–650.
47. Scheel, K.W., Eisenstein, B.L., and Ingram, L.A. 1985. Coronary, collateral, and perfusion territory responses to aortic banding. *Am. J. Physiol.* 246 (Heart Circ. Physiol.):H768–775.
48. Manohar, M., Thurmon, J.C., Tranquill, W.J., and Devous M.D. Sr., Theodorakis, M.C., Shawley, R.V., Reller, D.L., Benson, J.G. 1982. Regional myocardial blood flow and coronary vascular reserve in unanesthetized young calves with severe concentric hypertrophy. *Circ. Res.* 48:785–796.
49. Gascho, J.A., Mueller, T.M., Eastham, C., and Marcus, M.L. 1982. Effect of volume-overload hypertrophy on the coronary circulation in awake dogs. *Cardiovasc. Res.* 16: 288–292.
50. Chilian, W.M., Wangler, R.D., Peters, K.C., Marcus, M.L., and Tomanek, R.J. 1985. Thyroxine-induced left ventricular hypertrophy in the rat. Anatomical and physiological evidence for angiogenesis. *Circ. Res.* 57:591.
51. Mandache, E., Unge, G., and Ljungqvist, A. 1972. Myocardial blood capillary reaction in various forms of cardiac hypertrophy. An electron microscopical investigation in the rat. *Virchows. Arch. Abt. B. Zellpath.* 11:97–110.
52. Archie, J.P., Fixler, D.E., Ullyot, D.J., Buckberg, G.D., and Hoffman, J.I.E. 1974. Regional myocardial blood flow in lambs with concentric right ventricular hypertrophy. *Circ. Res.* 34:143–154.
53. Vlahakes, G.J., Turley, K., Verrier, E.D., and Hoffman, J.I.E. 1980. Greater maximal coronary flow in conscious lambs with experimental congenital right ventricular hypertrophy (abst). *Circulation* 62 (Supp. II):111.
54. Murray, P.A., Baig, H., Fishbein, M.C., and Vatner, S.F. 1979. Effects of experimental right ventricular hypertrophy on myocardial blood flow in conscious dogs. *J. Clin. Invest.* 64: 421–427.
55. Peters, K.G., Wangler, R.D., Tomanek, R.J., and Marcus, M.L. 1984. Effects of long-term cardiac hypertrophy on coronary vasodilator reserve in SHR rats. *Am. J. Cardiol.* 54: 1342–1348.
56. Marcus, M.L., Gascho, J.A., Mueller, T.M., Eastham, C., Wright, C.T., Doty, D.B., and Hiratzka, L.F. 1981. The effects of ventricular hypertrophy on the coronary circulation. *Basic Res. Cardiol.* 76:575–581.
57. Marcus, M.L., Doty, D.B., Hiratzka, L.F., Wright, C.B., and Eastham, C.L. 1982. Decreased coronary reserve. A mechanism for angina pectoris in patients with aortic stenosis and normal coronary arteries. *N. Engl. J. Med.* 307:1362–1366.
58. Hiratzka, L.F. Doty, D.B., Eastham, C.L., and Marcus, M.L. 1981. Pressure versus volume overload has different effects on coronary reserve (abst). *Circulation* 66(Supp. II):354.
59. Hultgren, P.B., and Bove, A.A. 1981. Myocardial blood flow and mechanisms in volume-overload-induced left ventricular hypertrophy. *Cardiovasc. Res.* 15:522–528.
60. Litten, R.Z. III, Martin, B.J., Low R.B., and Alpert, N.R. 1982. Altered myosin isozyme patterns from pressure overload and thyrotoxic hypertrophied rabbit hearts. *Circ. Res.* 50:856–864.
61. Tomanek, R.J., Wangler, R.E., and Bauer, C.A. 1985. Prevention of coronary vasodilator reserve decrement in spontaneously hypertensive rats. *Hypertension* 7:533–540.
62. Scheel, K.S., and Williams, S.E. 1985. Hypertrophy and coronary and collateral vascularity in dogs with severe chronic anemia. *Amer. J. Physiol.* 249 (Heart Circ. Physiol. 18):H1032–H1037.
63. Bell, R.D., and Rasmussen, R.L. 1974. Exercise and the myocardial capillary fiber ratio during growth. *Growth* 38:237–244.
64. Ljungqvist, A., and Unge, G. 1972. The finer intramyocardial vasculature in various forms of experimental cardiac hypertrophy. *Acta Pathol. Microbiol. Scand.* 80:329–340.
65. Alyond, D., Anderson, R.W. Parish, D.G., Dri, X. and Bache, R.J. 1986. Alterations of myocardial blood flow associated with experimental canine left ventricular hypertrophy secondary to valvular aortic stenosis. *Circ. Res.* 58:47–57.
66. Parrish, D.G., Ring, W.S., and Bache, R.J. 1985. Myocardial perfusion on compensated and failing hypertrophied left ventricle. *Am. J. Physiol.* 249 (Heart Circ. Physiol. 18):H534–H540.
67. Kannel, W.B. 1974. Role of blood pressure in cardiovascular morbidity and mortality. *Prog. Cardiovasc. Dis.* 17:5–17.
68. Kannel, W.B., Doyle, J.T., McNamara, P.M., Quickenton, P., and Gordon, T. 1975.

Precursors of sudden coronary death: Factors related to the incidence of sudden death. *Circulation* 51:606–615.

69. Kannel, W.B., Gordon, T., and Offutt, D. 1969. Left ventricular hypertrophy by electrocardiogram. Prevalence, incidence and mortality in the Framingham study. *Ann. Intern. Med.* 71:89–96.

70. Koyanagi, S., Eastham, C.L., Harrison, D.G., and Marcus, M.L. 1982a. Increased size of myocardial infarction in dogs with chronic hypertension and left ventricular hypertrophy. *Circ. Res.* 50:55–62.

71. Koyanagi, S., Eastham, C., and Marcus, M. 1982b. Effects of chronic hypertension and left ventricular hypertrophy on the incidence of sudden cardiac death after coronary artery occlusion in conscious dogs. *Circulation* 65:1192–1197.

72. Inou, T., Koyanagi, S., Harrison, D.G., Harbuzik, D., Eastham, C.L., and Marcus, M.L. 1983. Relative importance of hypertension versus left ventricular hypertrophy on infarct size and sudden cardiac death. (Abstract) *J. Am. Cell. Cardiol.* 1:660.

73. Inou, T., Lamberth, W., Koyanagi, S., Harrison, D., Lopez, A., Eastham, C., and Marcus, M.L. 1983b. Adverse effect of hypertension on infarct size and the incidence of sudden death in dogs with left ventricular hypertrophy. (Abstract) *Fed. Proc.* 42:1002.

74. Doty, D.B., Wright, C.B., Hiratzka, L.F., Eastham, C.L., and Marcus, M.L. 1984. Coronary reserve in volume-induced right ventricular hypertrophy from atrial septal defect *Am. J. Cardiol.* 54:1059.

75. Marcus, M.L. 1983. The coronary circulation in health and disease. New York: McGraw-Hill Book Co.

6. MICROCIRCULATION IN THE STRESSED HEART

KAREL RAKUSAN

Microcirculation is an integral part of the coronary blood flow. Most of the regulation of coronary blood flow, however, takes place at the level of the arterial bed preceding the coronary capillaries. Coronary blood flow in health and disease has been reviewed extensively in two recent publications [1, 2]. Therefore, it is not included in the present chapter. Similarly, two related and partly overlapping topics, capillary blood-tissue exchange in the heart and capillary permeability, have been reviewed comprehensively in a recent section on microcirculation in the *Handbook of Physiology* [3, 4].

This chapter is divided into three sections: studies of coronary capillaries in vivo, analysis of capillary structure and function based on studies of "frozen" sections of the heart, and studies based on histological methods.

IN VIVO STUDIES

It seems logical that the best approach for studying the effect of acute stress on coronary microcirculation would be to directly investigate changes in the terminal vascular bed in vivo. Unfortunately, in contrast to microcirculatory investigations in many other organs, the possibility of similar studies in heart muscle is limited, due to formidable technical difficulties. The use of in vivo capillaroscopy of the heart is confined to open-chest animals, hardly a physiological condition. In addition, the high speed and wide range of heart movement throughout the cardiac cycle hinders the clarity of the optical field and its recording. High-speed cinematography combined with transillumination has been used to investigate the vessel size, red-cell velocity, and pattern of flow in cat atria and turtle ventricles [5, 6].

Several authors have attempted to investigate the functional changes in microcirculation of mammalian ventricles by using the technique of epi-illumination. Such an approach is restricted to the most superficial layers of the epimyocardium, but has the advantage of enabling us to study functional alterations in the coronary capillary bed under various acute physiological and pathological conditions. However, this method does not yield unequivocal results. For instance, Martini and Honig [7] described the recruitment of resting capillaries after hyperoxia or hypoxia ($P_{a02} > 300$ mmHg or < 100 mmHg). After a prolonged hypoxia, a capillary reserve in close to 50% of the vessels was found. On the other hand, Steinhausen and coworkers [8] failed to find any changes in the functional intercapillary distance under hypoxic conditions, so they deny the existence of capillary recruitment in mammalian hearts. In our own experiments, we detected evidence of a moderate capillary recruitment of approximately 11% under hypoxic conditions, which was less pronounced in larger and older animals than in younger rats [9, 10] (see figure 6–1). Henquell and co-workers [11] reported capillary recruitment under normoxic conditions in hypertrophic hearts, which maintained the functional intercapillary distance within normal limits during the early stages of cardiac hypertrophy. In later stages, the mean functional intercapillary distance was greater than normal for the age of the animal.

In conclusion, coronary capillaries probably react to a hypoxic or hyperoxic environment by recruitment of additional, formerly resting capillaries. This capillary reserve, however, is relatively small, and it decreases even more in hearts of larger and older animals, as well as in cardiac hypertrophy. The minimal intercapillary distance obtained under anoxic conditions, and its changes during normal and pathological growth of the rat heart, are comparable to those obtained from morphometric determinations as described in the last portion of this chapter.

STUDIES ON THE "FROZEN" SECTIONS

Under this heading I would like to summarize the studies which analyze the in vivo situation on the basis of immobilized, ("frozen") samples. In most cases, these specimens are also frozen in a literal sense. Frozen samples were used, for instance, by Myers and Honig [12] to determine the capacity of the terminal vascular bed. They injected animals with a suspension containing red blood cells labeled with Cr^{51} and plasma labeled with I^{131}. By comparing the activity of the blood and the activity of the tissue samples containing no visible vessels, they obtained the tissue capillary blood content. We modified this method to estimate the capacity of the capillary bed and the capillary blood hematocrit in mammalian hearts subjected to various pathological conditions such as cardiac hypertrophy due to experimental aortic constriction, anemia, and polycythemia [13–15].

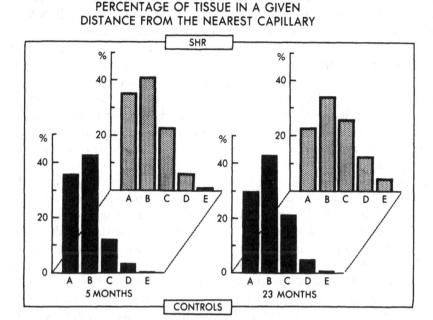

PERCENTAGE OF TISSUE IN A GIVEN
DISTANCE FROM THE NEAREST CAPILLARY

Figure 6–1. Frequency distribution of intercapillary distance under both normoxemic and hypoxemic conditions in the hearts from young and old rats (4–5 months versus 26 months). Difference between normoxemic and hypoxemic data is due to capillary recruitment. Reprinted from Rakusan and Korecky [10].

Cardiac hypertrophy was induced by experimental aortic constriction in adult rabbits and rats [13, 14]. In both species, the relative capacity of the terminal vascular bed in hypertrophic hearts, measured as capillary blood content per gram of tissue, was significantly lower than in normal hearts. This indicates a decreased capillary supply of hearts that were hypertrophied due to pressure overload. In contrast, the same pressure overload applied in young growing rabbits resulted in compensatory capillary growth. Therefore, when cardiomegaly was induced in young animals, the capillary supply was the same as in normal hearts [13]. In the study on rats, the hematocrit in terminal vessels of the hearts was also measured and found to be lower than the venous hematocrit in normal animals. In the hearts of rats with aortic constriction, this difference was even more pronounced and the hematocrit of the terminal vessels was significantly lower than in the hearts of normal rats [14].

We were also interested in capillary blood content and hematocrit in hearts of anemic and polycythemic rats [15]. Experimental anemia was induced in young rats by chronic feeding with a low iron diet, while polycythemia was a result of cobalt chloride injections. Cardiac weight in anemic rats increased considerably but no significant changes were found in polycythemic rats. The capacity of the capillary bed, per unit of tissue volume, was approximately the same in all experimental groups, despite a considerable degree of cardiomegaly in anemic animals. It was concluded that the cardiac growth induced in young rats by anemia is characterized by a proportional growth of the capillary bed. The capillary blood hematocrit was decreased in hearts from anemic rats and increased in hearts from polycythemic animals. However, the increase in the myocardial tissue hematocrit in the hearts from polycythemic rats was greater than the increase in hematocrit in large vessels, such as the femoral vein. In anemic animals, the decrease was approximately the same in both compartments. The results for hearts in anemic rats are in contrast to the results in most of the remaining organs in which the variations in tissue hematocrit during anemia and polycythemia were greater than those in venous blood (see figure 6–2).

Using a similar technique, Weiss and Cohen [16] studied changes in small-vessel blood content of the rat heart induced by hypercapnic and asphyxic conditions. Both pathological conditions were associated with an increased blood content indicating capillary recruitment. Scientists from the same laboratory also studied the effect of mild normovolemic hemodilution on small-vessel blood content in rabbit hearts subjected to acute coronary occlusion [17]. Occlusion increased small-vessel blood content (a measure of open capillaries) in the ischemic region. Hemodilution further significantly increased this volume in the occluded area, although the increase in the control region was not significant.

Frozen sections may also be used for microspectrophotometric determination of oxygen saturation of the hemoglobin present in small vessels. This approach, first introduced by Grunewald and Lubbers [18], can also yield the regional oxygen consumption, if the concomitant myocardial blood flow is known. Weiss and coworkers used a similar method to study the effect of various types of stress on regional myocardial blood flow, oxygen extraction, and oxygen consumption in canine hearts. In normal dogs, both myocardial blood flow and oxygen consumption were higher in the subendocardial region. In hearts stressed due to an arterio-venous shunt and to an acute valvular aortic stenosis or insufficiency, overall myocardial blood flow and oxygen consumption were increased and regional differences abolished. The limiting factor in these changes was probably the oxygen extraction in the subendocardial vessels, which was close to maximal [19–21]. A similar effect was also found with thyroxine-induced hypertrophy of the rabbit heart [22]. When subjected to hypoxia (8% O_2), control rabbits simply maintained a lower oxygen supply consumption ratio. In the thyroxine-treated animals, oxygen consumption was also maintained. This was coupled with an increased myocardial blood flow and a decreased oxygen extraction. Oxygen extraction in the T4-treated animals may have been maximal, and the hypoxic stress was met primarily by increased blood flow [23].

The final group of experiments included in this section forms a transition to the studies based on quantitative histology which will be reviewed subsequently. They deal mainly with the analysis of capillary perfusion patterns,

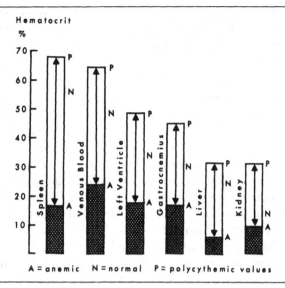

Figure 6–2. Hematocrit range in various blood compartments in normal (N), polycythemic (P) and anemic (A) rats. Note the differences in the extreme ranges when compared to normal values. Based on data from Rakusan and Rajhathy [15].

as proposed by Vetterlein and Schmidt [24]. Basically, this method consists of injecting macromolecules coupled with fluorochromes; the animals are then killed at various times after the dye application. In the histological sections, the dye-containing capillaries are subsequently identified and counted. After 5–10 seconds, virtually all capillaries are tagged, i.e., their numbers correspond to the anatomical counts and do not increase with longer intervals between the injections and heart excision, or with application of hypoxia. Therefore, it may be concluded that all capillaries were perfused by plasma within this period [25]. The speed of capillary plasma-filling depends on the velocity of plasma flow. When the metabolic demand on the heart is reduced by propranolol, coronary blood flow is decreased and complete filling occurs only after 40 seconds. In contrast, plasma-filling is accelerated by the infusion of epinephrine [26]. Similarly, the filling of the capillaries is accelerated by pharmacologically-induced coronary vasodilation [27]. The above results, obtained from the rat hearts, seem to indicate that all capillaries are perfused with plasma and any potential recruitment means only opening these vessels to the bolus flow of the red blood cells. Analogous results were also observed with isolated guinea pig hearts during normoxic and hypoxic perfusion [28]. In contrast, Weiss and Conway [29], using a similar approach and an even longer time interval between injection and killing, found a considerable capillary reserve in the rabbit heart (approximately 40%).

Finally, a similar approach has been used by Camilleri and co-workers [30] in their studies of capillary perfusion patterns during localized acute myocardial ischemia and after reperfusion in the rat heart. After permanent ischemia of 20 minutes duration, nonperfused areas were similar to the usual area of the infarctions obtained by this method in the rat. In reperfused ischemic myo-cardium, a nonuniform capillary labeling was also observed. The functional capillary density was significantly decreased after 1 minute of reperfusion and even more so after 15 min of reperfusion. Moreover, the heterogeneity of capillary plasma perfusion in the reperfused ischemic myocardium was greatly increased. These patterns are probably dependent upon the regional changes in cellular membrane permeability, which were studied simultaneously.

In conclusion, studies on the frozen sections did not solve the controversy concerning the coronary capillary reserve, as outlined in the previous section. Both the measurements of the capacity of terminal vessels and the studies of the plasma filling in coronary capillaries were used to investigate possible recruitment of coronary capillaries. Reported results varied from estimates of 40% of all capillaries being part of the capillary reserve, to a denial of the existence of capillary recruitment in cardiac muscle. This is the same situation as with the data from in vivo studies. Maximal capacity of the terminal vessels yielded reasonable estimates of cardiac capillarization; its changes in various experimental situations paralleled those derived from the in vivo measure-ments of intercapillary distances on the heart surface or from capillary counting in histological sections. The local hematocrit in these terminal vessels, however, was different from the overall blood hematocrit. It is also possible to measure the hemoglobin saturations inside the small coronary vessels and subsequently to estimate the local oxygen consumption. Oxygen extraction in the subendocardial vessels of hearts subjected to volume or pressure overload is close to maximal, which leads to a disappearance of regional differences in the oxygen consumption observed in normal hearts.

HISTOLOGICAL STUDIES

The Importance of Capillary Supply for Myocardial Oxygenation

In this section, we will concentrate on the quantitative morphology of terminal vessels in the stressed hearts. It may seem logical that the most important parameter in this case would be total capillary surface. Changes in the capillary surface area greatly influence the exchange processes between blood and tissue. Therefore, one would expect that the best indicator of tissue capillarization is capillary surface density, i.e., surface area per unit of tissue volume. Unfortunately, the situation is far more complicated. The exchange of respiratory gases, heat, and metabolites depends not only on the capillary surface density but also on its geometrical arrangement. Recently, we analyzed the effect of different geometrical distributions of the same capillary surface density on myocardial tissue PO_2 histograms [31]. The results are summarized in figure 6–3. A small decrease [15] in capillary surface density, due to a decreased number of capillaries, results in a moderate decline of the mean

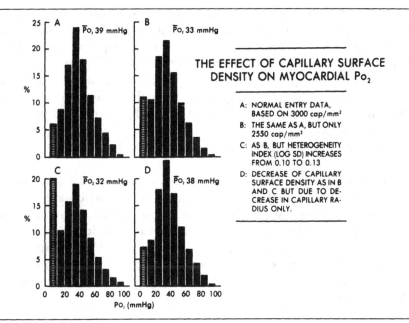

Figure 6-3. The effect of different geometrical arrangements of the same capillary surface density on calculated myocardial tissue PO_2 histograms. For more explanation, see text. Reprinted from Rakusan and Turek [31].

myocardial PO_2 (from 39 to 33 mmHg); but, more significantly, the percentage of tissue belonging to the class with the lowest PO_2 almost doubles (figure 6-3b). If, simultaneously, this decreased number of capillaries is distributed more irregularly, the mean myocardial PO_2 remains more or less unchanged but a sizable fraction of the tissue already lies in the lowest tissue PO_2 class, which is prone to hypoxia (figure 6-3c). In contrast, an identical decrease in capillary surface density, resulting from a decreased capillary radius, has only a marginal effect on myocardial oxygenation (figure 6-3d).

The above example stressed the importance of capillary supply for myocardial oxygenation. Three geometrical parameters, vital to the exchange processes, are the capillary density (number of capillaries per unit area of cross-section), the heterogeneity of capillary spacing, and the capillary radius. The data on capillary density in hearts subjected to various types of stress are abundant and they will be reviewed in this section. Methods for estimation of the heterogeneity in capillary spacing are relatively new, and few data from pathological situations are available. Usually, decreasing capillary density is accompanied by increasing heterogeneity of capillary spacing [32, 33]. Finally, the capillary radius has less influence on myocardial oxygenation, as demonstrated in the model situation described previously. Moreover, its values in morphological measurements are considerably influenced by the situation at the moment of killing and during the subsequent processing of the tissue samples. Therefore, the data on capillary radius are not included in this review.

As mentioned above, the data on myocardial capillarization in health and disease are abundant. To avoid overloading the bibliography of this chapter, all data published before 1970 are referenced in our 1971 review on the myocardial capillary supply [34]. The same review also contains a survey of methods used for visualization of capillaries. It is rather difficult to summarize the data succinctly because the response of the capillary bed will depend not only on the mechanism of stress and its duration, but also on the species, strain, and age of the organism. Moreover, capillary density and its changes may vary in different regions of the heart.

The absolute values of the capillary density in normal adult mammalian hearts vary from 2000 to 4000/mm², depending on the species, age, region, and method of capillary visualization. In this review, the concentration will be on relative changes of the capillary density due to stress overload. Most of this response is closely related to the response of the remaining tissue components. Thus, the typical reaction is cardiac hypertrophy characterized by an increase in the size of muscle cells, but no specific reaction from the capillary bed; this results in increased intercapillary distances.

Capillary Supply of Hearts Exposed to Pressure Overload

Changes in capillary density in mammalian hearts due to chronic exposure to pressure overload are summarized in table 6–1. Close examination of the results reveals that the characteristic response is a decreased capillary density associated with an unchanged capillary-to-myocyte ratio. This means that the major reaction is the hypertrophy of the individual cardiac muscle cells, while the total number of capillaries and myocytes does not change. As a result, the intercapillary distance is greater and the capillary density decreases. It seems that such a reaction appears first in the endomyocardium and only later is followed by similar changes in the rest of the heart [35]. This type of response is identical in all mammalian species examined. The only exception is an observation by Hort and Severidt [34] on newborn human hearts. In this case, the overload occurred during fetal development and in neonates. Capillary proliferation kept pace with the growth of muscle cells, so capillary density remained unchanged. This is similar to the observation mentioned in the previous section: cardiomegaly, produced by aortic constriction in newborn rabbits, was characterized by a normal capillary supply, while the same stimulus in adult rabbits resulted in a decreased capillary volume per unit of myocardial tissue [13].

Data on capillary density in hearts from rats with spontaneous hypertension (SHR) are not included in table 6–1, since the topic is covered elsewhere in this chapter, and this experimental model may not represent a simple pressure overload. It seems that cardiac hypertrophy often precedes the development of arterial hypertension in SHR. Reported results on SHR basically agree with

Table 6–1. Capillary density in hearts subjected to pressure overload.

Authors	Age	Region	CD	C/M	Remark
Man:					
Roberts and Wearn 1941 [34]	Adult	NA	decrease	no change	Various pathology, mainly pressure overload.
Hort and Severidt 1966 [34]	Newborn	various	no change	NA	Congenital heart disease, contains various malformations.
Cat:					
Breisch et al. 1984 [35]	Adult	endomyocardium	decrease	NA	Aortic constriction, changes in the
		epimyocardium	decrease	NA	endomyocardium appear earlier.
Rabbit:					
Shipley et al. 1937 [34]	Young	midsection	decrease	no change	Various models of experimental hypertrophy.
	Adult	midsection	decrease	no change	
Rat:					
Rakusan and Poupa 1966 [34]	Adult	endomyocardium	decrease	no change	Aortic constriction.
Lund and Tomanek 1978 [36]	Young adult	endomyocardium	decrease	NA	Aortic constriction.
		epimyocardium	decrease	NA	
Anversa et al. 1979 [37]	Adult	midsection	decrease	no change	Aortic constriction.
Wiener et al. 1979 [38]	Young adult	endomyocardium	decrease	no change	Renal hypertension.
		epimyocardium	decrease	no change	
Anversa et al. 1983 [39]	Adult	endomyocardium	decrease	NA	Renal hypertension.
		epimyocardium	decrease	NA	

CD = capillary density, C/M = capillary-to-myocyte ratio, NA = information is not available.
All the data refer to the measurements on the left ventricle.

results from animals with simple pressure overload, especially if one takes into account the usually modest degree of cardiomegaly encountered in this experimental model. The majority of studies reported a decreased capillary supply in the hearts of rats with spontaneous hypertension, with some authors finding a return towards normal values in older animals [32]. Lower capillary density in these hearts is reversible by running exercise [50]. Also, in hearts from senescent rats with spontaneous hypertension the degree of heterogeneity of capillary spacing was higher than in hearts from healthy controls [32].

Capillary Supply of Hearts Exposed to Volume Overload

Table 6–2 summarizes changes in myocardial capillary density due to chronic exposure to volume overload. The results are similar to those due to pressure overload described above. Characteristically, capillary density decreases, with the decrease being more pronounced mainly in the endomyocardial region of the heart. Obviously, the degree of change in capillary density is dependent on the concomitant hypertrophy of the muscle cells and the overall increase in cardiac mass. Once again, cardiomegaly induced in a young organism is characterized by normal, unchanged capillary density.

Perhaps we should also include here the observations of Kayar and Banchero [51] on myocardial capillarity in guinea pigs exposed to cold in the early stages of growth. Exposure to a cold environment caused a sustained elevation in cardiac output with resulted in a modest bilateral cardiac hypertrophy. Capillary density and the capillary-to-myocyte ratio were similar in both control and acclimated animals, which indicates a moderate compensatory capillary growth in young animals exposed to cold stress. Volume overload is probably also responsible for cardiac hypertrophy in hyperthyroidism, even though the direct influence of thyroid hormone cannot be excluded. Hyperthyroid-induced cardiac hypertrophy in adult rats was characterized by lower capillary density which was more pronounced in the endocardial region [52].

Capillary Supply of Hearts in Exercising Animals

Changes in capillarization of the heart from animals exposed to chronic exercise are presented in table 6–3. The results demonstrate that physical exercise does not necessarily lead to capillary proliferation or improved capillary supply to the heart, as is often described in the literature. The findings will apparently depend not only on the species, age, and sampling region, but also on the type of exercise and its regimen. An increased capillary-to-myocyte ratio does not necessarily imply a better capillary supply. If the increased ratio is associated with a concomitant hypertrophy of muscle cells, the overall capillary density may decrease. It can be clearly seen that myocardial capillary density rarely increases as a result of physical training. This occurs only when the exercise starts early in life [43, 47, 48]. In several reports, the capillary density was found to be unchanged in trained animals. If the cardiac mass did increase during the period of physical training, this might be interpreted as an

Table 6–2. Capillary density in hearts subjected to volume overload.

Authors	Age	Region	CD	C/M	Remark
Man:					
Roberts and Wearn 1941: see table 6–1; in some cases, results not different from pressure overload.					
Hort and Severidt 1966: see table 6–1; in some cases, results not different from pressure overload.					
Dog:					
Thomas et al. 1984 [40]	Adult	endomyocardium	decreased	NA	Arterio-atrial shunt.
		midsection	no change	NA	
		epimyocardium	no change	NA	
Rabbit:					
Shipley et al. 1937 [34]: see table 6–1; in some cases, results not different from pressure overload.					
Rat:					
Poupa et al. 1964 [34]	Young	endomyocardium	no change	no change	Anemia since the weaning period.
Rakusan et al. 1980 [41]	Adult	endomyocardium	decrease	NA	Aorto-caval fistula.
		midsection	decrease	NA	Decrease more pronounced in endomyocardium.

CD = capillary density, C/M = capillary-to-myocyte ratio, NA = information is not available.
All the data refer to the measurements on the left ventricle.

Table 6–3. Capillary density in hearts from animals subjected to exercise.

Authors	Age	Region	CD	C/M	Remark
Dog:					
Wyatt and Mitchell 1978 [42]	Adult	Septum	no change	NA	Running; subsequent deconditioning is associated with a decrease in CD.
Guinea pig:					
Frank 1950 [34]	Adult	NA	decreased	NA	Swimming.
Hakkila 1955 [34]	Adult	NA	decreased	no change	Running.
Rat:					
Tomanek 1970 [43]	Young	various fields combined	increased	increased	Running exercise started at 40 (young), 130 (adults) and 575 (old) days of age.
	Adult		no change	increased	
	Old		no change	increased	
Bell and Rasmussen 1974 [44]	prepubescent	NA	NA	increased	Swimming.
	postpubescent			increased	
Anversa et al. 1982 [45]	Young	right ventricle	decreased	no change	Strenuous running started at 35 days of age; right ventricular hypertrophy
		various fields combined			
Tharp and Wagner 1982 [46]	Young adult	NA	decreased	decreased	Running; 8 training regimes.
Anversa et al. 1983 [47]	Young	various fields combined	increased	no change	Moderate running started at 35 days of age; right ventricular hypertrophy.
		right ventricle	no change	no change	
		left ventricle	increased	increased	
Jacobs et al. 1984 [48]	prepubescent	NA	increased	increased	Running, two types of intensity, two time intervals.
	postpubescent	NA	no change	increased	
Loud et al. 1984 [49]	Young	various fields combined	no change	no change	Running, moderate exercise, strenuous, started at 35 days of age.
		right ventricle	no change	no change	
		left ventricle			

CD = capillary density, C/M = capillary-to-myocyte ratio, NA = information is not available. All the data refer to the measurements on the left ventricle unless specified otherwise.

indirect sign of compensatory proliferation of myocardial capillaries. Finally, in some cases even a decreased capillary density has been found in hearts from animals subjected to various types of strenuous exercise [34, 45, 46].

Capillary Supply of Hearts in Animals Exposed to Chronic Hypoxia

The effect of chronic exposure to hypoxia on myocardial capillarity is also not as obvious as it is usually represented in the literature. Similar to the situation with exercise, the widely held opinion regarding chronic exposure to hypoxia is that it leads to an increased myocardial capillary supply. Close examination of the available data, however, reveals that all possible outcomes, (i.e., an increase, no change, or a decrease in capillary density) have been reported in mammalian hearts after chronic exposure to hypoxia. (Older literature is summarized in 53; [see also 54 and 55].) One should keep in mind that in animals either born at high altitude or exposed to chronic hypoxia later in life, right ventricular hypertrophy develops. Therefore, the reports of normal capillarization in the hypertrophic right ventricle may be interpreted as a sign of compensatory capillary proliferation during hypertrophic growth of the muscle cells. The results follow the pattern seen in responses to various types of stress, as described previously; most of the capillary growth takes place early in life when the capacity for capillary proliferation is the highest [56]. Therefore, almost all reports of higher capillary density in hearts from animals exposed to chronic hypoxia involved exposure early in life.

Capillary Supply of Hearts with Acute or Chronic Necrosis

Two types of approaches employed for this topic should be mentioned briefly. First, chronic infarction is associated with hypertrophy of the remaining tissue. Accoring to studies on experimental infarction in adult rats, the capillary supply to the surviving hypertrophic cells is decreased [57, 58]. Second, the approach used by Factor and co-workers [59, 60] was to examine the capillary supply to the necrotic myocardium by identifying the terminal vascular bed with colored silicone rubber. They found that myocardial microcirculation is arranged in the form of discrete end-capillary loops and arcades, without interconnections among capillaries supplied by different large vessels. The same pattern persisted even in the border zone region of the myocardial infarction. As an extension of these studies, they documented evidence of microvascular spasm, both in hereditary cardiomyopathy of the Syrian hamster and in the acquired cardiomyopathy of the hypertensive-diabetic rat. They proposed that transient spasm of the myocardial microvessels may lead to focal necrosis and scarring.

SUMMARY AND CONCLUSIONS

Our knowledge about microvascular adjustments during acute exposure to stress is rather limited, due mostly to a methodological limitation of microcirculatory studies on the moving heart as explained earlier. We are still not sure if all the existing capillaries are perfused at any given time, either with plasma or with red blood cells. If some fraction of the terminal vascular bed is not perfused under resting conditions, can it be recruited in times of need, for instance on exposure to hypoxia? The studies described earlier report contradictory results; estimates of the capillary reserve varied from 0–40%. It is our belief that a coronary capillary reserve exists, but it is relatively small and becomes even smaller in larger and older hearts.

Analysis of the capillary blood content in frozen samples represents a simple alternative for estimation of the capillary supply to the heart. The results are similar to those obtained by histological methods. Obviously, the whole geometry of the vascular bed and any knowledge of the quantitative spatial relationships are missing when using this method. Studies on frozen samples also allow for estimates of the capillary blood hematocrit which may differ from the hematocrit obtained from larger vessels. They can also be used for appraisal of local oxygen extraction and consumption.

The capillary perfusion pattern may be investigated by histological analysis of hearts previously injected with dye. The effects of various drugs, ischemia, and perfusion were studied by this method and have been reviewed in this chapter.

The long-term effects of exposure to various types of stress were studied by the methods of quantitative morphology. Rarely, one can observe the effects of stress selectively influencing the capillary bed. Most of the response to chronic stress is in conjunction with the remaining components of the myocardial tissue, especially myocytes. Hypertrophy of cardiac myocytes is usually associated with an increased intercapillary distance and decreased capillary density, unless compensatory proliferation of the terminal vessels takes place. Even though the material has been arranged according to the various types of stress (mechanical pressure overload, volume overload, chronic exercise, chronic hypoxia, cardiac necrosis), the overall capillary pattern seems to be little influenced by the type of stress. Most cases of cardiac hypertrophy produced in the adult organism are characterized by decreased capillary density and greater intercapillary distance. There are regional differences in the response, with changes usually occurring earlier and being more pronounced in the endomyocardium. Cardiomegaly associated with a normal capillary supply is usually found in situations in which the stress has been introduced early in life. It is seldom that one can see an increase in capillary density in the mammalian heart. This has been reported in some, but by no means all, studies on the effect of chronic adaptation to exercise and hypoxia.

REFERENCES

1. Feigl, E. 1983. Coronary physiology. *Physiol. Rev.* 63:1–205.
2. Marcus, M.L. 1983. In *The coronary circulation in health and disease*, New York: McGraw Hill Book Company.

3. Crone, C., and Levitt, D.G. 1984. Capillary permeability to small solutes. In *Handbook of Physiology*, Section 2. *The cardiovascular system*, Volume IV. *Microcirculation*, Part 1, Renkin, E.M., and Michel, C.C., eds., pp. 411–466. Bethesda: American Physiological Society.

4. Rose, C.P., and Goresky, C.A. 1984. Interactions between capillary exchange, cellular entry, and metabolic sequestration processes in the heart. In *Handbook of Physiology*, Section 2. *The cardiovascular system*, Volume IV. *Microcirculation*, Part 2. Renkin, E.M., and Michel, C.C., eds., pp. 781–798. Bethesda: American Physiological Society.

5. Tillich, G., Mendoza, L., Wayland, H., and Bing, R.J. 1971. Studies of the coronary microcirculation of the cat. *Am. J. Cardiol.* 27:93–98.

6. Tillmanns, H., Ikeda, S., Hansen, H., Sarma, J.S.M., Fauvel, J.M., and Bing, R.J. 1974. Microcirculation in the ventricle of the dog and turtle. *Circ. Res.* 34:561–569.

7. Martini, J., and Honig, C.R. 1969. Direct measurement of intercapillary distance in beating rat heart in situ under various conditions of O_2 supply. *Microvasc. Res.* 1:244–256.

8. Steinhausen, M., Tillmans, H., and Thederanh. 1978. Microcirculation of the epimyocardial layer of the heart. *Pflugers Arch* 378:9–14.

9. Korecky, B., Hai, C.M., and Rakusan, K. 1982. Functional capillary density in normal and transplanted rat hearts. *Can. J. Physiol. Pharmacol.* 60:23–32.

10. Rakusan, K., and Korecky, B. 1982. The effect of growth and aging on functional capillary supply of the rat heart. *Growth* 46:275–281.

11. Henquell, L., and Odoroff, C.L., Honig, and C.R. 1977. Intercapillary distance and capillary reserve in hypertrophied rat hearts beating in situ. *Circ. Res.* 41:400–408.

12. Myers, W.W., and Honig, C.R. 1964. Number and distribution of capillaries as determinants of myocardial oxygen tension. *Am. J. Physiol.* 207:653–660.

13. Rakusan, K., Du Mesnil de Rochemont, W., Braasch, W., Tschopp, H., and Bing, R.J. Capacity of the terminal vascular bed during normal growth, in cardiomegaly, and in cardiac atrophy. *Circ. Res.* 21:209–215.

14. Rakusan, K. 1971. Vascular capacity and hematocrit in experimental cardiomegaly due to aortic constrictor in rats. *Can. J. Physiol. Pharmacol.* 49:819–823.

15. Rakusan, K., and Rajhathy, J. 1972. Distribution of cardiac output and organ blood content in anemia and polycythemic rats. *Can. J. Physiol. Pharmacol.* 50:703–710.

16. Weiss, H.R., and Cohen, J.A. 1978. Changes in small vessel blood content of the rat heart induced by hypercapnic, hyperoxic or asphyxic conditions. *Cardiology* 63:199–207.

17. Briden, K.L., Teltser, M., and Weiss, H.R. 1979. The effects of mild normovolemic hemodilution on regional blood flow, oxygenation, and small vessel blood content in the rabbit heart subjected to acute coronary occlusion. *Circulatory Shock* 6:223–233.

18. Grunewald, W.A., and Lubbers, D.W. 1976. Kryomicrophotometry as a method for analyzing the intracapillary HbO_2-saturation of organs under different O_2 supply conditions. In *Oxygen transport to tissue II*, Grote, J., Reneau, D., Thews, G., eds., pp. 55–64. New York, London: Plenum Press.

19. Briden, K.L., and Weiss, H.R. 1981. Effect of moderate arterio-venous shunt on regional extraction, blood flow, and oxygen consumption in the dog heart. *Cardiovasc. Res.* 15: 206–213.

20. Vinten-Johansen, J., and Weiss, H.R. 1980. Oxygen consumption in subepicardial and subendocardial regions of the canine left ventricle. The effect of experimental acute valvular aortic stenosis. *Circ. Res.* 46:139–145.

21. Vinten-Johansen, J., and Weiss, H.R., 1981. Regional O_2 consumption in canine left ventricular myocardium in experimental acute aortic valvular insufficiency. *Cardiovasc. Res.* 15:305–312.

22. Talafih, K., Briden, K.L., and Weiss, H.R. 1983. Thyroxine-induced hypertrophy of the rabbit heart. Effect on regional oxygen extraction, flow, and oxygen consumption. *Circ. Res.* 53:272–279.

23. Talafih, K., Grover, G.J., and Weiss, H.R. 1984. Effect of T_4-induced cardiac hypertrophy on O_2 supply-consumption balance extraction, flow, and oxygen consumption. *Am. J. Physiol.* 246:H374–H379.

24. Vetterlein, F., and Schmidt, G. 1980. Effects of isoprenaline on functional capillary density in the subendocardial and subepicardial layer of the rat myocardium. *Basic Res. Cardiol.* 75: 526–536.

25. Vetterlein, F., Dal Ri, H., and Schmidt, G. 1982. Capillary density in rat myocardium during timed plasma staining. *Am. J. Physiol.* 242:H133–H141.

26. Vetterlein, F., and Schmidt, G. 1984. Effects of propranolol and epinephrine on density of capillaries in rat heart. Am. J. Physiol. 746:H189–H196.

27. Schubothe, M., Vetterlein, F., and Schmidt, G. 1983. Density of plasma-perfused capillaries in the rat heart during carbocromene-induced vasodilation. Basic Res. Cardiol. 78:113–123.

28. Figulla, H.R., and Vetterlein, F. 1984. Capillary density in the isolated perfused guinea pig heart during normoxic and high-flow hypoxic perfusion. In Oxygen transport to tissue VI, Bruley, A., Bicher, H.I., and Beneau, D., eds., pp. 425–432. New York, London: Plenum Press.

29. Weiss, H.R., and Conway, R.S. 1985. Morphometric study of the total and perfused arteriolar and capillary network of the rabbit left ventricle. Cardiovasc. Res. 19:343–354.

30. Camilleri, J.P., Nlom, M.O., Joseph, D., Michel, J.B., Barres, D., and Mignot, J. 1983. Capillary perfusion patterns in reperfused ischemic subendocardial myocardium: experimental study using fluorescent dextran. Exp. Mol. Pathol. 39:89–99.

31. Rakusan, K., and Turek, Z. 1986. A new look into the microscope: proliferation and regression of myocardial capillaries. Can. J. Cardiol. 2:94–97.

32. Rakusan, K., Hrdina, P.W., Turek, Z., Lakatta, E.G., Spurgeon, H.A., Wolford, G.D. 1984. Cell size and capillary supply of the hypertensive rat heart: quantitative study. Basic Res. Cardiol. 79:389–395.

33. Turek, Z., and Rakusan, K. 1985. Heterogeneity of capillary spacing in developing and hypertrophic heart-comparison of two methods. The Physiologist 28:abstract 39.16.

34. Rakusan, K. 1971. Quantitative morphology of capillaries of the heart. Methods Achiev. Exp. Pathol. 5:272–286.

35. Breisch, E.A., White, F.C., and Bloor, C.M. 1984. Myocardial characteristics of pressure-overload hypertrophy. Lab. Invest. 50:333–342.

36. Lund, D.D., and Tomanek, R.J. 1978. Myocardial morphology in spontaneously hypertensive and aortic-constricted rats. Am. J. Anat. 152:141–151.

37. Anversa, P., Olivetti, G., Melissari, M., and Loud, A.V. 1979. Morphometric study of myocardial hypertrophy induced by abdominal aortic stenosis. Lab. Invest. 40:341–349.

38. Wiener, J., Giacomelli, F., Loud, A.V., and Anversa, P. 1979. Morphometry of cardiac hypertrophy induced by experimental renal hypertension. Am. J. Cardiol. 44:919–929.

39. Anversa, P., Olivetti, G., and Loud, A.V. 1983. Morphometric studies of left ventricular hypertrophy. Persp. Cardiovasc. Res. 8:27–39.

40. Thomas, D.P., Phillips, S.J., and Bove, A.A. 1984. Myocardial morphology and blood flow distribution in chronic volume-overload hypertrophy in dogs. Bas. Res. Cardiol. 79:379–388.

41. Rakusan, K., Moravec, J., and Hatt, P-Y. 1980. Regional capillary supply in the normal and hypertrophied rat heart. Microvasc. Res. 20:319–326.

42. Wyatt, H.L., and Mitchell, J. 1978. Influences of physical conditioning and deconditioning on coronary vasculature of dogs. J. Appl. Physiol. 45:619–625.

43. Tomanek, R.J. 1970. Effects of age and exercise on the extent of the myocardial capillary bed. Anat. Rec. 167:55–62.

44. Bell, R.D., and Rasmussen, R.L. 1974. Exercise and the myocardial capillary-fiber ratio during growth. Growth 38:237–244.

45. Anversa, P., Beghi, C., Levicky, V., McDonald, S.L., and Kikkawa, Y. 1982. Morphometry of right ventricular hypertrophy induced by strenous exercise in rat. Am. J. Physiol. 243:H856–H861.

46. Tharp, G.D., and Wagner, C.T. 1982. Chronic exercise and cardiac vascularization. Eur. J. Appl. Physiol. 48:97–104.

47. Anversa, P., Levicky, V., Beghi, C., McDonald, S.L., and Kikkawa, Y. 1983. Morphometry of exercise-induced right ventricular hypertrophy in the rat. Circ. Res. 52:57–64.

48. Jacobs, T.B., Bell R.D., and McClements J.D. 1984. Exercise, age and the development of the myocardial vasculature. Growth 48:148–157.

49. Loud, A.V., Beghi C., Olivetti G., and Anversa P. 1984. Morphometry of right and left ventricular myocardium after strenuous exercise in preconditioned rats. Lab. Invest. 51:104–111.

50. Crisman, R.P., Rittman B., and Tomanek, R.J. 1985. Exercise-induced myocardial capillary growth in the spontaneously hypertensive rat. Microvasc. Res. 30:185–194.

51. Kayar, S.R., and Banchero, N. 1985. Volume-overload hypertrophy elicited by cold and its effects on myocardial capillarity. Resp. Physiol. 59:1–14.

52. Gerdes, A.M., Callas, G., and Kasten, F.H. 1979. Differences in regional capillary distribution and myocyte sizes in normal and hypertrophic rat hearts. *Am. J. Anat.* 156: 523–531.
53. Rakusan, K., Turek, Z., and Kreuzer, F. 1981. Myocardial capillaries in guinea pigs native to high altitude (Junin, Peru, 4105m). *Pflugers Arch.* 391:22–24.
54. Kayar, S.R., and Banchero, N. 1985. Myocardial capillarity in acclimation to hypoxia. *Pflugers Arch.* 404:319–325.
55. Pietschmann, M., and Bartel, S.H. 1985. Cellular hyperplasia and hypertrophy, capillary proliferation, and myoglobin concentration in the heart of newborn and adult rats at high altitude. *Resp. Physiol.* 59:347–360.
56. Rakusan, K., and Turek, Z. 1985. Protamine inhibits capillary formation in growing rat hearts. *Circ. Res.* 37:393–399.
57. Turek, Z., Grandtner, M., Kubat, K., Ringnalda, B.E.M., and Kreuzer, F. 1978. Arterial blood gases, muscle fiber diameter, and intercapillary distance in cardiac hypertrophy of rats with an old myocardial infarction. *Pflugers Arch.* 376:209–215.
58. Anversa, P., Loud, A.V., Levicky, V., and Gulderi, G. 1985. Left ventricular failure induced by myocardial infarction. II. Tissue morphometry. *Am. J. Physiol.* 248:H883–H889.
59. Factor, S.M., Okun, E.M., Minase, T., and Kirk, E.S. 1982. The microcirculation of the human heart: end-capillary loops with discrete perfusion fields. *Circulation* 66:1241–1248.
60. Factor, S.M., and Sonnenblick, E.H. 1982. Hypothesis: is congestive cardiomyopathy caused by a hyperreactive myocardial microcirculation (microvascular spasm)? *Am. J. Cardiol.* 50:1149–1152.

7. PATHOLOGY AND PATHOPHYSIOLOGY OF THE CORONARY MICROCIRCULATION IN MYOCARDIAL ISCHEMIA

STEPHEN M. FACTOR

Historically, major interest in the coronary circulation has focused on the epicardial coronary vessels and their associated collaterals. These vessels can be visualized, instrumented, and perturbed in experimental preparations and in clinical situations to assess their role in obstructive disease leading to myocardial ischemia and infarction. Until recently, little attention was paid to the coronary microcirculation and its contribution in myocardial ischemia. Yet, it is clear that the primary determinant of whether an individual myocardial cell lives or dies, or in fact resides in a "twilight zone" of chronic ischemia, is the microcirculation and its ability to supply the cell with oxygenated substrate. Of late, this awareness of the intrinsic relationship between myocardial cell viability and the coronary microcirculation has stimulated a number of investigations of microvascular anatomy and function. These studies have provided new information addressing some of the major controversies of the past decade, particularly the presence of a lateral border zone around a myocardial infarction and the salvageability of the border zone tissue. Some of these new observations, as well as those pertaining to the no-reflow phenomenon, thromboembolic obstruction, and spasm of the micro-vasculature will be reviewed in this chapter. Although the purpose is not to provide a comprehensive review of all data in this field, the aim is to establish the importance of the microcirculation as it relates to our understanding of myocardial necrosis in both the experimental laboratory and in man.

NORMAL ANATOMY OF THE MICROCIRCULATION

Definition

The myocardium is supplied by a rich network of large and small vessels, as would be expected for an organ which constantly works even when the body is at rest. Only the arteries running on the epicardial surface along with their major primary, secondary, and tertiary branches, which enter the myocardium at right angles and then divide extensively, can be studied in vivo by angiographic techniques. The microcirculation, and even the smaller intramyocardial arteries cannot by resolved by these methods. Thus our knowledge of microcirculatory anatomy and pathology generally has depended on postmortem evaluations, although recent technical innovations have permitted direct visualization of the epicardial microcirculation in the beating heart [1]. In contrast to barium gelatin or latex rubber, which have been used to demonstrate the larger myocardial vessels but are too viscous to penetrate into the microcirculation, dyes or silicone rubber solutions can be used for this purpose.

The myocardial microcirculation consists of three components: arterioles, capillaries, and venules. A comparable lymphatic circulation is present, but for the purpose of this discussion it will not be considered. Arterioles are relatively thin-walled vessels composed of endothelium, basement membrane, and 1–3 layers of smooth muscle, important for modulation of the luminal diameter. Several different orders of arterioles ranging from 100–15 microns in diameter, are usually described in studies of the microcirculation, with terminal arterioles of approximately 15 microns giving rise to capillaries [2]. Venules generally have a greater luminal diameter than arterioles and absent to rare muscle coat [3], but they may be difficult to differentiate from arterioles morphologically, unless the direction of blood flow can be ascertained. Although theoretically, obstruction of venules could lead to myocardial cell damage, little is known about this potential problem, nor has the three-dimensional anatomy of these vessels been studied in any detail. Capillaries consist of endothelial cells surrounded by basement membrane material or basal lamina. It is these vessels which directly supply the myocardial cell with oxygenated substrate, and therefore the capillary may be intimately involved with the development of myocellular ischemia and necrosis.

Organization

Analysis of the myocardial microcirculation must take into account two very important features which have given rise to misinterpretation and artifacts. One feature is often overlooked when histopathologists examine tissue sections under the microscope: the microcirculation and the tissue supplied by it are spatially organized three-dimensionally. A failure to appreciate this simple fact has led to significant error in descriptions of myocardial infarction patterns, as will be discussed below. The second feature is more subtle, but I believe it also has given rise to misinterpretation: the microcirculation is so densely packed in the myocardium that attempts to analyze branching and interconnections when the vessels are filled with a perfusate of one color, will not allow for discrimination of individual vessels because of the superimposition of others. Many studies that have suggested the myocardial microcirculation was interconnected employed only perfusates of one color [4–6].

Although the weight of the older evidence implied that the microcirculation was interconnected, whether this is an established fact is not simply an academic question of little significance. It is clearly recognized that large coronary arteries and their major branches are interconnected by collaterals in the epicardium and superficial layers of the heart [7], but does this pattern persist down to the microcirculatory level? Does blood percolate through the myocardium diffusely, washing over all myocardial cells proportional to the upstream supply and pressure? If so, then occlusion of a large coronary artery might give rise to a central densely ischemic zone in the main territory supplied by that vessel, but as more and more microvascular interconnections fed blood into the tissue moving outwardly from the center, the tissue would become progressively less ischemic. This theoretical pattern is now generally recognized to be incorrect, at least when moving from the densely ischemic subendocardium toward the epicardium. Less than ten years ago gradated ischemia or a "bull's-eye" pattern was the commonly accepted view of myocardial infarction, giving rise to the concept of a moderately ischemic lateral border zone amenable to therapeutic interventions to keep the tissue from infarcting. As we shall see, this pattern is not consistent with the three-dimensional histology of myocardial infarctions, nor is it consistent with the anatomy of the myocardial microcirculation.

Diffuse interconnections of microcirculatory vessels are insufficient to keep small groups of myocardial cells viable, if all of the interconnecting vessels are being supplied by the same upstream coronary artery undergoing occlusion. However, several hypothetical patterns of the microcirculation could explain the existence of an ischemic border zone. For example, if two capillaries supplying a myocardial cell were derived from two different large vessels, then there would be a pattern of overlapping or alternating capillaries in a highly complex arrangement (figure 7–1). Thus occlusion of one large coronary artery could still allow the myocardial cell in that territory to obtain reduced substrate sufficient to keep it viable from the capillary supplied by the unoccluded coronary. A similar outcome could arise if there was a capillary pattern with each capillary supplied by blood from two different coronary arteries (figure 7–1). Again, myocardial cells could still obtain sufficient substrate to maintain viability, following occlusion of one artery.

To analyze the organization of the myocardial microcirculation, and to determine whether either of the two theoretical arrangements described above actually exist, it was necessary to perfuse the coronaries with more than a single-colored solution. We performed studies in both dog and human hearts

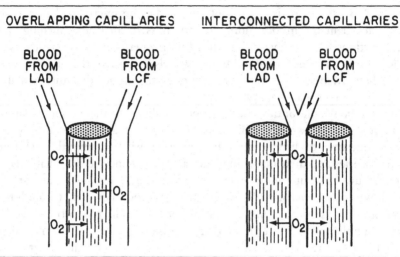

OVERLAPPING CAPILLARIES   INTERCONNECTED CAPILLARIES

BLOOD   BLOOD   BLOOD   BLOOD
FROM   FROM   FROM   FROM
LAD   LCF   LAD   LCF

Figure 7–1. Two hypothetical capillary anatomic patterns that could explain the existence of surviving but ischemic myocardium, at the lateral border of an acute myocardial infarction. On the left, each myocardial cell is intimately associated with interdigitating or overlapping capillaries, derived from separate large coronary arteries. Occlusion of one main vessel would allow the cell to be supplied by oxygenated blood from the patent artery in diminished amounts, compared to normal. On the right, capillaries derived from two major vessels are interconnected, so that occlusion of one coronary artery would allow cells to be partially supplied by the patent vessel. With both patterns, enough substrate might be provided from the nonoccluded vascular bed to keep the myocardial cells viable, though ischemic. LAD = left anterior descending coronary artery; LCF = left circumflex artery. (From Factor et al. [9]. Reproduced with permission of the American Heart Association, Inc., *Circulation* and the author.)

[8, 9] by perfusing two or three separate coronary arteries or their main branches with differently colored silicone rubber solutions. This material hardens after being perfused into the microcirculation, and since the colors can be identified when the tissue is examined with epi-illumination, the source of the vessel feeding a capillary can be determined. The silicone rubber solutions were perfused simultaneously and at the same pressure, to limit perfusion of the preformed epicardial large-vessel collaterals. The pressure falloff downstream would be such as to allow perfusion of microvascular collaterals, if they existed. Thus the color of the silicone rubber in any region of the myocardium would determine what coronary artery supplied that area; conversely, capillaries filled with different colors would demonstrate the nature of the microcirculation.

The observations in both the canine and human hearts provided unequivocal evidence that the microcirculation is discrete and not interconnected across two large coronary artery territories. We did not observe either of the two theoretical patterns postulated above; rather, we observed sharply delimited vascular regions, regardless of the size of the coronary vessel perfused. When we examined cleared myocardial tissue with epi-illumination from areas where two colors abutted, there was sharp demarcation along the border (figure

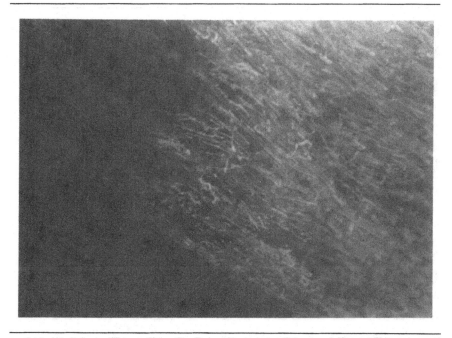

Figure 7–2. A simultaneous double perfusion of two coronary arteries with yellow (right) and red (left) silicone rubber. Note the sharp but irregular border between the two microcirculatory regions. Interconnections and capillaries filled with yellow-red perfusate are not seen. Along the border, many capillaries end as loops (Epi-illumination, × 63).

7–2). The border between the region was often irregular, composed of groups of vessels which invaginated into the opposite zone, but we saw no evidence of double-filled vessels or other interconnections. Close observation of the vessels showed that the capillaries filled with one color were organized as loops and branching arcades (figure 7–3). The loops at the border approached closely to loops filled with the other color, passing only several microns apart, but no connections were noted at the apex of the loops.

Two other observations supported the conclusion that the myocardial microcirculation is discrete. To rule out artifact, we perfused both brain and skeletal muscle with the same two-color technique. In both tissues, interconnections were easily demonstrated at the border between two perfusion fields, and vessels filled with two colors were observed. In the heart, several specimens were perfused with only one color per vessel, with the remaining vessels not perfused or perfused with saline. If the microcirculation was interconnected, one would expect that the perfusate would penetrate the tissue diffusely, and would end in a very irregular pattern. In fact, we observed sharp demarcation of the silicone rubber in a pattern similar to the double perfusion, with capillaries ending in loops along a well-defined border (figure 7–4).

These studies clearly showed that the coronary circulation is an end-vessel

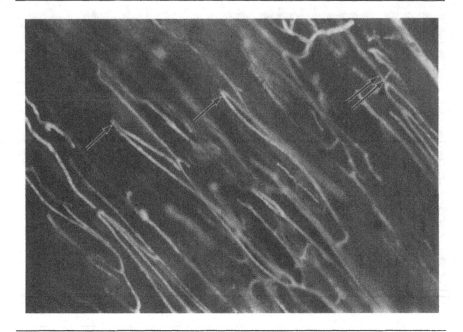

Figure 7–3. A high magnification of capillaries filled with silicone rubber along the border of a microcirculatory region. Note that many capillaries end with sharp hairpin loops (arrows), while several send out straight branches which extend into other loops, in the form of arcades (double arrows). (Epi-illumination × 150).

system, with specific territories supplied by discrete capillary beds. This finding has important implications for the anatomic pattern of myocardial ischemia or infarction, for it suggests that an end-capillary loop system would preclude a significant ischemic lateral border zone around a myocardial infarction. If a border zone is present (see below), something besides vascular mechanisms may explain its occurrence. The studies detailed in the next section, however, suggest that the lateral limits of an infarct are determined by the vascular anatomy, particularly at the microvascular level.

THE LATERAL BORDER ZONE OF MYOCARDIAL INFARCTION

As we have seen, the generally accepted view of acute myocardial infarction postulated a lateral region of ischemic tissue at risk for necrosis, surrounding a central zone of infarcted myocardium. This pattern was based on studies of the lateral region, which described levels of creatine kinase [10] and changes in the electrocardiogram [11–14] intermediate between those in the normal and the centrally necrotic zones. Semiquantitative analyses, involving measurement of changes in large volumes of tissue, may give rise to two opposite conclusions:

1. All of the tissue in the region is affected relatively equally, and therefore an

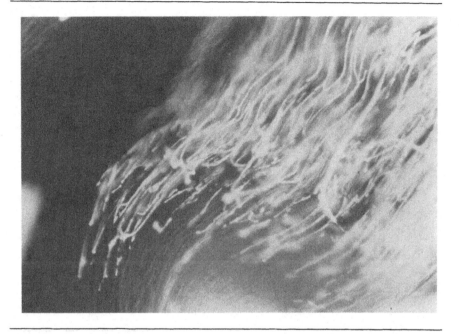

Figure 7–4. A human heart in which one coronary artery was perfused with silicone rubber, while the others were vented to atmosphere. The capillaries terminate along a sharp but irregular border, with many loops apparent (here seen obliquely). The perfusate does not penetrate into the surrounding vascular territory, as it would if the capillaries from all coronary arteries were interconnected. (Epi-illumination, × 63).

intermediate level of some marker of damage is representative of homogeneous alterations; or,

2. The region is composed of discrete admixtures of normal myocardium and ischemic or infarcted myocardium in a complex arrangement that will not permit separation by methods that are either too gross or insensitive. In the latter case, therefore, intermediate levels of a marker represent an average value which does not indicate a border zone is present. In fact, studies performed by Hirzel and colleagues [15], in which ischemic and normal tissue was differentially marked with radioactive microspheres and then analyzed for creatine kinase content, showed that there was apparently a sharp border between the infarcted and the surrounding normal myocardium with the absence of a lateral border zone.

As we have suggested previously, myocardial tissue and its vasculature is organized three-dimensionally, and therefore must be analyzed spatially. A common histologic observation, when sections are examined from the border of an acute myocardial infarction, is to see isolated islands of normal myocardium in a "sea of necrosis" (figure 7–5). This finding has been considered a manifestation of myocardium that is ischemically damaged and at

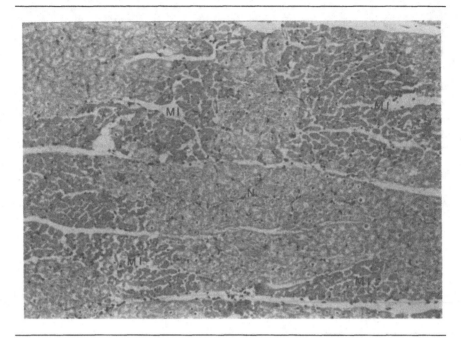

Figure 7–5. An acute 24-hour-old canine myocardial infarction sectioned along the lateral border. A central paler zone of histologically normal muscle (N) is completely surrounded by darker staining (hypereosinophilic) necrotic myocardium (MI), creating the appearance of an island. Parenthetically, the necrotic muscle is also surrounded by normal tissue making it into an island as well. Serial sections, however, showed that both the normal and infarcted myocardial islands became confluent with homologous tissue, thereby demonstrating that the islands were, in fact, peninsulas. The lateral border between the normal and the infarcted myocardium is discrete but very irregular, and is remarkably interdigitated. (Hematoxylin-eosin, × 63).

risk for necrosis, but that receives sufficient blood supply to survive in a precarious "twilight zone" [16]. We demonstrated that this observation was an artifact of two-dimensional sectioning of a three-dimensional process, by serially reconstructing the border region of canine infarctions employing hundreds of histological sections [17]. When individual "islands" of normal or necrotic myocardium were followed sequentially, they were shown to connect with the homologous region of unaffected or infarcted tissue respectively. Thus the border or interface between the two tissues was very discrete and was composed of "peninsulas" of interdigitating myocardium. The degree of interdigitation along the border suggested that any relatively gross sampling from this region would lead to averaging of normal and necrotic myocardium, thereby giving rise to intermediate levels of some marker.

Other studies performed with care to analyze either small volumes of tissue or the spatial geometry of the lateral border have demonstrated that there is essentially no large region of ischemic but viable myocardium outside of the central infarct zone [18–21]. Yellon and Hearse [18, 22] have shown that metabolic and flow characteristics of the border region are not compatible with an intermediately ischemic zone when very small pieces of muscle are rapidly removed with multiple bioptomes. Similarly, Marcus and co-workers [21] have demonstrated that cutting tissue into small segments to analyze radioactive microsphere-measured blood flow does not reveal a gradual falloff from the lateral to the central area at risk. Clearly, the smaller the volume of myocardium sampled, the less likely that there will be an admixture of heterogeneous tissue; however, it is obvious that relatively gross techniques of analysis cannot separate normal from abnormal myocardium down to the cell and capillary level.

To study the border region at the cellular level, and to correlate the presence of a sharp but irregular histological border with the microvascular supply to the tissue, we perfused silicone rubber into 24-hour-old canine myocardial infarctions [23, 24]. By combining histology of the acute infarction with epi-illumination of the vascular supply feeding the normal and necrotic muscle, we were able to correlate the degree of concordance of the two along the border. In other words, the presence of viable muscle in the lateral border supplied by the occluded artery would support the existence of an intermediate ischemic border zone. However, the results of this study demonstrated a high degree of correlation between the necrotic tissue and the vascular perfusion field of the occluded coronary artery, with the closely abutting normal tissue along the lateral border supplied by the unoccluded vessel (figure 7–6). The number of discordant vessels and the distances involved (generally less than 50 microns) could be accounted for by simple diffusion of substrate from the normal zone into the area at risk, thereby maintaining a thin rim of myocytes viable. This study demonstrated the absence of a significant lateral ischemic border at 24 hours, and showed that the boundaries between normal and necrotic myocardium were extremely sharp, and were determined by the microvascular supply. Furthermore, the study also showed that irregular peninsulas along the border were supplied by congruous vessels, thus confirming the histological reconstructions previously described.

TEMPORAL PROGRESSION AND THE AREA AT RISK

A potential criticism of the previously cited study would be that a completed infarct at 24 hours may not have the same spatial geometry in relation to the lateral vascular perfusion field as a developing infarct at an earlier time. If this is valid, then interventions shortly after infarct onset may salvage significant volumes of lateral muscle not available for salvage at later time periods. The classical studies of Reimer and Jennings [25, 26] have firmly established the concept that myocardial infarction is a temporal event in which a wavefront of necrosis extends from subendocardium to subepicardium with progressive time. What is less well-established is whether the enlargement of the infarct in an endocardial-epicardial direction is fixed laterally, or whether some lateral extension also may occur with time. A corollary of their studies is that myocardial infarction occurs within a specific vascular territory. This territory

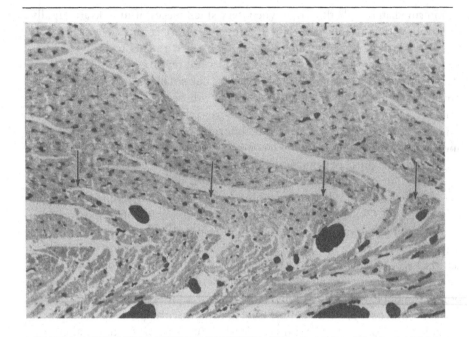

Figure 7–6. The border of a 24-hour-old canine infarction in which the occluded coronary artery has been perfused with white silicone rubber, and the adjacent artery has been perfused with red. With transillumination both perfusates appear black; however, epi-illumination permits differentiation of the two colors. The infarcted zone (below arrows) is perfused solely by the occluded vessel. Both the vascular and the histologic border correspond closely without significant overlap. Note the diminished number of perfused vessels in the infarcted tissue and the extravasation of perfusate, secondary to the "no-reflow" phenomenon. (Hematoxylin-eosin, × 63).

is the myocardial area at risk: the region of muscle supplied by any vessel, and jeopardized when coronary occlusion occurs, but a region which does not undergo necrosis uniformly or instantly following the onset of hypoperfusion. The volume of the area at risk may include the entire region supplied by a large coronary artery, and may progress down to the microcirculation, depending on the level and extent of the collateral supply, if any. The smallest area at risk would be that group of myocardial cells supplied by one arteriole branching into a single arcade of capillaries. As we shall see, such an arteriolar area at risk may account for extremely small regions of necrosis occurring within the myocardium.

EXTENSION OF ACUTE MYOCARDIAL INFARCTION

Although studies of myocardial infarction at 24 hours show a tight correlation between the vascular supply and histological necrosis within the area at risk, investigations at earlier time periods after coronary occlusion are fraught with difficulty, since the tissue does not have overt histological features of necrosis until at least 6–12 hours have passed. To circumvent this problem, it is

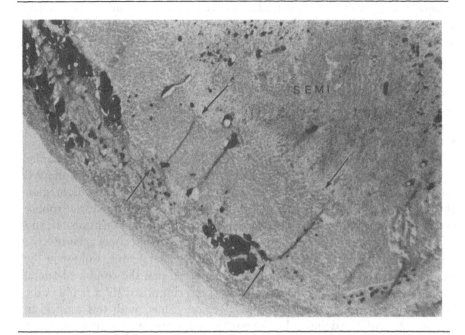

Figure 7–7. A one-week-old subendocardial myocardial infarction (SEMI) due to transient coronary artery occlusion, demarcated from a thick zone of previously preserved immediately subendocardial myocardium (arrows). Within this subendocardial zone there is now acute necrosis, following permanent occlusion of the same coronary artery. The black material is silicone rubber. There is extensive acute hemorrhage and silicone rubber extravasation in the endocardial tissues. (Hematoxylin-eosin, × 63).

necessary to do temporary coronary occlusions, with reperfusion of the tissue for a time sufficient to allow for histological necrosis to be evident. This technique can also be combined with subsequent complete occlusions of the same vessel to gauge how, and in what direction, the region of necrosis extends. This model has the additional advantage of being relevant to human transient coronary artery occlusion causing a subendocardial infarction, with eventual complete occlusion of the same vessel leading to transmural infarction.

In two studies employing this model [27, 28], our group has demonstrated some specific and quantitative aspects of acute myocardial infarction and its direction of extension. In one study [27], we showed that there was a rather large zone (8 ± 1%) of immediately subendocardial tissue preserved after a transient 40 minute coronary artery occlusion. This zone was infarcted when the same coronary vessel was permanently occluded (figure 7–7), leaving only a few preserved cell layers immediately under the endocardium. By using silicone rubber perfusions, we were able to show that the initially preserved muscle was within the microvascular region at risk, and was supplied by the occluded coronary artery. We postulated that the preserved layers in the subendocardium obtained sufficient substrate from the ventricular cavity to maintain viability during the period of transient occlusion, but that permanent coronary occlusion caused the tissue to undergo necrosis. The fact that we identified a number of human subendocardial infarctions with new necrosis in the subendocardial zone, following transmural extension due to coronary occlusion, suggested that the pathophysiology of this event in the dog and human is similar. Although this relatively small region of jeopardized muscle (a minute subendocardial border zone within the region at risk) may have little importance functionally, it may be a significant source of post-infarct arrhythmias.

The second study [28] directly addressed the question of the lateral border zone at early time periods. By using the same model of a transient, followed by a permanent, coronary occlusion, and by defining the microvascular region at risk as well as the normal zone with differently colored silicone rubber solutions, we could track the degree of lateral infarct extension, if any occurred. Morphometric methods were employed to precisely quantify the volume of new muscle necrosis, occurring in the lateral zone, following the permanent coronary artery occlusion. We showed that the combined lateral extension (on both sides of the central infarction) comprised $1.7 \pm 0.1\%$ of the cross-sectional area of the vascular risk region. Thus, with this model, an extremely small, but definite, border zone was demonstrated, but one that was insignificant in terms of salvageable, functionally important myocardium.

Even the estimate of salvageability in the prior experiment may be too high due to inherent errors of the techniques used to define the lateral borders. (Because of endocardial curvature and irregularity, the perpendicular margins of the lateral border are not easily ascertained). A recent study by Murdock and associates [29] analyzed chronically instrumented dogs with serial post-mortem angiograms following acute coronary artery occlusion. They demonstrated that the "border zone" was limited to a narrow region immediately inside the perfusion field of the occluded vasculature (area at risk). Furthermore, when they used a microsphere exclusion technique to separate the vascular perfusion fields, they found that reduction of blood flow at the border of the ischemic zone resulted from an admixture of normal and necrotic myocardium. Thus, even at extremely early time periods, the boundary between normal and ischemic tissue appears to be sharp, with well-defined microvascular territories determining the area at risk. The intermediately ischemic lateral border zone is apparently an artifact of insensitive measuring techniques.

NO-REFLOW PHENOMENON

Definition

When a coronary artery is occluded for at least 20 minutes, progressive, irreversible damage is produced focally in subendocardial myocytes, which extends, with time, toward the epicardium. As shown by Jennings and colleagues [30], reperfusion of the tissue, prior to 20 minutes, salvages virtually all jeopardized myocytes, while reperfusion during subsequent time periods salvages fewer cells. In addition to myocyte damage, there is also ischemic damage to capillary endothelial cells. Blebbing and swelling of the endothelium may lead to obstruction of the microvasculature, or marked increases in capillary permeability [31]. The failure to achieve uniform reperfusion, which in experimental canine infarctions occurs within about 90 minutes of occlusion time, is known as the "no-reflow" phenomenon [30]. When this phenomenon was described in ischemic myocardium, it was of pathophysiologic interest with little clinical relevance; however, today with a pronounced trend toward early intervention to open or bypass obstructed coronary arteries during acute myocardial infarction, this problem may be of practical significance.

Significance

The "no-reflow" phenomenon manifests itself as an inability to reperfuse myocardial tissue after a period of coronary artery occlusion. The phenomenon leads to a progressive, relative absence of blood within the affected territory, often surrounded by a zone of hemorrhage. The latter is secondary to permeability changes in perfusable capillaries. Myocardium within the no-reflow area develops typical coagulation necrosis, whereas irreversibily damaged tissue accessible to reperfused blood shows signs of contraction-band necrosis. The "no-reflow" phenomenon can be demonstrated experimentally with silicone rubber perfusions of the microcirculation. Tissues so affected have a marked diminution in the number of perfusate filled vessels, and often demonstrate extravasation of material, even when the perfusion was done at physiological pressures (figure 7–6).

A major question has been whether the "no-reflow" phenomenon is the primary cause of irreversible ischemic myocyte damage, or whether it is a concurrent or subsequent process. Clearly, this is a significant issue, because attempts to reinstitute perfusion prior to the onset of "no-reflow" might salvage jeopardized myocardium, if "no-flow" was the cause of the necrosis; whereas, if "no-reflow" followed as a secondary event, such attempts would be of no benefit. Studies by Jennings and colleagues [31] and Kloner et al. [32] have demonstrated that the ultrastructural evidence of microvascular damage (which correlated with "no-reflow") lagged behind the myocellular injury, suggesting it is not the primary cause of the damage. However, Tillmanns and Kubler [2] have argued recently that functional disturbances of the microcirculation which may precede the onset of structural changes in the vessels, may be the primary cause of myocellular death. This issue is still not completely resolved, but it appears that the evidence favors "no-reflow" as a secondary event.

Pathogenesis

The cause of the "no-reflow" phenomenon has been ascribed to several mechanisms which may act independently or concurrently to obstruct the microcirculation. Ischemic endothelial damage affects the structural integrity of the microvasculature, with swelling and blebbing of cells leading to luminal obstruction. Lipasti et al. [33] have suggested that ventricular contracture occurring with hypoxic perfusion of the myocardium may compress the intramural vessels so that flow is limited. McDonagh [34] proposed that damage due to oxygen-free radicals and plugging, secondary to platelets or granulocytes, may be involved in the vessel obstruction. Recently, Fukuyama et al. [35] also suggested that extravasation of blood from damaged, permeable vessels may contribute to the phenomenon.

Clinical Implications

Regardless of the precise cause of "no-reflow," most of the current evidence supports the view that if the microcirculation cannot be perfused, the myocardium served by those vessels will die. The morphology of the infarction may be altered (hemorrhagic rather than bland, contraction band rather than coagulative necrosis), but there is no firm indication that this has any adverse consequences for the patient. Therefore, attempts to reperfuse myocardial tissue early in the infarction period by coronary angioplasty, streptokinase infusion, or coronary bypass should not be halted because of concern over the "no-reflow" phenomenon.

OBSTRUCTION OF THE MICROCIRCULATION

Thrombotic Occlusion

Although the area at risk, as described earlier, is usually thought to be the region supplied by a large coronary artery, the end-loop pattern of the cardiac microcirculation has given rise to the concept of multiple microscopic areas at risk. Thus, occlusion of the vasculature at any pre-capillary level, can, under the appropriate circumstances, lead to myocellular necrosis. Theoretically, even capillary obstruction, if sufficient numbers of capillaries were involved, could cause myocellular necrosis; however, single capillary occlusion does not lead to overt myocyte damage, because each muscle cell is supplied by more than one capillary. This is shown by an absence of damage when the microcirculation is embolized with 9 or 15 micron diameter microspheres to measure myocardial blood flow in experimental preparations.

A number of recent studies suggest that microcirculatory occlusion may be a significant event with clinical implications. In most cases, the microcirculation is obstructed with platelet aggregates, although admixtures of fibrin and cells may be seen. It may be difficult to ascribe direct effects on the myocardium to an isolated arteriole occluded by a platelet microthrombus, as may be seen in disseminated intravascular coagulopathy. However, when large numbers of vessels are involved, as in thrombotic, thrombocytopenic purpura (figure 7–8) unequivocal myocardial changes may be identified. Haerem [36] has shown that platelet aggregates in intramyocardial vessels, even in patients

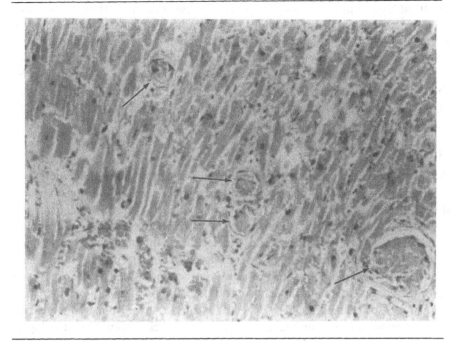

Figure 7–8. A section of myocardium from a patient with thrombotic, thrombocytopenic purpura. Several arterioles are partially or completely occluded by fibrin-platelet microthrombi (arrows), and the surrounding myocardium shows focal fragmentation and necrosis. (Hematoxylin-eosin, × 150).

without major acute abnormalities in the epicardial coronary arteries, may be seen in sudden coronary death. Whether the obstruction of the microcirculation is a primary or secondary event is not known, and additional study is necessary to address this question.

Experimentally, the administration of catecholamines to animals may result in focal contraction-band necrosis of myocytes, which is considered to be due to the direct effects of the drugs on the myocardium. Although several different mechanisms may play a role in the development of tissue damage, the localized nature of the necrosis can be explained on a vascular basis because the changes occur in contiguous, grouped myocytes. If the catecholamine was affecting myocytes individually, one would expect to see multiple and scattered necrotic cells throughout the myocardium. The microvascular changes induced by the catecholamine may be vasospastic (see below), but Haft et al. [37] have demonstrated platelet aggregates in the myocardium, have associated them with cardiovascular injury [38], and have prevented catecholamine-induced myocardial necrosis with platelet aggregate inhibitors [39].

As we have described already, obstruction of the microcirculation may be involved in the "reflow" phenomenon during acute myocardial infarction. Recently, McNamara and co-workers [40] demonstrated that platelet trapping occurs at the margins of acute experimental myocardial infarctions and can be inhibited with aspirin pretreatment. What influence this may have on the ultimate size of the infarction was not apparent from their study. Many otherwise healthy individuals are taking aspirin prophylactically for its antiplatelet effects. Although there is no convincing evidence to date that such therapy is beneficial, it is equally true that in individuals without aspirin allergy or peptic ulcer disease, an aspirin regimen may have positive effects on the coronary arteries and the cardiac microcirculation.

Microvascular Spasm

As suggested in the previous section, thrombotic obstruction of the microcirculation, particularly by platelets, may have adverse effects on the myocardium. Platelet aggregates in the microcirculation may result from damage to the vascular endothelium, due to mechanical, ischemic, toxic, or infectious etiologies. Among the mechanical processes which can cause platelets to aggregate, arteriolar spasm may be significant. Although platelet aggregates themselves may lead to smooth muscle contraction, secondary to release of thromboxane, vasospasm can damage endothelial cells and result in adherence of platelets to subendothelial collagen. There is now extensive evidence, derived from direct visualization of in vivo vessels, from pharmacologic interventions, and from microvascular perfusion studies, that microvascular spasm is a real pathophysiologic process.

A recent study from our laboratories demonstrated both the morphologic effects of microvascular obstruction and the prevention of these effects by anti-vasospastic therapy [41]. Embolization of 25 micron-sized microspheres into myocardial arterioles led to the development of multiple foci of acute contraction-band necrosis (figure 7–9). The contraction-band changes suggested the possibility that the lesions were secondary to microvascular obstruction and reperfusion. Accordingly, phentolamine, a rapidly acting alpha adrenergic blocking agent, was administered 10 minutes prior to microsphere embolization. Despite the fact that microspheres were present in arterioles for 24 hours and the effects of the drug had worn off, no necrosis was identified in multiple sections of myocardium. Similarly, the calcium-blocking agent verapamil was effective in preventing necrosis. Based on these observations we concluded that microvascular embolization with arteriolar-sized microspheres was insufficient to produce myocardial damage simply by obstruction, but that arteriolar vasospasm soon after embolization caused the focal lesions. The implications of these findings may be significant with regard to the development of focal myocardial lesions, and, as we shall see in the next section, they may be important in other forms of specific myocardial disease.

Microvascular Spasm and Congestive Cardiomyopathy

Recent evidence suggests that at least three and possibly several other experimental congestive cardiomyopathies have demonstrable microvascular

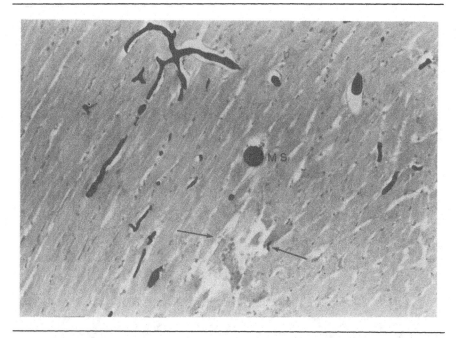

Figure 7–9. A 25 micron microsphere (MS) has been embolized into the microcirculation of this heart. A discrete focal area of contraction-band myocardial necrosis is adjacent to the microsphere (arrows). Incomplete perfusion of the microvasculature with silicone rubber is also apparent. (Hematoxylin-eosin, × 150).

spasm as a potential cause of the focal myocardial lesions typical of these conditions [42–44]. The cardiomyopathic Syrian hamster, a hereditary model of cardiomyopathy and muscular dystrophy, develops focal cardiac necrosis, which with time leads to progressive ventricular dysfunction and death [42]. Silicone rubber perfusion studies early in the course have demonstrated microvascular spasm (figure 7–10). Treatment of the animals with verapamil, or the alpha adrenergic-blocking drug prazosin, completely prevents the development of microvascular spasm and the associated myocardial degeneration [42, 45]. The fact that vasodilators can inhibit the disease, when ordinarily 100% of the animals are affected, supports the hypothesis that microvascular vasospasm plays an important role in its pathogenesis.

Similarly, we have recently demonstrated the presence of microvascular spasm in two acquired forms of cardiomyopathy: the hypertensive and diabetic rat [43], and the Trypanosoma cruzi-infected mouse with acute Chagasic cardiomyopathy [44]. Both are models of human disease, and both have similar features to the hamster, in that focal myocardial necrosis and subsequent fibrosis are prevalent. Microvascular perfusion studies with silicone rubber have revealed typical focal areas of constriction and aneurysm formation consistent with spasm. To date, vasodilator therapy has not been attempted.

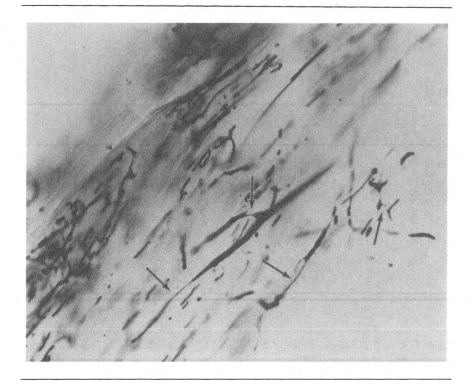

Figure 7–10. A cleared section of myocardium from a cardiomyopathic Syrian hamster reveals multiple vessels in the microcirculation with changes consistent with microvascular spasm (arrows). (Transillumination, × 150).

Although it may be premature to generalize from animal models to human disease, the presence of focal necrosis leading to discrete microscopic regions of fibrosis is a characteristic feature of both experimental and clinical congestive cardiomyopathy. Although the pathogenesis may be variable, it is appealing to speculate that microvascular spasm may be a cause of myocardial micronecrosis in humans, and that, as in the Syrian hamster, it may be preventable with appropriate early therapy.

SMALL VESSEL DISEASE

Although the purpose of this chapter has been to describe some aspects of the coronary microcirculation and myocardial ischemia, brief mention should be made of the so-called small vessels of the heart. For one thing, despite the fact that these vessels are much larger in caliber (100–1000 microns) than the microcirculation, some investigators place them in the same category. Second, it is true that there is a certain arbitrary and artificial separation between small intramyocardial muscular arteries and arterioles, in that both have contractile resistance properties, and may suffer pathological lesions leading to myocar-

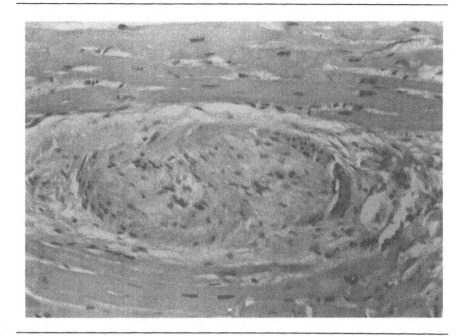

Figure 7-11. A small muscular artery from a patient with alcoholic cardiomyopathy. There is pronounced intimal and medial smooth muscle proliferation virtually occluding the lumen. Perivascular fibrosis surrounds the vessel. (Hematoxylin-eosin, × 400).

dial damage. On the whole, then, it appears reasonable to consider the small muscular arteries as being along a continuum with the microcirculation, and potentially important in the development of focal myocardial ischemia and necrosis.

The pathological alterations of the small arteries are too extensive to describe in any detail here. Among the degenerative changes which may occur are intimal and medial proliferative lesions (figure 7-11) which may significantly affect the luminal patency of the vessel. Myocardial necrosis and fibrosis may occur in association with these changes, along with arrhythmias, conduction system abnormalities, and sudden death [46, 47]. Small vessel disease is particularly prevalent in cardiomyopathies, of both the congestive and hypertrophic type. Severe lesions can be seen in chronic alcoholic cardiomyopathy [48]. The degenerative features of small vessel disease may be observed in association with epicardial coronary artery atherosclerosis, but primary small vessel lesions leading to symptomatic ischemic heart disease can occur as an isolated abnormality. Atypical chest pain can occur as a consequence of small vessel obliteration. Recent use of endomyocardial biopsies to investigate patients with anginal symptoms and normal coronary arteries, has revealed a subset of individuals with highly abnormal intramyocardial vessels as the only alteration (figure 7-12). These findings are too preliminary to fully

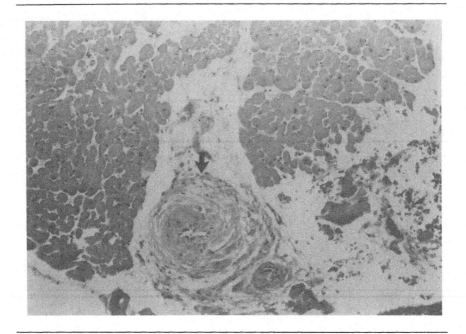

Figure 7–12. A section from an endomyocardial biopsy performed on a patient with atypical angina and normal coronary arteries. The myocardium is unremarkable. The only abnormality noted is a severely narrowed muscular artery (arrow) with sclerosis of the intima and media, and perivascular fibrosis. Several other vessels from the same biopsy showed similiar changes. (Hematoxylin-eosin, × 150).

ascribe patients' symptoms to the vasculopathy as yet. However, further studies are being performed.

CONCLUSIONS

Recent investigations have provided strong evidence for implicating the cardiac microcirculation in a variety of pathological states leading to myocardial ischemia or necrosis. The anatomy of the microcirculation, though still not worked out in detail, has an important bearing on the volume and geometry of myocardium undergoing infarcton following coronary artery occlusion. Pathological changes in the microcirculation, due to ischemia, may prevent reperfusion of the myocardium ("no-reflow" phenomenon) and may change a bland infarct into a hemorrhagic one. The microcirculation has been shown to develop functional abnormalities (spasm) in experimental models which may contribute to or cause cardiomyopathy; the lessons learned in the animal laboratory may apply to man. The microcirculation also may develop occlusive obstruction which can cause focal, generally microscopic regions of myocardial necrosis. Lesions in the small arterial vessels may reflect unique abnormalities, or they may reflect functional or morphological disturbances within the entire intramyocardial vascular tree.

Future trends, based on the experience of the past decade, suggest that investigation of the microcirculation will become more important. Undoubtedly, techniques will be developed or improved to assess the microcirculation in clinical situations. Therapeutic interventions to maintain microvascular patency or to prevent spasm will be employed to a greater extent. Clinical study of morphological changes in the microcirculation using the endomyocardial biopsy will be applied to selected patients whose atypical symptoms cannot be explained by large coronary artery disease. Since we now know that the microvessels supplying the individual myocytes play a significant role in normal myocardial function and in disease states, it is likely that the next decade will see even greater advances in this field.

REFERENCES

1. Steinhausen, M., Tillmanns, H., and Thederan, H. 1978. Microcirculation of the epimyocardial layer of the heart. *Pflugers Arch* 378:9–14.
2. Tillmans, H. and Kubler, W. 1984. What happens in the microcirculation? In *Therapeutic approaches to myocardial infarction size limitation*, Hearse, D.J., and Yellon, D.M., eds., pp. 107–124. New York: Raven Press.
3. Sherf, L., Ben-Shaul, Y., Leiberman, Y., and Neufeld, H.N. 1977. The human coronary microcirculation: An electron microscopic study. *Am. J. Cardiol.* 39:599–607.
4. Gross, L. 1921. *The blood supply to the heart in its anatomical and clinical aspects*, pp. 77–92. New York: Paul B. Goeber.
5. Brown, R.E. 1965. The pattern of the microcirculatory bed in the ventricular myocardium of domestic mammals. *Am. J. Anat.* 116:355–374.
6. Ludwig, G. 1965. Capillary pattern of the myocardium. *Methods Achiev. Exp. Pathol.* 5:238–271.
7. Fulton W.F.M. 1965. *The coronary arteries: Arteriography, microanatomy and pathogenesis of obliterative coronary artery disease.* pp. 72–128. Springfield, Illinois: Charles C. Thomas.
8. Okun, E.M., Factor, S.M., and Kirk, E.S. 1979. End-capillary loops in the heart: An explanation for discrete myocardial infarctions without border zones. *Science* 206:565–567.
9. Factor, S.M., Okun, E.M., Minase, T., and Kirk, E.S. 1982. The microcirculation of the human heart: End-capillary loops with discrete perfusion fields. *Circulation* 66:1241–1248.
10. Kjekshus, J.K., and Sobel, B.E. 1970. Depressed myocardial creatine phosphokinase activity following experimental myocardial infarction in rabbit. *Circ. Res.* 27:403–414.
11. Kjekshus, J.K., Maroko, P.R., and Sobel, B.E. 1972. Distribution of myocardial injury and its relation to epicardial ST-segment changes after coronary artery occlusion in the dog. *Cardiovasc. Res.* 6:490–499.
12. Lie, J.J., Pairolero, P.C., Holley, K.E., McCall, J.T., Thompson, H.K., Jr., and Titus, J.L. 1975. Time course and zonal variations of ischemic-induced myocardial cationic electrolyte derangements. *Circulation* 51:860–866.
13. Ross, J. Jr. 1976. Electrocardiographic ST-segment analysis in the characterization of myocardial ischemia and infarction. *Circulation* 52 (Suppl. I):1–73.
14. Hillis, L.D., Askenuzi, J., Braunwald, E., Radvany, P., Muller, J.E., Fishbein, M.C., and Masoko, P.R. 1976. Use of changes in the epicardial QRS complex to assess interventions which modify the extent of myocardial necrosis following coronary artery occlusions. *Circulation* 54:591–598.
15. Hirzel, H.D., Sonnenblick, E.H., and Kirk, E.S. 1977. Absence of a lateral border zone of intermediate creating phosphokinase depletion surrounding a central infarct 24 hours after acute coronary occlusion in the dog. *Circ. Res.* 41:673–683.
16. Edwards, J.E. 1957. Correlations in coronary arterial disease. *Bull. N.Y. Acad. Med.* 33:199–217.
17. Factor, S.M., Sonnenblick, E.H., Kirk, E.S. 1978. The histologic border zone of acute myocardial infarction: Islands or peninsulas? *Am. J. Pathol.* 92:111–120.
18. Yellon, D.M., Hearse, D.J., Crome, R., Grannell, J., Wyse, R.K.H. 1981. Characterization

of the lateral interface between normal and ischemic tissue in the canine heart during evolving myocardial infarction. *Am. J. Cardiol.* 47:1233–1239.

19. Harken, A.M., Barlow, C.H., Harden, W.R., and Chance, B. 1978. Two-and three-dimensional display of myocardial ischemic "border zone" in dogs. *Am. J. Cardiol.* 42: 954–959.

20. Janse, M.J., Cinca, J., Morena, H., Fiolet, J.W.T., Kleber, A.G., DeVries, G.P., Becker, A.E., and Durrer, D. 1979. The "border zone" in myocardial ischemia. An electrophysiological metabolic, and histochemical correlation in the pig heart. *Circ. Res.* 44:576–588.

21. Marcus, M.L., Kerber, R.E., Ehrhardt, J., and Abboud, F.M. 1975. Three dimensional geometry of acutely ischemic myocardium. *Circulation* 52:254–263.

22. Hearse, D.J., and Yellon D.M. 1982. The three-dimensional geometry of regional myocardial ischemia: The role of the coronary microcirculation in determining patterns of injury. In *Microcirculation of the heart*, Tillmanns, H., Kubler, W., and Zebe, H. eds. pp. 149–161. Berlin: Springer-Verlag.

23. Factor, S.M., Okun, E.M., and Kirk, E.S. 1981. The histological lateral border of acute canine myocardial infarction. A function of microcirculation. *Circ. Res.* 48:640–649.

24. Factor, S.M., and Kirk, E.S. 1982. Microcirculatory determints of infarct dimensions. In *Microcirculation of the heart*, Tillmanns, H., Kubler, W., and Zebe, H. eds., pp. 141–148. Berlin. Springer-Verlag.

25. Reimer, K.A., Lowe, J.E., Rasmussen, M.M., and Jennings, R.B. 1977. The wave front phenomenon of ischemic cell death. I. Myocardial infarct size vs. duration of coronary occlusion in dogs. *Circulation* 56:786–794.

26. Reimer, K.A., and Jennings, R.B. 1979. The "wavefront phenomenon" of myocardial ischemic cell death. II. Transmural progression of necrosis within the framework of ischemic bed size (myocardium at risk) and collateral flow. *Lab. Invest.* 40:633–644.

27. Forman, R., Cho, S., Factor, S.M., and Kirk, E.S. 1983. Acute myocardial infarct extension into a previously preserved subendocardial region at risk in dogs and patients. *Circulation* 67:117–124.

28. Forman, R., Cho, S., Factor, S.M., and Kirk, E.S. 1985. Lateral border zone: Quantitation of lateral extension of subendocardial infarction in the dog. *J. Am. Coll. Cardiol.* 5:1125–1131.

29. Murdock, R.H. Jr., Harlan, D.M., Morris, J.J., III, Pryor, W.W. Jr., and Cobb. F.R. 1983. Transitional blood flow zones between ischemic and nonischemic myocardium in the awake dog: Analysis based on distribution of the intramural vasculature. *Circ. Res.* 52:451–459.

30. Kloner, R.A., Ganote, C.E., and Jennings, R.B. 1974. The "no-reflow" phenomenon after temporary coronary occlusion in the dog. *J. Clin. Invest.* 54:1496–1508.

31. Jennings, R.B., Kloner, R.A., Ganatoe, C.E., Hawkins, H.K., and Reimer, K.A. 1982. Changes in capillary fine structures and function in acute myocardial ischemic injury. In *Microcirculation of the heart*, Tillmanns, H., Kubler, W., and Zebe, H. eds., Berlin: Springer-Verlag.

32. Kloner, R.A., Rude, R.E., Carlson, N., Maroko, P.R., DeBoer, L.W.V., and Braunwald, E. 1980 Ultrastructural evidence of microvascular damage and myocardial cell injury after coronary artery occlusion: Which comes first? *Circulation* 62:945–952.

33. Lipasti, J., Nevalainen, T.J., and Alanen, K. 1981. Effect of hypoxia on the microvascular function in insolated rat hearts. *Exp. Path.* 20:73–78.

34. McDonagh, P.F. 1983. The role of the coronary microcirculation in myocardial recovery from ischemia. *Yale J. Biol. Med.* 56:303–311.

35. Fukuyama, T., Sobel, B.E., and Roberts, R. 1984. Microvascular deterioration: implications for reperfusion. *Cardiovasc. Res.* 18:310–320.

36. Haerem, J.W. 1972. Platelet aggregates in intramyocardial vessels of patients dying suddenly and unexpectedly of coronary artery disease. *Atherosclerosis* 15:199–213.

37. Haft, J.I., and Fani, K. 1973. Stress and the induction of intravascular platelet aggregation in the heart. *Circulation* 48:164–169.

38. Haft, J.I. 1974. Cardiovascular injury induced by sympathetic catecholamines. *Prog. Cardiovasc. Dis.* 17:73–86.

39. Haft, J.I., Gershengorn, K., Kranz, P.D., and Oestreicher, R. 1972. Protection against epinephrine-induced myocardial necrosis by drugs that inhibit platelet aggregation. *Am. J. Cardiol.* 30:838–843.

40. Ruf, W., McNamara, J.J., Suehiro, A., Suehiro, G., and Wickline, S.A. 1980. Platelet

trapping in myocardial infarct in baboons: Therapeutic effect of aspirin. *Am. J. Cardiol.* 46:405–412.

41. Eng., C., Cho, S., Factor, S.M., Sonnenblick, E.H., and Kirk, E.S. 1984. Myocardial micronecrosis produced by microsphere embolization: Role of an alph-or-adrenergic tonic influence on the coronary microcirculation. *Circ. Res.* 54:74–82.

42. Factor, S.M., Minase, T., Cho, S., Dominitz, R., and Sonnenblick, E.H. 1982. Microvascular spasm in the cardiomyopathic Syrian hamster: A preventable cause of focal myocardial necrosis. *Circulation* 66:342–354.

43. Factor, S.M., Minase, T., Cho, S., Fein, F., Capasso, J.M., and Sonnenblick, E.H. 1984. Coronary microvascular abnormalities in the hypertensive-diabetic rat: A primary cause of cardiomyopathy? *Am. J. Pathol.* 116:9–20.

44. Factor, S.M., Cho, S., Wittner, M., and Tanowitz, H. 1985. Abnormalities of the coronary microcirculation in acute murine Chagas' disease. *Am. J. Trop. Med. Hyg.* 34:246–253.

45. Sole, M.J., Factor, S.M. 1985. Hamster cardiomyopathy: A genetically-transmitted sympathetic dystrophy? In *Pathogenesis of stress-induced heart disease*, Beamish, R.E., Panagia, V., Dhalla, N.S. eds., pp. 34–43. Boston: Martinus Nijhoff Publishing.

46. James, T.N. 1977. Small arteries of the heart. *Circulation* 56:2–14.

47. Rahlf, G. 1982. Small vessel disease, morphology. In *Microcirculation of the heart*, Tillmanns, H., Kubler, W., Zebe, H., eds., pp. 231–252. Berlin: Springer-Verlag.

48. Factor, S.M. 1976. Intramyocardial small-vessel disease in chronic alcoholism. *Am. Heart J.* 92:561–575.

8. THE BIOCHEMISTRY OF MYOCARDIAL FAILURE

LOUIS A. SORDAHL AND CLAUDE R. BENEDICT

Almost twenty years ago, Richard Bing and colleagues [1] addressed the question, "What is cardiac failure?" These authors concluded that we had no answer to this question, partly because of limitations in our techniques, but more likely because there is not one single answer to the complex array of changes associated with the heart's failure to pump blood. Recently, McCall and O'Rourke [2] noted that the relationship between biochemical changes and depressed myocardial contractility associated with failure remain unclear and a subject of continuing investigation. Despite tremendous advances in techniques and knowledge, our understanding of the fundamental biochemical mechanisms underlying myocardial contractile function and its regulation is still limited. These limitations make the understanding of myocardial failure all the more difficult and congestive heart failure continues to be a major clinical problem [3]. Although major deficiencies still exist in our knowledge of cause and effect relationships between biochemical "defects" and myocardial failure, it is clear that prolonged hemodynamic stress leads to decreased myocardial contractility [4]. Sustained hemodynamic stress can be caused by a variety of factors including hypertension, valvular heart disease and loss of functional myocardium following ischemic injury. Clinical congestive heart failure, in the vast majority of cases, results from hypertensive or coronary artery disease (ischemic injury). The focus of this chapter will be on those biochemical changes related to these two general types of hemodynamic stress. A great deal of experimental investigation, involving animal models [5] has been on the effects of pressure and volume overload on the heart. We will summarize these biochemical changes and attempt to relate these experimental observations to the clinical aspects of congestive heart failure.

MYOCARDIAL ULTRASTRUCTURE

A brief review of the ultrastructural anatomy (figure 8–1) and function in the normal heart will provide a framework for subsequent discussions of the pathophysiological changes in myocardial contractility. The primary, functional unit of heart muscle is the sarcomere, which is composed of actin (thin) and myosin (thick) filaments (figure 8–1). This is the essential contractile system which converts chemical energy (ATP) into mechanical work (contraction). Two other major proteins, tropomyosin and troponin, are the regulatory proteins of the myofibrillar or contraction apparatus. These four proteins constitute the basic unit of contraction of the heart muscle. Contraction (systole) can be considered to be initiated with the binding and subsequent hydrolysis of ATP by the myosin head units or crossbridges (myosin ATPase). This "activates" the myosin crossbridges so that they are ready to bind to the actin filament. In order for this binding to take place, the tropomyosin molecule that "masks" or covers the actin binding site must be shifted so as to expose the actin binding site for myosin. This is accomplished by the binding of calcium to a subunit (troponin C) of the troponin protein which is in close association with the tropomyosin. Calcium binding to troponin rearranges the troponin-tropomyosin complex, exposing the actin binding site, allowing myosin to bind to actin and contraction (systole) occurs. In order for relaxation (diastole) to occur, calcium must now be removed from the troponin-tropomyosin complex. Relaxation occurs by removal of calcium from the troponin by the sarcoplasmic reticulum (SR), which is a network of membranes wrapped around the myofibrillar elements (figure 8–1). The uptake of calcium by the SR is driven by a Ca-ATPase pump. It is evident from the above discussion that calcium ion plays a significant role in the excitation-contraction coupling process of heart muscle. Calcium enters the myocardial cell during membrane depolarization in an electrogenic fashion, i.e., "the slow inward current." This entering calcium does not immediately affect the contractile apparatus, but is held in an "activator pool," located on the inner surface of the sarcolemmal membrane, possibly the terminal cisternae. The terminal cisternae are contiguous with the SR and lie in close approximation to the T-tubules which are periodic invaginations of the sarcolemmal membrane. It is thought that the depolarization of the sarcolemmal membrane, extending to the T-tubules, triggers the release of the activator calcium from the terminal cisternae, making it available to bind to troponin and initiate contraction. It is further speculated that the calcium taken up by the SR during relaxation is subsequently transported back to the terminal cisternae or "activator pool" of calcium. The sarcolemmal membrane contains

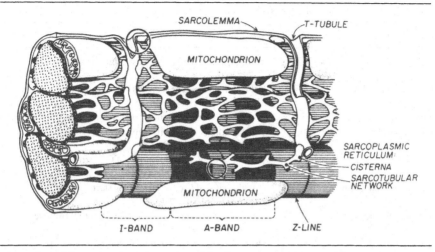

Figure 8-1. Diagrammatic representation of the ultrastructural anatomy of the myocardium. The sarcomere, composed of actin (thin) and myosin (thick) filaments, is differentiated as the contractile unit from one Z-line to the next. (Reprinted by permission from *The New England Journal of Medicine*, 293:1184, 1975.)

a Na-Ca exchange pump over which calcium can leave the heart cell during sodium influx. The sarcolemmal membrane also contains the Na, K-ATPase system which maintains ionic homeostasis between the intracellular and extracellular compartments. The adenylate cyclase enzyme complex is also located in the sarcolemmal membrane and linked to the B-receptors through which the catecholamines can act to modify cardiac function. All of these membrane systems (SR, terminal cisternae, sarcolemma and T-tubules) are involved in calcium metabolism in the myocardial cell and can be considered to be regulators of myocardial contractility. These systems which contain active pumping mechanisms (ATPases) to translocate ions, as well as the myosin ATPase involved in contraction, can generally be classified as energy-utilizing systems.

THE MITOCHONDRION

Mitochondria constitute the principal energy-producing (ATP) system of the myocardial cell. These organelles occupy 35-40% of ventricular cell volume and represent approximately 25% of the total protein of the heart muscle cell. Mitochondria produce ATP through oxidative metabolism and account for 95-98% of myocardial oxygen consumption. The preferential substrates for heart mitochondrial oxidation are fatty acids which are taken up from the blood, coupled in the cystosol with coenzyme A to form acyl CoA esters, and transported into the mitochondria where they undergo the process of β-oxidation resulting in the formation of acetyl CoA which then enters the Krebs citric acid cycle. The process of oxidative phosphorylation in mitochondria

Table 8–1. Subcellular components of myocardial cell

Component	Function
Actin	Binding sites for myosin crossbridges, contraction initiated.
Myosin Head Units	ATP splitting enzyme converting chemical energy to mechanical via cross-bridges.
Troponin C	Ca^{2+} receptor of the contractile proteins (actin).
Mitochondria	ATP synthesis via substrate oxidations; possible Ca^{2+} "sink".
Sarcoplasmic reticulum	Release of Ca^{2+} to and removal of Ca^{2+} from troponin C; storage of Ca^{2+}.
Subsarcolemmal cisternae	Possible sites of Ca^{2+} release at the start of systole (initiation of contraction).
Sarcotubular network	Possible site where Ca^{2+} is accumulated to terminate systole (relaxation).
Sarcolemma	Propagation of action potential; control of ion fluxes in and out of cell.
Transverse tubular system	Conduction of action potention to interior of cell.

produces significantly greater amounts of ATP than glycolysis. However, the obligatory requirement for molecular oxygen in the terminal step of this process makes the heart an essentially aerobic organ. The myocardial cell is capable of limited glycolytic activity (anaerobic), but cannot sustain the energy (ATP) requirements of heart for any length of time through this metabolic pathway.

In summary, ATP and calcium are essential for active contraction and relaxation of the myocardial cell. A number of other subcellular structures and enzyme systems (mitochondria, sarcoplasmic reticulum, sarcolemma, etc.) actively participate in the regulation of ATP and calcium homeostasis in the intracellular compartment. These various systems and their function are summarized in table 8–1. Comprehensive reviews are available for those who wish to pursue selected areas in greater detail [4–10]. In the past twenty years, a great deal of intensive investigation has been directed not only to elucidating the mechanisms controlling ATP and calcium metabolism in the myocardial cell, but to identifying changes in these systems that would be the primary "biochemical lesion" underlying decreased myocardial contractility or heart failure. To date, no single alteration or change in the biochemical processes associated with heart failure has been identified as a primary, causative factor. It may be that no single factor is causative, but rather multiple compensatory changes and adjustments ultimately result in functional failure.

BIOCHEMISTRY OF MYOCARDIAL HYPERTROPHY

In order to understand the biochemistry of myocardial failure, it is necessary to begin with cardiac hypertrophy, since it is very likely that the mechanisms underlying failure, at least in part, start here. Marked increases in protein synthesis occure in the heart as a result of increased aortic pressure, and the stretch of the ventricular wall appears to be the mechanical parameter most closely correlated with this response [11]. Cardiac hypertrophy due to pressure overload results in a depressed rate of isometric force development, decreased velocity of unloaded shortening, and decreased myosin ATPase activity. These changes have led to intensive studies that suggest that alterations in cardiac myosin isoenzymes are a major causative agent in depressed myocardial contractility associated with hypertrophy failure [12]. Initial studies of isolated muscle from pressure-overloaded hearts showed that with myocardial hypertrophy there was a concomitant decrease in myocardial contractility [13]. Subsequently, it was shown that, depending on the stimulus, hypertrophy can lead to a wide spectrum of physiologic and biochemical changes [14], with enhanced [15–17], normal [18, 19], or depressed performance [20–23]. The hypertrophy spectrum has been called physiologic at one end and pathologic at the other [14].

Biochemical Changes in Hypertrophy and Failure.

A considerable amount of information exists, based on experimental studies, regarding biochemical changes associated with myocardial hypertrophy and failure. A number of these studies conflict [15–23], probably because of the wide range of experimental variables involved. These include: the type of hemodynamic stress that was imposed, the point along the hypertrophy-to-failure spectrum where tissue was taken for biochemical studies, and the methods used to assay the biochemical systems. The latter variable is not as contentious a point as it used to be, now that many experimental methods are more standardized and accepted. In general, a number of biochemical changes can be related to hypertrophied-failing hearts subjected to pressure and volume overload conditions. It is now reasonably established that cardiac myosin exists in three isoenzyme forms designated V_1, V_2, and V_3. The V_1 form has the highest myosin ATPase activity and is associated with fast tension development [12]. The V_3 form has the lowest ATPase activity and appears associated with cardiac contractility that is slower in tension development. The V_2 form is intermediate between the V_1 and V_3 forms. In man and several other mammalian species, the V_3 form is the predominant cardiac myosin isoenzyme. Pressure-overload hypertrophy results in decreased myosin ATPase activity, which correlates with decreased rates of isometric tension development and crossbridge cycling rates, which increase the economy of force production [12]. The implication of these observations is that an enhanced synthesis of V_3 isoenzyme occurs in response to the hemodynamic stress of pressure overload and these changes underlie the fundamental decreases in contractility. It is well known that protein synthesis is signficantly increased in cardiac hypertrophy. Morgan et al. [11] have demonstrated that acccelerated ribosome formation is an early and important factor in the hypertrophic response. Further studies are still necessary to identify the types and steps of new ribosome formation that are increased in cardiac enlargement and the types of changes in myosin isoenzymes that determine the adaptation of the heart to various stresses.

Altered Function of the Sarcoplasmic Reticulum

Altered regulation of intracellular calcium by the sarcoplasmic reticular (SR) system as a causative agent in the onset of myocardial failure became the focus of intensive studies almost 20 years ago [4, 8, 27]. Although the initial microsomal preparations that were used were "contaminated" with various subcellular membranes, a number of studies reported depressed rates and total uptake of calcium in SR preparations obtained from hypertrophied and failing hearts [8, 27]. These observations led to the speculation that reduced calcium transport by the SR was a primary cause of decreased myocardial contractility. The central role played by calcium in the excitation-coupling process makes this an attractive hypothesis. To date, no definitive studies exist which demonstrate a direct correlation between reduced myocardial contractility and decreased SR calcium-handling as a primary mechanism in heart failure. It may very well be that decreased activity in the subcellular calcium transport systems is secondary to other changes associated with the hypertrophic process (e.g., pH, decreased high energy phosphates, cAMP dependent processes related to catecholamines) [4].

Alterations in the Sarcolemmal Membrane

Documented changes in the sarcolemmal membrane, associated with decreased myocardial contractility in hypertrophy failure, have been equivocal [4, 8, 27]. Structural changes in membrane composition, alterations in the relative densities of membrane pumps, and changes in sodium pump activities (Na^+, K^+-ATPase) have all been suggested as possible sources of depressed function during hypertrophy and failure [8, 27]. The Na^+, K^+-ATPase has attracted considerable interest because it is selectively inhibited by cardiac glycosides and is thought to be the pharmacologic receptor for glycoside action on the heart (i.e., positive inotropy). Inhibition of this sodium pump mechanism can result in increased intracellular sodium which, in turn, increases intracellular calcium and consequently enhances activation of the troponin-tropomyosin complex, causing a greater force of contraction. However, it has not been established that reduced Na^+, K^+-ATPase activity occurs in either hypertrophy or failure [4, 8, 27]. Other functional properties of the sarcolemmal membrane, such as adrenergic receptor-site activity or density, adenylate cyclase-cAMP activity and sodium-calcium exchange pumps remain the subject of intense investigation. Changes in these membrane systems associated with cardiac hypertrophy and failure have been reported, but their role in cardiac dysfunction remains unclear.

Impaired Energy Metabolism in Failure

The singular dependence of cardiac muscle on mitochondrial oxidative phosphorylation for its energy (ATP) supply has resulted in many studies aimed at demonstrating impaired energy metabolism as a primary cause of heart failure [8, 10, 12, 27]. Pressure-overload hypertrophy initially produces rapid increases in the synthesis of cardiac mitochondrial protein [12, 27, 42]. However, at the point of overt failure in experimental models, mitochondria exhibit normal efficiency in ATP production (ADP: 0 ratios) and *apparently* normal values for rates of phosphorylating respiration (state 3 respiration; a quantitative index of mitochondrial ATP-producing capacity). Similar results have been obtained in two separate studies on mitochondria obtained from failing human hearts [8]. In general, the consensus in the literature would suggest that energy production is not impaired or a primary causative factor in heart failure. Rather, "defects" or dysfunction in the energy-utilizing systems (myosin, sarcoplasmic reticulum, sarcolemma) are the potential causative factors in myocardial contractile failure.

VENTRICULLAR DYSFUNCTION IN MYOCARDIAL FAILURE

In adults, hypertrophy normally implies an increase in cell volume. The stimulus inducing the process of hypertrophy appears to be an increase in wall stress on cardiac fibers that are required to increase their workload [24]. The maximal amount of hypertrophy occurs in the basal and subendocardial regions of the heart where wall stress is maximal. This effect of increased wall tension on myocardial cells may lead to local hypoxia or hypercapnia and may be a stimulus for norepinephrine release. Administration of norepinephrine in doses that do not cause hypertension can also produce left ventricular hypertrophy [25]. Cardiac performance of normal and hypertrophied hearts, as determined by the velocity of contraction, is at least partially related to the rate of hydrolysis of ATP by myosin [26]. Preferential synthesis of one of the myosin isoenzymes can lead to enhanced [16] or decreased myosin ATPase activity [20–22]. The rate of uptake and binding of calcium by sarcoplasmic reticulum is decreased in congestive heart failure [8, 27]. The slower rate of calcium uptake by the sarcoplasmic reticulum during diastole leads to a lengthening of the relaxation period. Altered synthesis of contractile proteins with misalignment of actin with myosin and/or increased production of collagen by hyperplasia of connective tissue may also contribute to ventricular dysfunction [14]. Increased collagen leads to an increase in diastolic stiffness of the ventricle [19, 28–30]. This may also lead to an increase in internal resistance to shortening of the sarcomere [30]. Finally, the increased collagen that is laid down may prevent the myocardium from returning to normal function after the hemodynamic burden is corrected [28]. In summary, ventricular hypertrophy may be thought of in terms of a spectrum. Pressure overload that occurs abruptly does not invariably, but is likely to, lead to a depression in ventricular performance. In contrast, volume overload first causes hyperfunction and subsequently hypofunction. When ventricular hypertrophy is produced by intermittent volume overload, as in exercise conditioning, it leads to an improvement of cardiac function [17]. Therefore, the new sarcomeres enable the heart to distribute an increased workload over more contractile units in order to normalize the stress. The contractile performance of these new units depends on the pattern of protein synthesis, especially myosin isoenzymes, as well as the architecture of the cardiac pattern assumed. The major determinant of the latter are ventricular volume, wall thickness and deposition of collagen.

Segmental loss of myocardial contractile elements (ischemic injury) imposes an increased workload on the remaining myocardial cells. When the undamaged cells are unable to sustain these increased demands, clinical manifestations of congestive heart failure appear. Studies in several models of heart failure show a poor correlation between the magnitude of structural derangement, and decreased cardiac function [31, 32]. In patients with cardiac failure, Baandrup et al. [31] found no correlation between quantitative morphology, which included measurements of muscle fiber diameter and volume fraction of collagen tissue, and angiographically determined ejection fraction. Similarly Gvozdjak et al. [32] measured the hydroxyproline content as an index of the amount of fibrosis in biopsies taken from patients with nonischemic cardiomyopathy. They found that less than 2% of the total effective myocardial mass was replaced by fibrosis and concluded that myocyte replacement with fibrotic tissue was probably not the main reason for the development of left ventricular failure. They speculated that metabolic disturbances at the cellular or subcellular level may be responsible for myocardial failure [32]. A significant amount of experimental data from models of heart muscle disease, especially animal models of myocardial infarction, support the concept that ventricular function is perserved until a critical degree of myocardial damage occurs [33–35]. In general, when the damage is limited to 20% or less of the left ventricular mass, the function remains within normal range. When a greater area of left ventricle is damaged, the ability to compensate is overcome with subsequent deterioration of function [34, 35]. Using a canine model of myocardial infarction, Hood et al. [34] correlated the changes in left ventricular filling pressure with stroke index and used these measurements as an index of left ventricular function. They showed that there were no significant changes in the left ventricular end-diastolic pressure in dogs with infarcts that impaired less than 20% of the total left ventricular mass. Larger infarcts resulted in left ventricular end-diastolic pressures greater than 10 mmHg. They found infarcts that constituted greater than 36% of the left ventricular mass to be incompatible with life. When animals with myocardial infarction were given isoproterenol, the control animals demonstrated an improvement in left ventricular function while those with infarct and stable left ventricular function showed little or no improvement in left ventricular function. This implies an already maximally utilized myocardial reserve. Opherk and associates [35] assessed left ventricular end-diastolic pressure and dP/dt as indices of left ventricular function in dogs with acute myocardial ischemia and found function deterioration when ischemia compromised more than 15% of the left ventricular mass [35]. Smaller lesions did not produce significant LV dysfunction.

The nonlinear "critical damage" nature of the structure-function relationship conflicts with the predictions based on theoretical models [36]. For example, the ejection fraction should decrease in direct proportion to the loss in myocyte contractile units. In the theoretical model of left ventricular function following myocardial infarction in humans, Swan et al. [36] predicted that ejection fraction will decline as a linear function of the amount of remaining, normally functioning left ventricular myocardium. However, this has not been supported by actual experimental observation. The poor correlation between myocardial structure and function described in most clinical pathology studies [31, 32], and the nonlinear relationship observed in other models of cardiomyopathies [33–35, 37], suggest that compensatory mechanisms are capable of preserving myocardial function in the face of mild to moderate structural damage. Some of the mechanisms responsible for the nonlinear structure function relationship have been elucidated. Hood was among the first to attribute the increased contractility of the noninfarcted muscle in dogs subjected to experimental infarcts to the Frank Starling mechanism [38].

Meerbaum and co-workers demonstrated the increase in contractility of the myocardial noninfarcted segment by measuring the regional lactate metabolism, potassium loss and increased oxygen extracted from the noninfarcted areas of infarcted dog hearts [3]. Mathes and Gudbjarnason extended this observation and correlated the increased contractility with the Frank-Starling mechanism and with the depletion of myocardial norepinephrine stores, thereby invoking a role for increased plasma catecholamines as a second possible mechanism for increased contractility in normal tissue [40, 41]. Yoran et al. [33] studied the role of catecholamines in increasing the contractility of nonischemic myocardium in infarcted hearts. A series of dogs were treated with reserpine to deplete the catecholamines from the myocardium before producing an infarction. They found a linear correlation between the mass of infarcted ventricular tissue and left ventricular stroke volume when the amount of damaged tissue ranged from 20.3–39.8% of total left ventricular mass. These data suggest that catecholamines may play a role in maintaining the structure-function relationship when less than a critical amount of tissue is destroyed [33].

MYOCARDIAL FAILURE AND CATECHOLAMINES

An alteration in sympathetic neurotransmitter metabolism in hypertrophied and failing hearts was first documented by Chidsey et al. [42] and Meerson et al. [43] in 1963. These observations were subsequently confirmed in several animal models of heart failure [44–47]. The marked loss of norepinephrine cannot be accounted for by the process of hypertrophy alone, as the decrease is seen in both ventricles regardless of which ventricle is subjected to hemo-dynamic stress. Similar depletion of myocardial catecholamines are also seen in other models of cardiac failure. In experimentally induced myocardial infarction and failure, there is release of catecholamines from the ischemic myocardial tissue. Activation of nervous reflexes arising from the sites of infarct triggers the release of epinephrine and norepinephrine from the adrenal medulla [48]. In addition, there may be an enhancement of norepinephrine release from postganglionic sympathetic nerve endings in the heart [48]. In the Syrian hamster model of cardiomyopathy, there is an increased turnover of myocardial catecholamine stores, resulting in eventual depletion of these compounds [49]. These observations suggest that the initial source of increased catecholamine concentrations at the myocardial receptor site are the adrenergic nerve terminals of the heart. As heart failure worsens, this source is depleted. This depletion of norepinephrine stores in the heart probably has physiological relevance. Stimulation of cardiac sympathetic nerves during congestive heart failure in dogs is not reflected by an appropriate increase in heart rate or myocardial contractility [50]. In patients with heart failure [51], there is a paradoxical change in heart rate response to exercise, upright tilt or hypo-tension, not altered by the administration of atropine [52]. This impairment of intrinsic sympathetic support of the heart is probably compensated for by an increase in plasma norepinephrine levels [53]. Chidsey et al. described an increase in urinary excretion of norepinephrine in patients with congestive heart failure reflecting an increase in sympathetic activity [54]. In a recent study, Cohn et al. correlated the functional status and prognosis of patients with congestive heart failure with the degree of increased plasma norepine-phrine concentrations [55]. Several other studies have also reported a positive relationship between the presence of congestive heart failure and an increase in plasma catecholamines [48, 53, 56]. A decrease in cardiac output reflexively stimulates the sympathetic nervous system with increased inotropic stimula-tion and vasoconstriction at the periphery with increased peripheral resistance. Eventually, the increased sympathetic activity fails to compensate for de-creases in ejection fraction. In addition, the increased peripheral resistance against which the myocardium has to pump also impairs the ability of the heart to empty. This leads to further decreases in cardiac output. Therefore, the elevated concentrations of plasma catecholamines may, in part, contribute to the deterioration in cardiac function that occurs after a critical mass of myocardium is damaged.

With cardiac failure, the catecholamine induced augmentation of cardiac performance cannot be maintained for long, due to down-regulation of receptor sensitivity. Thomas and Marks speculated that myocardial beta-adrenergic receptors become desensitized to elevated plasma concentrations of catecholamines [53]. Colucci, et al. [57] measured the beta-receptor density on lymphocytes and found that it decreased in patients given the orally effective catecholamine Pirbuterol which correlated with the development of tolerance to this agent. These authors also described a significant decrease in the number of beta-receptors on lymphocytes in patients with heart failure when compared with normal controls. Bristow, et al. [58] have confirmed the down-regulation of beta-receptors in failing human hearts and have documented that the receptor loss leads to decreased adenylate cyclase responsiveness and decreased catecholamine stimulation of mechanical function.

Studies in animal models reveal a similar subsensitivity phenomenon in catecholamine-induced hypertrophy and in nonischemic areas of infarcted hearts [59]. Thus, although the adrenergic nervous system is capable of providing compensatory support to the failing myocardium, this mechanism is at least partially self-limited by depletion of myocardial catecholamine stores and by the decrease in sensitivity of beta-adrenergic-receptors. Many studies point to the persistent stimulation of the heart by catecholamines as a potential cytotoxic mechanism [60]. This suggests that the eventual effect of this compensatory process may cause further cardiac dysfunction or damage.

THE TRANSITION FROM MYOCARDIAL COMPENSATION TO FAILURE

Despite our understanding of the hemodynamic and biochemical changes that are involved during the end stage of congestive heart failure, we do not understand the pathogenesis of the mechanisms that lead to the development of ventricular failure. It is well established that many forms of heart failure are due to the deterioration in ventricular function in response to a hemodynamic load rather than to an increase in the severity of that burden. Ventricular myocardium is capable of functioning normally while sustaining an excessive load for many months or years. However, at some point ventricular function becomes impaired and the chronically stressed ventricle begins to fail. Although there are many studies of the biochemical, physiological and pathological changes that occur in the myocardium shortly after the imposition of stress and in the very late stages of congestive heart failure, far less is known about the conversion of normal ventricular function to early ventricular dysfunction. There are many reasons why identification of the mechanisms of pathogenesis and conversion from normal function to the decompensated early stage are difficult to investigate and appreciate clinically. First, patients generally present only late in the course of the disease with symptoms of congestive heart failure, atypical chest pain; the ability to identify patients in the early stages of the disease is limited. However, with widespread use of noninvasive techniques and the increased clinical acceptance of endomyocardial biopsies, it is likely that, in the future, diagnoses, may be made more often at the onset of the process. Second, the histopathology of the dilated, failing heart is essentially similar, even when the initial etiology may be different [61, 62]. The heart has limited responses to injury and the focal scarring and myocellular hypertrophy that are characteristic of late stage cardiomyopathy give only a few clues to the process or processes that may lead to these changes. Finally, the number of animal models that permit sequential investigation of pathogenesis has been limited [5] and often there has been controversy over the relevance of these models to the human counterpart. Therefore, due to the lack of well-defined knowledge of pathogenesis, clinical emphasis has been placed on the symptoms of cardiomyopathy and their treatment, rather than on the prevention of the onset of cardiac failure.

Congestive cardiac failure, secondary to myocardial failure, is generally not clinically apparent in the early compensated stages nor is it associated with segmental loss of a large mass of myocardium. This indicates that there may be an extended period of time between the onset of myocardial injury and the development of clinically apparent ventricular dysfunction and congestive heart failure. Sequential endomyocardial biopsies provide a possible means to follow the progression from initial injury to a clinically overt cardiac failure. Patients with an acute myocarditis diagnosed by biopsy of the myocardium develop congestive heart failure over a variable period of time [63–66]. This progression of myocardial failure is also variable from patient to patient. This variability is probably due to the different putative etiologic agents that damage the myocardium and the point along the natural history curve when the patient is identified. Early mortality is probably due to a greater degree of myocardial damage in which the heart shows greater cardiac enlargement, low ejection faction, and higher end-diastolic pressures [67]. Although these features may be suggestive of severe myocardial damage, this may also be a reflection of late identification of the patient at the lower end of a prolonged survival curve. Prognosis in cardiac failure probably depends on three partially related factors:

1. the myocardial reserve
2. the rate of myocardial cell damage or loss
3. compensatory hypertrophy

Massive necrosis of myocardial cells, which may occur with myocarditis or extensive loss of heart muscle due to a large transmural myocardial infarction, may rapidly exhaust myocardial reserve and not leave a sufficient time interval for compensatory hypertrophy to develop, leading to early death from ventricular failure. Conversely, a less severe form of injury, or a small segmental infarction, may allow the remaining myocytes enough time to hypertrophy and increase the number of contractile elements available for ventricular function and to compensate for the loss of cells.

The evidence of hypertrophy following myocardial damage, as assessed by an increase in wall thickness, has recently been claimed to have a favorable effect on prognosis in congestive cardiac failure [68]. However, wall thickness may not correlate with the degree of myocellular hypertrophy depending on the extent of cell loss. Clinical manifestations in cardiac failure may either be related to the loss of myocardial reserve due to progressive myocardial damage or may be secondary to inadequate compensatory hypertrophy. It is not known whether the compensatory hypertrophy occurring in response to myocardial injury in itself contributes significantly to ventricular dysfunction. Meerson [69] has suggested that cardiac hypertrophy caused by a number of different factors represents a stable, compensatory, and adequate response to cellular deficiency of high energy phosphates. Similarly, the ventricular hypertrophy in the spontaneoulsy hypertensive rat is believed to be an adaptive response [70]. There is very little evidence to suggest that this form of compensatory hypertrophy, in the absence of other myocardial stress or injury, can lead to ventricular dysfunction and eventual myocardial failure.

MYOCARDIAL FAILURE: A HOMOGENEOUS OR HETEROGENOUS PROCESS?

It is generally believed that congestive heart failure results from a diffuse process that affects the myocardial cells equally throughout the ventricle. This presumed homogeneity of the process provides the reason for performing biochemical analysis on the whole ventricles or on significant number of unselected myocardial cells. If the changes are diffuse, any observed biochemical changes should reflect what is occurring at the level of the individual cell. Yet it appears that few consistent biochemical changes have been identified. Alterations in mitochondrial oxidative phosphorylation, sarcoplasmic calcium flux, myosin ATPase, sarcolemmal phospholipid composition, myosin subtypes, and lysosomal enzyme activity have been described by some investigators and disputed by others [71]. The contradictions that exist may reflect not only the different models employed at variable stages of disease, but also the possibility that the congestive heart failure process is heterogeneous. Similar problems exist with ultrastructural studies of myocardium in congestive heart failure in which mitochondrial, sarcoplasmic reticulum, and lysosomal abnormalities have been identified, but these generally nonspecific changes may have questionable relevance to the pathogenesis of congestive heart failure.

It is generally accepted that at least some forms of human and experimental congestive cardiomyopathies have heterogeneous and focal histopathologic changes [72]. An unusual feature of focal pathology in congestive cardiomyopathy is the frequency with which contraction-band or myocytolytic necrosis is observed as the main form of myocellular damage [72]. It is important to note that contraction-band necrosis is the characteristic histopathology seen in myocardium with administration of high doses of exogenous norepinephrine or with pheochromocytomas [73]. Although the mechanism of the catecholamine-induced changes is not clear, it is thought to lead to increased calcium flux across the sarcolemma, thereby causing hypercontraction of individual myocytes [74]. Why this may occur in small discrete zones may be explained by the findings of Factor et al. [75]. They demonstrated microvascular spasm in left ventricular microcirculation in 150-day-old Syrian hamsters, prior to the development of cardiac failure. There intermittent episodes of recurrent ischemia may induce myocardial necrosis, as shown by Geft et al. [76]. However, it is believed that cardiac microcirculation is organized into a system of anastomosing vessels at the microcirculatory level. This makes it difficult to understand how transient obstruction of these vessels could lead to necrosis of the tissue supplied by the vessel. Recently, it was shown that in dogs [77] as well as in humans [78], the microvasculature is organized into a pattern of end-capillary loops without intercapillary connections. This may provide the necessary anatomy for the development of small foci of cardiac necrosis if the supplying vessel is occluded. Eng et al. [79] have shown that embolization of the coronary microcirculation of dogs with 25 or 50 μm microspheres leads to focal contraction-band necrosis similar to that seen in cardiomyopathies. When the animals were pretreated with phentolamine prior to embolization, there was no evidence of necrosis, despite the presence of the beads [79]. These data suggest that microvascular spasm rather than anatomic obstruction by microspheres was the cause of contraction band necrosis. This vasospasm appears to be induced by a β-adrenergic mechanism. This may be the link by which increased sympathetic nervous activity may either precipitate or aggravate pre-existing myocardial dysfunction and failure.

THE SEQUENCE OF MYOCARDIAL RESPONSE TO STRESS

Figure 8–2 summarizes the events following the onset of hemodynamic stress on the heart. Pressure overload can result from a primary effect of hypertension or from peripheral hormonal effects, which could give rise to increased catecholamines (? norepinephrine), which in turn would exert an increased workload on the heart. The increased vascular tone, associated with hypertension, could also produce microvascular spasm, resulting in diffuse focal necrosis in the myocardium. The other major stress addressed in this chapter involves the onset of volume overload following ischemic injury due to coronary artery disease (CAD, segmental cell loss). These stresses produce the hypertrophic response indicated in the center of figure 8–2. It is very likely that early adaptive biochemical changes begin to occur with the onset of hemodynamic stress leading to hypertrophy. Although not depicted on the arrow leading from hemodynamic stress to overt hypertrophy, these changes may be those referred to as physiologic by some investigators. It is also possible that physiological or biochemical changes due to some types of hemodynamic stress (e.g., exercise training) do not follow this same axis of change and constitute a separate, nonpathologic response to hemodynamic stress [80]. Diffuse focal necrosis could occur as a primary etiologic agent associated with hypertension. In this case, the net loss of myocytes may produce the same effect as that seen following ischemic injury due to coronary

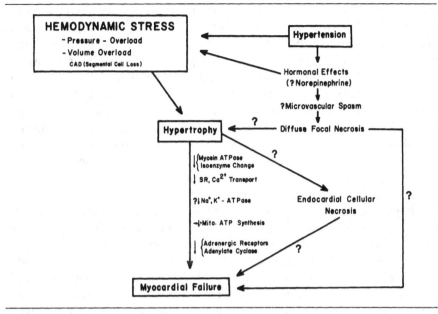

Figure 8–2. Schematic representation of the factors leading from hemodynamic stress to myocardial failure. See text for details.

artery disease. The pressure-overload hypertrophy resulting from the hypertension would be exacerbated by loss of myocardium, imposing an additional volume-overload burden on the heart. Finally, it has been suggested that during hypertrophy, the increasing wall thickness results in increasing transmural pressures (elevated LVEP) that cause underperfusion of the endocardium with resultant ischemia and cellular necrosis. This would occur in the latter stages of the hypertrophic response as a secondary process. Nevertheless, this implies that ischemic injury becomes a contributory factor in producing myocardial failure in severe hypertrophy.

As depicted in figure 8–2, the biochemical changes leading from hypertrophy to myocardial failure can be characterized in terms of decreased contractile protein activity, depressed calcium transport kinetics, possible decreases in sodium, potassium ion transport, which in turn affects cellular calcium and ionic homeostasis, altered energy metabolism, and decreased adrenergic receptor and adenylate cyclase activity, which impacts the responsiveness of the heart to inotropic and chronotropic control. The apparent "normal" levels of high energy phosphates and mitochondrial function in overt myocardial failure do not necessarily obviate a compromised energy supply as a causative mechanism in myocardial failure. Sordahl [27, 81] has pointed out that if marked increases in mitochondrial ATP production are observed during compensatory hypertrophy, then control or "normal" values, seen in overt failure stages, suggest that energy-producing capacity has failed to keep pace with energy utilization. Recently, Ingwall et al. [82] reported decreased MM creatine kinase activity (CPK) and total creatine content in hypertrophied human ventricular myocardium. Similar results were also obtained in ischemic myocardium, leading these investigators [82] to speculate that pressure-overload hypertrophy and ischemia bring about alterations in the myocardial CPK system through a common stimulus. Increased MB CPK was also observed in these studies [82]. These data offer an additional interpretation regarding energy supply in the hypertrophic myocardium, namely a compartmentalization of the relative supply of ATP to various energy utilizing systems. Thus, "normal" levels of whole tissue, high energy phosphates may not accurately reflect the availability of energy to select cellular systems in the hypertrophied or failing myocardium.

A number of years ago, Katz [83] suggested that biochemical "defects" or decreases associated with hypertrophy failure may reflect a compensatory process to reduce the work of the chronically overloaded heart. The many studies that have been reported since Katz's original suggestion [83] add validity to this concept. Decreased myosin-ATP utilization, with enhanced synthesis of the slower contracting (more economical ?) isoenzyme (V_3), is an early response to hemodynamic stress. It would follow that a "tuning-down" or decreases in the calcium transport systems, energy producing, and utilizing systems, and the chronotropic and inotropic regulatory systems, should occur. It is conceivable that once these changes are set into motion, the down regulation of multiple biochemical processes supporting myocardial contractility are summated such that the heart becomes unable to respond to a hemodynamic load and overt myocardial failure ensues. If multiple biochemical systems are impaired, modification of one of them may not be helpful and may, in fact, aggravate the overall biochemical derangement. This suggests that effective clinical intervention to prevent or ameliorate the loss of myocardial function should be instituted before these multiple changes have placed the heart in an irreversible state. This means that we need to identify patients during the early stages of development of myocardial failure, if we are to treat them effectively.

REFERENCES

1. Bing, R.J., Bottcher, D., and Cowan, C. 1968. What is cardiac failure? *Amer. J. Cardiol.* 22: 2–6.
2. McCall, D., and O'Rourke, R.A. 1985. Congestive heart failure. *Mod. Concept Cardiovasc. Dis.* 54:55–59.
3. Smith, W.Mc.F. 1985. Epidemiology of congestive heart failure. *Amer. J. Cardiol.* 55:3A–8A.
4. Katz, A.M. 1975. Congestive heart failure role of altered myocardial cellular control. *N. Eng. J. Med.* 293:1184–1191.
5. Smith, H.J., and Nuttall, A. 1985. Experimental models of heart failure. *Cardiovasc. Res.* 19:181–186.
6. Neely, J.R., and Morgan, H.E. 1974. Relationship between carbohydrate and lipid metabolism and the energy balance of heart muscle. *Ann. Rev. Physiol.* 36:413–459.
7. Dhalla, N.S., Ziegelhoffer, A., and Harrow, J.A.C. 1977. Regulatory role of membrane

systems in heart function. *Can. J. Physiol. Pharmacol.* 55:1211–1234.
8. Dhalla, N.S., Das, P.K., and Sharma, G.P. 1978. Subcellular basis of cardiac contractile failure. *J. Mole. Cell. Cardiol.* 10:363–385.
9. Williamson, J.R. 1979. Mitochondrial function in the heart. *Ann. Rev. Physiol.* 41:485–506.
10. Crass, M.F., and Sordahl, L.A. eds. 1979. *Metabolic and morphologic correlates in cardiovascular function.* Texas Reports on Biol. Med. 39.
11. Morgan, H.E., Gordon, E.E., Kira, Y., Siehl, L., Watson, P.A., and Chua, B.A.L. 1985. Biochemical correlates of myocardial hypertrophy. *Physiologist* 28:18–27.
12. Alpert, N.R., ed. 1983. *Myocardial hypertrophy and failure, Perspectives in cardiovascular research* 7. New York: Raven Press.
13. Braunwald, E., Ross, J., Jr., and Sonnenblick, E.H., eds. 1967. *Mechanisms of contraction of the normal and failing heart.* Boston: Little, Brown.
14. Wikman-Coffelt, J., Parmley, W.W., Mason, D.T. 1979. The cardiac hypertrophy process. Analyses of factors determining pathological vs. physiological development. *Circ. Res.* 34:697–707.
15. LeWinter, M.M., Engler, R.L., and Karliner, J.S. 1980. Enhanced left ventricular shortening during chronic volume overload in conscious dogs. *Am. J. Physiol.* 238:H126–133.
16. Morkin, E. 1979. Stimulation of cardiac myosin adenosine triphosphatase in thyrotoxicosis. *Circ. Res.* 44:1–7.
17. Scheuer, J., and Bhan, A.K. 1979. Cardiac contractile proteins, adenosine triphosphate activity and physiological function. *Circ. Res.* 45:1–12.
18. Sasayama, S., Ross, J. Jr., Franklin, D., Bloor, C.M., Bishop, S., and Dilley, R.B. 1976. Adaptations of the left ventricle to chronic pressure overload. *Circ. Res.* 38:172–178.
19. Williams, J.F., and Potter, R.D. 1974. Normal contractile state of hypertrophied myocardium after pulmonary artery constriction in the cat. *J. Clin. Invest.* 54:1266–1272.
20. Grossman, W., Braunwald, E., Mann, T., McLaurin, L.P., and Green, L.H. 1977. Contractile state of the left ventricle in man as evaluated from end-systolic pressure-volume relations. *Circulation* 56:845–852.
21. Lompre, A.M., Schwartz, K., d'Albis, A., Lacombe, G., Van Thiem, N., and Swynghedauw, B. 1979. Myosin isoenzyme redistribution in chronic heart overload. *Nature* 282: 105–107.
22. Maughan, D., Low, E., Litten, R. III., Brayden, J., and Alpert, N. 1979. Calcium-activated muscle from hypertrophied rabbit hearts. *Circ. Res.* 44:279–287.
23. Newman, W.H., and Webb, J.G. 1980. Adaptation of left ventricle to chronic pressure overload: response to inotropic drugs. *Am. J. Physiol.* 238:4134–4143.
24. Vandenburgh, H., and Kaufman, S. 1979. In vitro model for stretch-induced hypertrophy of skeletal muscle. *Science* 203:265–268.
25. Laks, M.M. 1977. Norepinephrine, the producer of myocardial cellular hypertrophy and/or necrosis and/or fibrosis. *Am. Heart J.* 94:394–399.
26. Delcayre, C., and Swynghedauw, B. 1975. A comparative study of heart myosin ATPase and light subunits from different species. *Pfluegers Arch.* 355:39–47.
27. Schwartz, A., Sordahl, L.A., Entman, M.L., Allen, J.C., Reddy, Y.S., Goldstein, M.A., Luchi, R.J., and Wynborny, L.E. 1973. Abnormal biochemistry in myocardial failure. *Am. J. Cardiol.* 32:407–422.
28. Pinsky, W.W., Lewis, R.M., Hartley, C.J., and Entman, M.L. 1979. Permanent changes of ventricular contractility and compliance in chronic volume overload. *Am. J. Physiol.* 237:H575–583.
29. Grossman, W., McLauren, L.P., and Stefadouros, M.A. 1974. Left ventricular stiffness associated with chronic pressure end volume overloads in man. *Circ. Res.* 35:793–800.
30. Natarajan, G., Bove, A.A., Coulson, R.L., Carey, R.A., and Spann, J.F. 1979. Analysis of oxygen diffusion from anteriolar networks. *Am. J. Physiol.* 237:H676–680.
31. Baandrup, V., Florio, R.A., Rehan, M., Richardson, P.J., and Olsen, E.G. 1981. Critical analysis of endomyocardial biopsies from patient suspected of having cardiomyopathy II: Comparison in histology and clinical haemodynamic information. *Br. Heart J.* 45:487–493.
32. Gvozdjak, J., Bada, V., and Niederland, T.R.. 1969. The role of myocardial fibrosis in the development of cardiac insufficiency in cardiomyopathies. *Cor Vasa* 11:229–234.
33. Yoran. C., Sonnenblick, E.H., and Kirk, E.S. 1982. Contractile reserve and left ventricular function in regional myocardial ischemia in the dog. *Circulation* 66:121–128.

34. Hood, W.B., McCarthy, B., and Lown, B. 1967. Myocardial infarction following coronary ligation in dogs. *Circ. Res.* 21:191–199.

35. Opherk, D., Finke, R., Mittmann, U., Muller, J.H., Wirth, R.H., and Schmier, J. 1977. The influence of the size of acute ischaemic myocardial lesions on coronary reserve and left ventricular function in the dog. *Basic Res. Cardiol.* 72:402–410.

36. Swan, H.J., Forrester, J.S., Diamond, G., Chatterjee, K., and Parmley, W.W. 1972. Hemodynamic spectrum of myocardial infarction and cardiogenic shock. *Circulation* 45: 1097–1110.

37. Bristow, M.R., Mason, J.W., Billingham, M.E., and Daniels, J.R. 1981. Dose effect and structure-function relationships in doxorubicin cardiomyopathy. *Am. Heart J.* 102:709–718.

38. Hood, W.B., Jr. 1970. Experimental myocardial infarction 3. Recovery of left ventricular function in the healing phase. Contribution of increased fiber shortening in noninfarcted myocardium. *Am. Heart J.* 79:531–538.

39. Meerbaum, S., Lang, T.W., Corday, E., Rubins, S., Hirose, S., Costanini, C., Gold, H., and Dalmastro, M. 1974. Progressive alterations of cardiac hemodynamic and regional metabolic function after acute coronary occlusion. *Am. J. Cardiol.* 33:60–68.

40. Mathes, P., Romig, D., Sack, D., and Erhardt, W. 1976. Experimental myocardial infarction in the cat. I. Reversible decline in contractility of noninfarcted muscle. *Circ. Res.* 38:540–546.

41. Mathes, P., and Guabjarnason, S. 1971. Changes in norepinephrine stores in the canine heart following experimental myocardial infarction. *Am. Heart J.* 81:221–229.

42. Chidsey, C.A., Braunwald, E., Morrow, A.G., and Mason, D.T. 1963. Myocardial norepinephrine concentration in man. Effects of reserpine and of congestive heart failure. *New Engl. J. Med.* 269:653–658.

43. Meerson, F.Z., Manukhin, B.N., Pshenichnikova, M.G., and Rozanova, L.S. 1963. On mediator metabolism of the myocardium in compensatory hyperfunction and hypertrophy of the heart. *Patologischeskaya Fiziologiya i eksperimentalnaya terapia* 7:32–36.

44. Chidsey, C.A., Kaiser, G.A., Sonnenblick, E.H., Spann, J.F., and Braunwald, E. 1964. Cardiac norepinephrine stores in experimental heart failure in the dog. *J. Clin. Invest.* 43: 2386–2393.

45. Spaan, J.F., Chidsey, C.A., Pool, P.E., and Braunwald, E. 1965. Mechanism of norepinephrine depletion in experimental heart failure produced by aortic constriction in the guinea pig. *Circ. Res.* 17:312–321.

46. Fischer, J.E., Horst, W.D., and Kopin, I.J. 1965. Norepinephrine metabolism in hypertrophied rat hearts. *Nature* (Lond) 207:951–953.

47. Spann Jr., J.F., Buccino, R.A., Sonnenblick, E.H., and Braunwald, E. 1967. Contractive state of cardiac muscle obtained from cats with experimentally produced ventricular hypertrophy and heart failure. *Circ. Res.* 21:341–354.

48. Staszewska-Barczak, J. 1971. The reflex stimulation of catecholamine secretion during the acute stage of myocardial infarction in the dog. *Brit. Heart J.* 41:419–439.

49. Lund, D.D., Schmid, P.G., Bhatnagar, R.K., and Roskoski Jr., R. 1982. Changes in parasympathetic neurochemical indices in hearts of myopathic hamsters. *J. Auton. Nerv. Sys.* 5:237–246.

51. Covell, J.W., Chidsey, C.A., and Braunwald, E. 1966. Reduction of the cardiac response to postganglionic sympathetic nerve stimulation in experimental heart failure. *Circ. Res.* 19:51–56

51. Goldstein, R.E., Beiser, G.D., Stampfer, M., and Epstein, S.E. 1975. Impairment of autonomically mediated heart rate control in patients with cardiac dysfunction. *Circ. Res.* 36:561–578.

52. Higgins, C.B., Vatner, S.F., Eckberg, D.L., and Braunwald, E. 1972. Alterations in the baroreceptor reflex in conscious dogs with heart failure. *J. Clin. Invest.* 51:715–724.

53. Thomas, J.A., and Marks, B.H. 1978. Plasma norepinephrine in congestive heart failure. *Am. J. Cardiol.* 41:233–243.

54. Chidsey, C.A., Braunwald, E., Morrow, A.G. 1965. Catecholamine excretion and cardiac stores of norepinephrine in congestive heart failure. *Am. J. Med.* 39:442–451.

55. Cohn, J.N., Levine, T.B., Olivari, M.T., Garberg, V., Lura, D., Francis, G.S., Simon, A.B., and Rector, T. 1984. Plasma norepinephrine as a guide to prognosis in patients with chronic congestive heart failure. *New Eng. J. Med.* 311:819–823.

56. Vogel, J.H., and Chidsey, C.A. 1969. Cardiac adrenergic activity in experimental heart failure

assessed with both receptor blockade. *Am. J. Cardiol.* 24:198–208.
57. Colucci, W.S., Alexander, R.W., Williams, G.H., Rude, R.E., Holman, B.L., Konstam, M.A., Wynne, J., Mudge, G.H., and Braunwald, E. 1981. Decreased lymphocyte beta-adrenergic-receptor density in patients with heart failure and tolerance to beta-adrenergic agonist pirbutol. *New Engl. J. Med.* 305:185–190.
58. Bristow, M.R., Ginsburg, R., Minobe, W., Cubicciotti, R.S., Sagemen, W.S., Lurie, K., Billingham, M.E., Harrison, D.C., and Stinson, E.B. 1982. Decreased catecholamine sensitivity and beta-adrenergic receptor density in failing human hearts. *New Engl. J. Med.* 307:205–211.
59. Baumann, G., Riess, G., Erhardt, W.D., Felix, S.B., Ludwig, L., Blumel, G., and Blomer, H. 1981. Impaired beta-adrenergic stimulation in the uninvolved ventricle post-acute myocardial infarction: reversible defect due to excessive circulating catecholamine-induced decline in number and affinity of beta-receptors. *Am. Heart J.* 101:569–581.
60. Rona, G., Chappel, C.I., and Bazaza, T. 1959. *Archives of Pathology* 45:99.
61. Roberts, W.C., and Ferrans, V.J. 1979. Pathologic anatomy of the cardiomyopathies: Idiopathic dilated and hypertropic types, infiltrative types and endomyocardial disease with and without eosinophilia. *Hum. Pathol.* 6:287–342.
62. Olsen Jr., E.G. 1979. The pathology of cardiomyopathies: A critical analysis. *Amer. Heart.* 98:385–392.
63. Johnson, R.A., and Palacios, I. 1982. Dilated cardiomyopathies of the adult. *New Engl. J. Med.* 307:1051–1058; 1119–1126.
64. Kawai, C. 1971. Idiopathic cardiomyopathy: A study on the infectious-immune theory as a cause of the disease. *Jap. Circ. J.* 35:765–770.
65. Waterson, A.P. 1978. Virological investigations in congestive cardiomyopathy. *Postgrad. Med. J.* 54:505–507.
66. O'Connel, J.B. 1983. Evidence linking viral myocarditis to dilated cardiomyopathy in humans. In *Myocarditis: Precursor of cardiomyopathy*, Robinson, J.A., and O'Connel, J.B., eds., pp. 93–108. Lexington, MA:Collamore Press.
67. Fuster, V., Gersh, B.J., Giuliani, E.R., Tajik, A.J., Brandenburg, R.O., and Frye, R.L. 1981. The natural history of idiopathic dilated cardiomyopathy. *Am. J. Cardiol.* 47:525–531.
68. Benjamin, I.J., Schuster, E.H., and Bulkley, B.H. 1981. Cardiac hypertrophy in idiopathic dilated congestive cardiomyopathy. A cliniciopathologic study. *Circulation* 64:442–447.
69. Meerson, F.Z. 1974. Development of modern components of the mechanism of cardiac hypertrophy. *Circ. Res.* 35:58–63.
70. Pfeffer, M.A., and Pfeffer, J.M. 1983. Cardiac hypertrophy in the spontaneously hypertensive rat: adaptation or primary myopathy? In *Perspectives in cardiovascular research*, vol. 8, Tarazi, R.C., and Dunbar, J.B., eds., pp. 193–200. New York: Raven Press.
71. Entman, M.L., Van Winkle, W.B., Tate, C.A., and McMillan-Wood, J.B. 1982. Pitfalls in biochemical studies of hypertrophied and failing myocardium. In *Congestive heart failure: current research and clinical applications*, Braunwald, E., Mock, M.B., and Watson, J., eds. pp. 51–64. Orlando, FL: Grune and Stratton.
72. Factor, S.M., and Sonnenblick, E.H. 1985. The pathogenesis of clinical and experimental congestive cardiomyopathies: recent concepts. *Progress in Cardiovascular Diseases* 27:395–420.
73. Reichenback, D.D., and Benditt, E.P. 1970. Catecholamines and cardiomyopathy: the pathogenesis and potential importance of myofibrillar degeneration. *Hum. Pathol.* 1:125–150.
74. Bloom, S., and Cancilla, P.A. 1969. Myocytolysis and mitochondrial calcification in rat myocardium after low doses of isoproterenol. *Am. J. Pathol.* 54:373–391.
75. Factor, S.M., Minase, T., Cho, S., Dominitz, R., and Sonnenblick, E.H. 1982. Microvascular spasm in the cardiomyopathic Syrian hamster: a preventable cause of focal myocardial necrosis. *Circulation* 66:342–354.
76. Geft, I.L., Fishbein, M.C., Ninomiy, K., Hashida, J., Chaux, E., Yano, J., Y-Rit, J., Genov, T., Shell, W., and Ganz, W. 1982. Intermittent brief periods of ischemia have a cumulative effect and may cause myocardial necrosis. *Circulation* 66:1150–1153.
77. Okum, E.M., Factor, S.M., and Kirk, E.S. 1979. Endcapillary loops in the heart. An explanation for discrete myocardial infarction without border zones. *Science* 206:565–567.
78. Factor, S.M., Okum, E.M., Minase, T., and Kirk, E.S. 1982. The microcirculation of the human heart. End-capillary loops with discrete perfusion fields. *Circulation* 66:1241–1248.
79. Eng, C., Cho, S., Factor, S.M., Sonnenblick, E.H., and Kirk, E.S. 1984. Myocardial

micronecrosis produced by microsphere embolisation: Role of an alpha-adrenergic tonic influence on the coronary microcirculation. *Circ. Res.* 54:74–82.
80. Stone, H.L., and Sordahl. L.A. 1984. Exercise and pressure-overload-induced hypertrophy in dog. In *Functional aspects of the normal, hypertrophied and failing heart*, Abel, F.L., and Newman, W.H. eds., pp. 239–252. Boston: Martinus Nijhoff/Kluwer Academic.
81. Sordahl, L.A. 1983. Mitochondrial changes in pressure-overload hypertrophy and failure. In *Perspectives in cardiovascular research*, Alpert, N.R., ed. pp. 535–540. New York: Raven Press.
82. Ingwall, J.S., Kramer, M.F., Fifer, M.A., Lorell, B.H., Shemin, R., Grossman, W., and Allen, P.D. 1985. The creatine kinase system in normal and diseased human myocardium. *N. Engl. J. Med.* 313:1050-1054.
83. Katz, A.M. 1973. Biochemical "defect" in the hypertrophied and failing heart. *Circulation* 47:1076–1079.

9. FORCE-INTERVAL RELATIONSHIP AND ACTIVATOR CALCIUM AVAILABILITY: SIMILARITIES OF SYMPATHETIC STIMULATION AND HYPERTROPHY AND HEART FAILURE

PAGE A.W. ANDERSON

The properties of the sarcoplasmic reticulum (SR) and sarcolemma, which are important in the control of cytosolic calcium [1–9], are among the many aspects of the myocardium that are affected by hypertrophy and heart failure. In this chapter, the effects of disease on the modulation of activator calcium are examined by means of the "force-interval relationship," which expresses the dependence of the force of contraction on the temporal pattern of stimulation [10].

PHYSIOLOGY OF THE FORCE-INTERVAL RELATION AND CALCIUM CONTROL

The effects of hypertrophy and heart failure on membrane function are manifest in the force-interval relationship. These effects will be described and will be compared to the effects of α- and β-stimulation on the normal myocardium. The remarkable qualitative similarity of some of the effects of α-stimulation and of hypertrophy, and of β-stimulation and heart failure, on the modulation of activator calcium suggest causal relationships.

The similarity of the effects of α-stimulation and of hypertrophy on the force-interval relationship is especially interesting in view of findings that

This work was supported in part by National Heart, Lung, and Blood Institute Grants HL-20749, HL-33680, HL-12486; and by a Grant-in-Aid from the American Heart Association, with funds contributed in part by the North Carolina Heart Association Affiliate.

169

α-stimulation induces hypertrophy [11–13]. The similarity of the effects of β-stimulation to some of the effects of heart failure may indicate the presence of chronic β-stimulation during heart failure [14]. The presence of such chronic stimulation has raised questions as to its possible deleterious effect on the heart, as compared to its usefulness in maintaining the output of the failing heart [14–18].

Contraction and relaxation of the heart require the integration of the functions of the membrane systems and of the contractile apparatus of the cardiac myocyte. Although many aspects of this process have been explored, a coherent and accepted model, which explains and integrates all the various experimental results, has not yet been advanced. The increase in cytosolic calcium concentration following activation occurs through transsarcolemmal inward movement of calcium and the release of calcium from the sarcoplasmic reticulum [1–9]. The modulation of this release of calcium controls contractility. The mechanisms of control of these systems, and their messengers, are still being investigated. How activation depends on the history of the myocardium and the previous and ongoing neurohumoral and hormonal signals needs to be established.

Our focus will be on the modulation of activator calcium and its effects on the ability of the myocardium to contract as a function of time: the *force-interval relationship* [10]. The discussion will not explain nor attempt to integrate all the findings and hypotheses which relate to the control of activator calcium [10, 19–28]. Indeed, I do not deal impartially with all hypothetical mechanisms that have been put forward to explain membrane-controlled alterations in cytosolic calcium, instead I select only a few, in an attempt to provide a possible explanation of how the membrane systems of the sarcolemma and sarcoplasmic reticulum control calcium, thereby altering contractility in the normal and diseased myocardium. What I have to say rests on observations that hypertrophy and heart failure induce alterations in the force-interval relationship, demonstrating that these disease processes alter the function of these cell systems and their richly complex interaction.

Reasons for Use of the Force-Interval Relationship

The relationship between the strength of contraction and the pattern of stimulation has been given many names [10]—the "force-interval relationship," the "interval-strength relationship," the "force-frequency relationship." The relationship has long been considered to be a manifestation of the process of excitation-contraction coupling and the modulation of activator calcium.

The sarcoplasmic reticulum and the sarcolemma are considered to be major components of the system that modulates activator calcium. The function of the sarcoplasmic reticulum control of activator calcium will be discussed at length in view of the effects of ryanodine, an inhibitor of calcium release from cardiac sarcoplasmic reticulum [29, 30], on activator calcium and on the force-interval relationship [31], and, in view of the effects of calcium, caffeine, and inositol on calcium release from the sarcoplasmic reticulum [3, 32–34].

Hypertrophy and heart failure have been shown to alter significantly the function of the sarcoplasmic reticulum and the sarcolemma: e.g., the rate of calcium uptake by the SR and Na^+-K^+-ATPase [35–46]. Indeed, stress-induced derangement of the control of calcium activator availability can ultimately become so severe that a blunting of the excitation-induced release of cytosolic calcium may occur [3]. This depressed level of calcium would produce a weakened force of contraction and the clinical syndrome of heart failure.

The rate and amount of calcium uptake from the cytosol by the sarcoplasmic reticulum can become abnormal before mechanical function reaches the profoundly depressed levels of heart failure. Indeed, in the presence of hypertrophy, no measurable fall may be noted in the rate and amount of calcium uptake by sarcoplasmic reticulum vesicles [47–54]. It seems reasonable that more subtle alterations in the membrane control of calcium could be revealed by examining how the force-interval relationship has been altered as a consequence of the disease process. Because of the large changes in activator calcium which bring about the force-interval relationship and the way in which activator calcium is thought to be controlled by the sarcoplasmic reticulum and sarcolemma, such changes would, indeed, be expected.

An enormous range of mechanical responses is elicited by altering the pattern of stimulation. These include post-extrasystolic potentiation, the positive and negative staircases which occur with a change in rate, and the steady-state responses at various rates [16]. Any attempt to examine how a disease process alters each aspect of the force-interval relationship, let alone how normal myocardium produces these responses, would require a consideration of essentially every component of the systems that control contraction. As will be discussed later, changes in the physiologic aspects of systems which require hundreds of contractions to express themselves will in general not be considered, allowing us to focus on those which produce large beat-to-beat changes in activator calcium.

The Components of the Force-Interval Relationship

The strength of contraction of cardiac muscle (figure 9–1) is markedly altered simply by varying the pattern of stimulation. Such a relationship between force and stimulus interval, common to all mammalian myocardium, is intrinsic to the cardiac cell. In other words, these variations in the force of contraction do not require interventions, such as a change in muscle length or the exposure of the muscle to an inotropic agent, which are known to modulate the force of contraction.

Two components of the force-interval relationship have been identified: the short-term and the long-term component [10].

The *short-term component* of the force-interval relationship consists of the

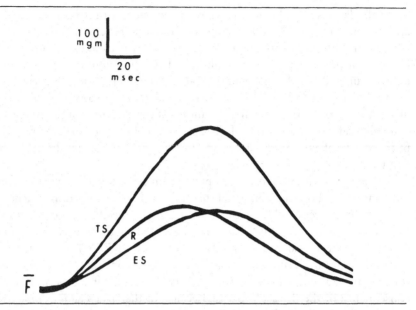

Figure 9–1. The response of an isolated rabbit papillary muscle to the introduction of an extrasystole. The response of a contraction at the basic rate (R), the subsequent extrasystole (ES) and post-extrasystole (TS) are superimposed. Force, $\bar{F}$.

large alterations in the force of contraction that occur within the first few beats after a perturbation of a basic rate of stimulation: for example, the beat-to-beat changes in force which occur when an extra stimulus is interposed during a constant rate of stimulation (see figure 9–1). The force of the extrasystole is small, and the force of the subsequent contraction is potentiated. Another example is the large increase in force that occurs in the first few contractions, following an increase in the rate of stimulation.

The *long-term component* of the force-interval relationship is composed of the small beat-to-beat changes in force which occur over hundreds of beats following a change in rate. Typically, an initial quasi-steady-state level of force is achieved in the first ten or twenty contractions following a change of rate, after which force continues to change gradually until a final steady-state response at the new rate is established. This is illustrated in figure 9–2. Note that there is a gradual increase in force over the hundreds of contractions following the initial fall to a quasi-steady-state value when the pacing rate is decreased. Conversely, a slow decrease in force follows the initial rise in the case of an increase in rate.

The long-term and short-term components of the force-interval relationship have been demonstrated in both the isolated muscle and the heart of the intact animal [10, 55]. The changes are reproducible and are expressed in the presence of muscarinic and β-agonist blockade. The presence of the two components in the intact animal preparation, as well as in the isolated muscle, implies

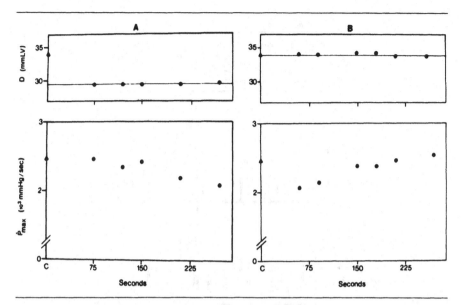

Figure 9–2. The effect of increasing pacing rate (A, 90 to 140 beats/minute) and decreasing rate (B, 140 to 90 beats/minute) on the maximum rate of rise of pressure (P_{max}) in a chronically instrumented adult dog. After the initial quasi plateau, the maximum rate of rise of left ventricular pressure gradually changes with either an increase or a decrease in rate. After a rate increase (A), P_{max} gradually falls from its plateau to a final steady state. After a decrease in rate (B), P_{max} gradually rises from the initial quasi plateau to a level which is equal to P_{max} measured prior to the rate changes. Note that the end-diastolic dimension (D) was the same for each group of systoles.

that a rapidly and a slowly equilibrating change are both intrinsic to cell function.

Interpreting Changes in Myocardial Function Using the Force-Interval Relationship

The changes in force in the long-term component of the force-interval relationship must derive from the many cellular events which occur during the time required for the long-term component to reach a steady state: e.g., changes in the intracellular amounts of calcium, sodium, and potassium, and the compartmentalization of calcium. The characteristics of the long-term component must also be affected by the superimposed effects of such variables as substrate availability in the isolated muscle and the effects of cardiovascular reflexes on the function of the heart in situ.

The short-term component of the force-interval relationship is composed of large and rapidly equilibrating changes in force which must, in contrast, reflect the function of systems within the cell, which themselves rapidly equilibrate. The changes in force during the short-term component are associated with large changes in cytosolic calcium [31]. See figure 9–3. These large beat-to-beat changes allow responses to be examined before there is any significant superimposition of the effects of other systems (e.g., reflexes in the intact animal). For this reason, the short-term component of the force-interval

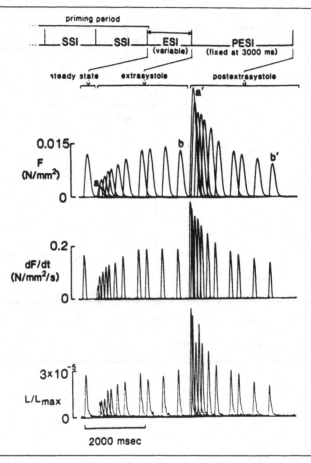

Figure 9–3. Original records illustrating restitution and post-extrasystolic potentiation. The stimulation protocol is shown at the top. Traces show tension (F, top), rate of tension development (dF/dt, middle), and aequorin luminescence (L/Lmax, bottom), from steady state, extrasystolic, and post-extrasystolic beats respectively. Records have been aligned in time to superimpose steady state responses. Responses a and a' are from an extrasystole and subsequent post-extrasystole obtained with an extrasystolic interval, ESI, of 450 ms; b and b' correspond to ESI = 3000 ms. The basic pacing interval, SSI, was 1500 ms, and $(Ca^{2+})_0 = 0.7$ mM. Traces are averages of 16 to 32 sweeps. [Reproduced with permission from W.G. Weir and D.T. Yue, Intracellular calcium transients underlying the short-term force-interval relationship in ferret ventricular myocardium. *Journal of Physiology*, in press].

relationship will be used here to evaluate cell function in the normal and in the diseased heart.

The Short-Term Component of the Force-Interval Relationship: Restitution of Contractility

One component of the force-interval relationship, called "the restitution of contractility" by Braveny and Kruta [56], describes how contractility recovers with time, following a contraction at a basic pacing interval (figure 9–4). This component is present in all mammalian myocardium [10, 57].

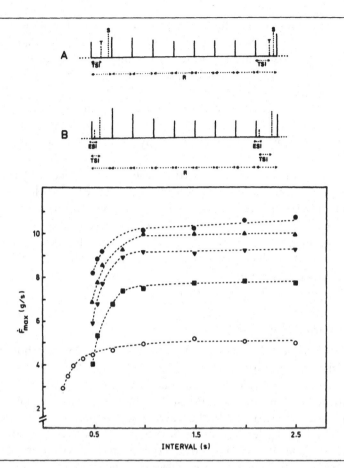

Figure 9–4. Typical results obtained from the two-stage experiment used to analyze the short-term force-interval relationship (F_{max}, the maximum rate of rise of force). The pacing protocol is illustrated in A and B. The muscle is stimulated at a constant rate (R), and a test stimulus (T) interpolated after every n stimuli (n = 8 in this figure). In the first stage, which describes the restitution of contractility after a contraction at the basic rate (A), F_{max} of test contractions in response to a stimulus at various intervals following the preceding stimulus at the basic rate (extrasystolic interval, TSI) are measured (open circles). In the second stage, which describes restitution after an extrasystole (B), an extra stimulus (ES) is inserted at a fixed extra systolic interval (ESI) after every eighth stimulus at the basic rate, and F_{max} of the post-extrasystolic contractions in response to a test stimulus (T) are measured (filled symbols). The values of F_{max} obtained by repeating the second stage of the experiment with four different fixed extra stimulus intervals (sold symbols, 200 ms ●, 225 ms ▲, 250 ms ▼, and 300 ms ■) are the four upper curves. F_{max} of the previous regular contraction was the same for all test contractions (5.0 g/s). Curves drawn by hand. Basic rate, 0.33 Hz. Rabbit papillary muscle.

In the isolated papillary muscle, the interposition of an additional stimulus in a regular pacing interval soon after the preceding contraction (a short extrasystolic interval) produces an extrasystole which develops a relatively small force in comparison to the force at the basic rate (figures 9–1 and 9–4). When extrasystoles are introduced at increasingly longer extrasystolic intervals, as the extrasystolic interval approaches that of the basic rate, the extrasystole's force increases until the extrasystole becomes equal to the contraction at the basic rate. In short, contractility is depressed immediately after a contraction and increases with time until it reaches a plateau value which is maintained for some seconds.

The restitution curve differs from one basic pacing rate to another. For most mammalian myocardia, a faster pacing rate produces a more forceful contraction, shown in the restitution curve by a greater plateau value at faster rates.

When contractions following an extrasystole are examined, the restitution curve is different from those at the basic rate [10] (figure 9–4). The curve rises faster and to a higher plateau in post-extrasystolic contractions. The timing of the extrasystole alters the plateau of the subsequent restitution of contractility; the more premature the extrasystole, the greater the post-extrasystolic potentiation or, equivalently, the higher the plateau of the restitution curve. Rate also affects potentiation. For the same extrasystolic interval, the faster the rate, the less the amount of potentiation. (figure 9–5).

The Single Cardiac Cell

The single cardiac cell has been used to assess how sarcomere shortening is altered by the temporal pattern of stimulation [58–60]. This approach has the virtue of examining the effects of pacing interval on sarcomere shortening, free of the extracellular matrix, of cell-to-cell connections, and of the complex geometry of the whole tissue. In the studies by Nassar et al. [58, 59] on cells from the rabbit ventricle, sarcomere shortening was altered by varying the pacing pattern. The effects of the introduction of an extrasystole are illustrated in figure 9–6. In this premature extrasystole, the amount and velocity of sarcomere shortening are much less than in the contraction at the basic rate. Post-extrasystolic potentiation of sarcomere shortening occurs in the subsequent contraction. These changes in sarcomere shortening of the rabbit myocyte are qualitatively similar to those observed in the force waveform of the rabbit papillary muscle (figure 9–1).

The Restitution of Contractility in the Single Cardiac Cell

The characteristics of the restitution of contractility of the isolated cell, as representd by sarcomere shortening, are similar to those described by measurements of force in the isolated muscle [58–60]. The most premature extrasystole which could be elicited produced the smallest amount and slowest velocity of sarcomere shortening. When the extrasystole was elicited at increasingly longer intervals after the previous contraction, the extent and velocity of extrasystolic sarcomere shortening increased until a plateau response equal to the contraction at the basic rate was achieved.

The restitution of contractility after an extrasytole was examined in the

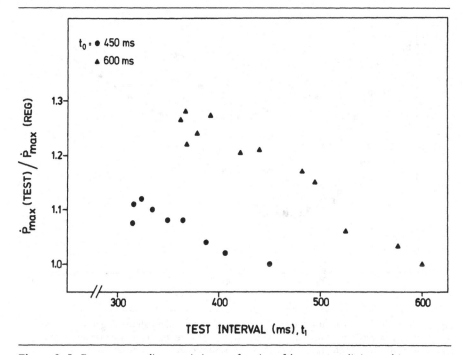

Figure 9–5. Post-extrasystolic potentiation as a function of the extrasystolic interval (test interval, t_1). The data were obtained from a child with a residual ventricular septal defect and left ventricular hypertrophy during cardiac catheterization one year following repair of Tetralogy of Fallot. Potentiation is described by the ratio of the maximum rate of rise of left ventricular pressure, $\dot{P}_{max}$, of the post-extrasystole divided by $\dot{P}_{max}$ of the previous systole at the basic rate for a given extrasystolic interval, where the end-diastolic dimensions of these two systoles were the same. Two different basic pacing intervals, $t_0=450$ ms (●), $t_0=600$ ms (▲) were used (see figure 9–4 for definitions). The force-interval ration increased as t_1 was decreased and for a given t_1 the ratio was greater at the slower rate. [Reproduced by permission from Page A.W. Anderson, Andres Manring, Gerald A. Serwer, D. Woodrow Benson, Sam B. Edwards, Brenda E. Armstrong, Richard J. Sterba, and Richard D. Floyd, IV. 1979. The force-interval relationship of the left ventricle. *Circulation* 60:2, 334–348].

single cell by Nassar et al. [58, 59], using a pacing pattern similar to figure 9–4.

When a post-extrasytole is elicited early after an extrasystole, sarcomere shortening is slower and smaller in amount than at the basic rate. When the contraction is elicited at longer intervals following the extrasystole, sarcomere shortening of the post-extrasystole becomes greater, rising to a plateau which exceeds the response at the basic rate. As noted in regard to force the more premature the extrasystole, the higher the plateau and the faster the rise to the plateau. These responses are reproducible.

In addition to the similarity of the effects of variations in the pacing pattern on the amount and velocity of sarcomere shortening and on the amount and rate of rise of force, the changes induced in contraction duration are the same in the isolated cell and in the isolated muscle (figures 9–1 and 9–6).

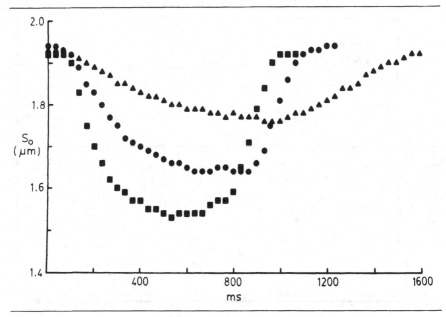

Figure 9-6. The effects of introducing an extrasystole on sarcomere shortening in an isolated single cell. These waveforms were obtained from a rabbit ventricular myocyte that was paced using the protocol similar to figure 9-4. The cell was shortening against no external load. The response at the basic rate, circles, the extrasystole, triangles and the post-extrasystole, squares (S_0, sarcomere length). The basic rate was 0.25 Hz, and the extrasystole was introduced 1100 ms following the preceding stimulus at the basic rate.

The Dependence of the Action Potential on the Pattern of Stimulation

The changes in the duration of contraction in response to alterations of the pattern of stimulation serve as a reminder that the action potential is affected by the pacing pattern [10].

Take the rabbit myocardium for example. Just as the premature extrasystole has a longer duration than the contraction at the basic rate, so the action potential of the extrasystole is much longer than at the basic pacing rate. The fact that the duration of the action potential and of the contraction, induced by varying the pattern of stimulation, both change in the same direction has led to the hypothesis that changes in the action potential cause, or are at least related to, the changes in force of the concomitant and following contraction.

Species Variation and the Dependence of the Action Potential on the Pattern of Stimulation

Prominent changes in the action potential configuration in response to variations of the pattern of stimulation have been described in a wide range of species [10]. However, the changes in the action potential in response to the same pattern of stimulation can be directionally opposite from one species to another, while the changes in force are, qualitatively, the same.

For example, the restitution of contractility and post-extrasystolic potentiation are common to the rabbit, guinea pig, and chicken ventricular myocardium [10]. In the rabbit, the area under the action potential waveform of the premature extrasystole is always larger than at the basic rate; in the guinea pig, it may be about the same; and in the chicken it is always smaller than at the basic rate [10]. In the rabbit, the area under the action potential of the post-extrasystole may be less than, equal to, or greater than at the basic area, yet force is enhanced in all three cases [10]. A straightforward correlation of action potential to force cannot be obtained merely by describing the effects of varying the pacing pattern. It is of interest that a correlation likewise cannot be found when the action potential of the hypertrophied or failing myocardium is compared to that of the normal one [61–63].

Restitution of Contractility and Membrane Function

Although the velocity of sarcomere shortening in cardiac muscle depends on many factors intrinsic to the cell (e.g., myosin ATPase), the changes in sarcomere shortening velocity, seen for instance during the restitution of contractility, must be attributed to those aspects of cell function which change more rapidly than cell proteins can. The rapid changes in the contractile response must be based on the function of membrane systems that modulate activator calcium, such as the sarcolemma and the sarcoplasmic reticulum.

Activator Calcium and the Modulation of Contraction

A variety of evidence can be advanced to support the contention that the complexity of the relationship between the temporal pattern of stimulation and the resultant sarcomere shortening is dependent on the modulation of activator calcium concentration. Some of the evidence is rather indirect. The calcium concentration in the bathing medium affects the sarcomere length of the isolated single cell from which the membranes have been removed by detergent treatment. Increasing calcium concentration induces sarcomere shortening, and the amount of shortening depends on the concentration of calcium (personal observation).

In the isolated intact single cell, an increase in extracellular calcium concentration increases the velocity and the amount of sarcomere shortening in response to electrical stimulation just as force is increased in the isolated muscle. In view of the effect of calcium on sarcomere length in the absence of membranes, the enhancement of sarcomere shortening in the intact cell suggests that activator calcium concentration is increased by the elevation in extracellular calcium concentration through such mechanisms as trans-sarcolemmal-calcium movement via the calcium channel or Na-Ca exchange.

Alterations in Cytosolic Calcium as Shown by Aequorin Luminescence

A more direct approach to relating the effects of alterations of the pattern of stimulation to activator calcium was pursued by Weir and Yue [31] and by Yue

[64] who injected aequorin into the cells of papillary muscles isolated from the ferret and the rabbit. The beat-to-beat changes in the luminescence of aequorin were used as indicators of change in the cytosolic calcium bathing the contractile apparatus.

The restitution of contractility, expressed in terms of the peak value of the time derivative of force, had the same characteristics in both species. As described earlier, contractility increased from a small value immediately following the previous contraction to a plateau (figures 9–3 and 9–4). A similar relationship was observed between luminescence and time following the previous contraction (figure 9–3). The amplitude of the luminescence was least in the earliest extrasystole and became greater at longer intervals until a plateau equal to the luminsecence in the contraction at the basic rate was achieved. The marked similarity of the temporal courses of the restitution of contractility and of the luminescence strongly suggest that the restitution of contractility is intimately related to the availability of activator calcium.

In examining the relationship between the post-extrasystolic potentiation of force and the aequorin luminescence [31, 64] it was found that the more premature the extrasystole, the greater the luminescence in the post-extrasystole (figure 9–7). Indeed, post-extrasystolic potentiation was directly related to the increases in luminescence.

This finding is well demonstrated by the following [31, 64]: an index of post-extrasystolic potentiation was defined as the ratio of the peak value of the first time derivative of isometric tension of the potentiated contraction to the peak value of the time derivative of tension of the previous contraction at the basic rate. The ratio of peak luminescence of the potentiated beat (the post-extrasystolic contraction) to the peak luminescence of the contraction at the basic rate (calibrated to calcium concentration) was also determined. When this ratio was compared to the index of post-extrasystolic potentiation, they were found to be the same for any pattern of pacing (figure 9–7). These findings indicate that the modulation of force through alterations in the pacing pattern are mediated directly through changes in activator calcium availability.

Calcium Availability and Myocardial Ultrastructure

After having demonstrated a close relationship between changes in force and aequorin luminescence in response to perturbations in rhythm, the question then arises: what is the ultrastructural basis for such time- and pattern-dependent availability of activator calcium which results in the various aspects of the force-interval relationship? One likely candidate is the sarcoplasmic reticulum.

Vesicles of sarcoplasmic reticulum take up large amounts of calcium relatively rapidly, and release calcium in response to such stimuli as caffeine [6]. The uptake and release of calcium by the sarcoplasmic reticulum is thought to be reflected in the temporal course of aequorin luminescence in mammalian ventricular myocardium [32–34]. In the mechanically skinned

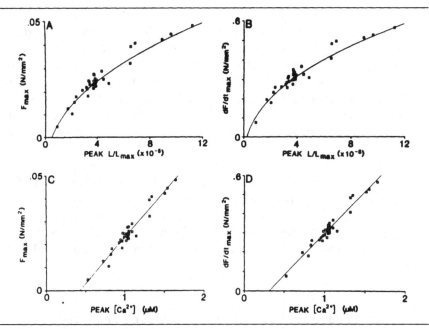

Figure 9–7. Relation of peak aequorin luminescence (L/LP_{max}) to peak tension (F_{max}, A), and to maximum rate of rise of tension (dF/dt_{max}, B) derived from variably restituted and potentiated beats. The solid curves in A and B represent $y = G\,[(L/L_{max})^{1/2,37}] + H$. Panels C and D show the same relations after peak L/L_{max} has been calibrated to peak $(Ca^{2+})_i$. The solid lines in C and D are linear regressions. [Reproduced with permission from W.G. Weir and D.T. Yue, Intracellular calcium transients underlying the short-term force-interval relationship in ferret ventricular myocardium. *Journal of Physiology*, in press].

cardiac cell, release of calcium from the SR occurs on exposure to an increase in calcium concentration or to caffeine, as measured by the development of force and by aequorin luminescence [32]. Pharmacological interventions, which inhibit the uptake of calcium and prolong its release from the sarcoplasmic reticulum, prolong the aequorin signal, while those which increase the release of calcium increase the luminescence [33]. In the presence of ryanodine, which is thought to block the release of calcium from cardiac sarcoplasmic reticulum, post-extrasystolic potentiation is blunted and the post-extrasystolic enhancement of luminescence is eliminated [31, 64]. Caffeine, which releases calcium from the SR, prolongs the duration of the luminescence signal and isoproterenol enhances its amplitude. Thus, the alterations in luminescence which occur with alterations of the rate and pattern of stimulation can describe how the sarcoplasmic reticulum controls cytosolic calcium.

The Sarcoplasmic Reticulum (SR) and its Organization

In adult mammalian ventricular myocardium, the SR is composed of longitudinal, junctional, and corbular components which together make up a prominent, repetitive, well-organized cellular system of membranes [65].

The longitudinal SR extends from Z-disc to Z-disc, forming a rete around the myofilaments. The lumen of this longitudinal network is connected directly to the junctional and corbular SR which are located at the level of the Z-disc. Foot processes extend from the surface of the junctional SR toward the surface sarcolemma and from the surface of the corbular SR into the cytosol. The intimate and specialized relationship between the junctional SR and the transverse tubular system or surface sarcolemma is found in all mammalian myocardium.

The different locations of SR structures along the sarcomere have been related to different functional characteristics of these components [22]. The electron-dense material in the lumen of the corbular and junctional SR contains calsequestrin. The lumen of the longitudinal SR does not [66]. In contrast, the wall of the longitudinal SR is rich in the ATP-dependent calcium pump and the associated protein, phospholamban, while the junctional and corbular SR have little [6].

Relationship between Structure and Function of the SR Components

The functional and structural properties of the different components of the SR imply that the sites containing calsequestrin are the calcium-release sites, while the sites of the calcium pump are the sites of calcium uptake. These relationships can be integrated into a model of excitation and contraction, as follows.

The close anatomic relationship between the junctional SR and the sarcolemma is desirable if, with activation, the foot processes of the junctional SR transduce the changes in membrane potential to the SR and bring about calcium release from the junctional SR; and, through a longer intracellular pathway, the foot processes of the corbular SR (e.g., in response to trans-sarcolemmal movement of calcium) induce calcium release from the corbular SR. The messenger might be calcium, or perhaps inositol triphosphate or something else [3, 34]. During the action potential, additional calcium would enter the cell from extracellular space through calcium channels and by Na-Ca exchange.

The longitudinal SR and the sarcolemma are the membrane systems which lower cytosolic calcium concentration and bring about relaxation. Calcium would be extruded from the cell through the sarcolemma and calcium would be taken up by the longitudinal SR via the calcium ATPase-dependent pump.

This model, which separates the intracellular release sites—the junctional and corbular SR—from the uptake sites, the longitudinal SR, is predicated in part on the concept that calcium moves within this system from uptake to the release site before it is available for release with the next activation. This intracellular movement of calcium would provide an explanation for the time required for the restitution of activator calcium availability, as described by aequorin luminescence and by the strength of contraction (figure 9–3).

Soon after a contraction, little calcium will have reached the release site, but with time, the calcium within the longitudinal SR fills the junctional and corbular SR. The increased availability of calcium results in an increase in contractility and in the luminescence signal.

The explanation of an additional characteristic of the SR follows from the work of Fabiato [67], and may also be an explanation of the restitution of contractility. The SR may not be able as readily to release Ca immediately after a contraction, even if calcium is available within the release site. Following a contraction, the ability to release calcium would return gradually to the basic rate.

Whether these time-dependent processes control restitution, the maintenance of a sustained plateau of contractility, following the process of restitution, indicates that the same amount of calcium is retained in a releasable form for many seconds before its availability declines (e.g., by moving to some other intracellular compartment or by loss from the cell), as described in the rested-state contraction [68].

The Basis of Post-Extrasystolic Potentiation

If this model is correct, we would expect that post-extrasystolic potentiation would result from an increase in activator calcium made available through these same structures.

Various models which incorporate aspects of the uptake and release of activator calcium by the sarcoplasmic reticulum and the associated trans-sarcolemmal movement of calcium during the extrasystole and post-extrasystole have been proposed [10, 20–28]. One group of models relates post-extrasystolic potentiation to the amount of calcium available within the release site or to the ability of the site to release it. For example, when an extrasystole is elicited, the calcium which has been taken up by the longitudinal SR is still being transported from its uptake to its release site. Less calcium is then available at the release site when the extrasystole is elicited, leaving calcium within the SR to be released during the next contraction. The ability of the site to release the calcium is also a function of time, so the sooner activation occurs after the previous action potential, the less calcium is released [67]. If these two mechanisms exist, they would result in some increase in activator calcium during the post-extrasystole.

Post-extrasystolic potentiation can also be brought about by increases of intracellular stores of calcium as a result of the inward trans-sarcolemmal movement of calcium during the extrasystole, e.g., trans-sarcolemmal inward movement through the calcium channel and voltage-dependent sodium-calcium exchange. During the most premature extrasystole, more calcium would cross the sarcolemma than during the action potential at the basic rate because the lower cytosolic calcium during the premature extrasystole would result in the calcium channel turning off later. Hiraoka and Sana [69] have demonstrated that the calcium current decreases with time following the previous depolarization. The decrease in inward calcium movement with time, following the previous action potential, would occur because calcium would increase in the extrasystoles as the extrasystolic interval increased (figure 9–3). The movement of this larger amount of calcium through the sarcoplasmic reticulum to the release sites would produce the enhanced post-extrasytolic restitution of contractility and post-extrasystolic potentiation (see figures 9–1, 9–3, 9–4).

However, these suggested mechanisms cannot easily explain the marked potentiation in force which can be seen in the rabbit papillary muscle. If Yue and Weir [31, 64] are correct in observing that the aequorin signal (calibrated to calcium concentration) and the peak rate of rise of force have a linear relationship, then the fourfold potentiation seen occasionally in the rabbit papillary muscle [70] requires that the release of calcium also be four times greater during such a post-extrasystole than during the contraction at the basic rate. Since it is thought that the amount of calcium which enters the cell is not sufficient for a maximal contraction [32], some other system must be invoked to explain the marked increase in activator calcium which can become available during the post-extrasystole.

As an alternative to enhanced cellular stores, a possible model for post-extrasystolic potentiation follows from the hypothesis that the calcium which enters the cell during a contraction is available to the myofilaments during that contraction. Such a mechanism would account for the observation that an interval-dependent depletion of extracellular calcium occurs in mammalian ventricular myocardium during activation. Such calcium movement has been considered electroneutral; hence its size cannot be estimated by current measurements [25, 71]. Variations in the force of contraction, in response to alterations of the pattern of stimulation, have almost always been found to be related to the extent of the depletion of extracellular calcium. This suggests that the extrasystole alters the membrane characteristics, such that trans-sarcolemmal movement of calcium is enhanced during the subsequent post-extrasystolic contraction. In this model, the more premature the extrasystole, the greater the extent of inward calcium movement during the subsequent post-extrasystolic contraction, and so the greater the potentiation of force.

Based on available experimental data, the increase in activator calcium, which produces post-extrasystolic potentiation, can be considered to be the result of some combination of the following: greater intracellular stores, an enhanced ability of the SR to release calcium, and greater trans-sarcolemmal movement of calcium.

Phylogenetic Differences in the Control of Activator Calcium

The control of activator calcium appears to differ markedly across the vertebrate phyla. Frog ventricular myocardium, which has cells with small diameters and thus short diffusion distances and sparse SR, is strongly dependent on trans-sarcolemmal movement of calcium [4]. Among mammals whose myocardium is replete with SR, differences appear to exist in the response of the SR to intracellular messengers that induce calcium release. Fabiato [72] found that the calcium-induced calcium release system is much more prominent in rat myocardium than in rabbit.

Whatever the reason for these phylogenetic differences, they may affect the characteristics of the restitution of contractility. Differences in restitution among species can therefore be seen as the result of differences in how calcium is kept available for release. For example, phylogenetic differences in the ability to retain calcium within its release sites could explain why restitution in one species rises to a sustained plateau, while in another, over a comparable period of time, restitution rises and then falls [57]. Similarly, the prominent post-extrasystolic potentiation seen in many mammals, and its almost complete absence in others (e.g., the rat), may be an important clue as to how differences in the morphology and function of the membrane systems alter their control of cytosolic calcium.

Quantitative Models of the Force-Interval Relationship

Several mathematical models have been developed to represent how alterations of the temporal pattern of stimulation affect the force of contraction [10, 27, 28]. Since the force-interval relationship has long been considered to describe basic cellular processes, such a quantitative model would be a useful adjunct in seeking the mechanisms which are the basis of excitation-contraction coupling. In order to incorporate the force-interval relationship, some models have required two variables, others have four or more. Unfortunately, a model whose solutions fit the observations obtained in all preparations, known to represent real mechanisms, is not yet available. The general application of these models to testing how disease processes alter the control of activator calcium is therefore limited.

Observations obtained from the isovolumically contracting isolated dog heart have been the basis for one such quantitative model [27, 28]. Restitution curves obtained at different pacing rates could be fitted by a monoexponential function, and the curves were found merely to be scaled versions of one another, with different amplitudes but the same time constant. If the variables within the model correspond to physical quantities, the marked similarity from one rate to another suggests that the underlying basic cellular processes which control restitution are unaffected by rate. This has important practical consequences. For example, the absence of an affect of rate would allow comparisons of these cellular processes in the same heart at different times, and possibly between different hearts, to be made regardless of differences in the heart rate. Unfortunately, the constancy of the restitution of contractility obtained at different rates or following extrasystoles is not common to all tissues and preparations [23, 24, 73]. See figure 9–8.

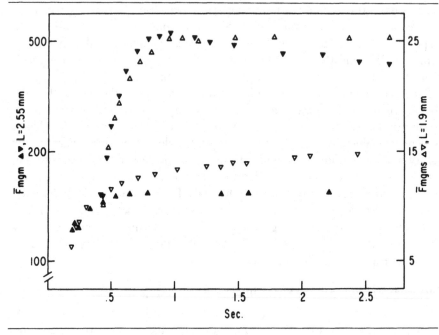

Figure 9–8. Peak isometric force ($\bar{F}$) of test contractions obtained at two muscle lengths using the pacing protocol of Figure 9–4. The contractions which provided these values of force are the same as in Figure 9–9. The muscle lengths were 2.5 mm (solid symbols) and 1.9 mm (open symbols). Note the difference in the ordinate scales: scale for data at 2.5 mm on the left and that for data at 1.9 mm on the right. [Reproduced by permission of the American Heart Association, Inc. from Page A.W. Anderson, Andres Manring, and Edward A. Johnson. 1973. Force-frequency relationship: A basis for a new index of cardiac contractility? *Circulation Research* 33].

Criteria for an Index of Contractility

Recognizing that the force-interval relationship is a manifestation of basic cellular processes (figures 9–6 and 9–7), several studies have examined whether descriptions of the relationship could be found to qualify as an index of contractility. If so, the force-interval relationship would be a very useful approach to the assessment of the effects of disease states or pharmacological interventions on myocardial function.

An index of contractility must satisfy the following criteria:

1. be independent of preload
2. be independent of afterload
3. be sensitive to a change in inotropy.

Effect of Preload

The force-interval relationship has been found to be independent of length of isolated muscle, and independent of ventricular enddiastolic volume in the

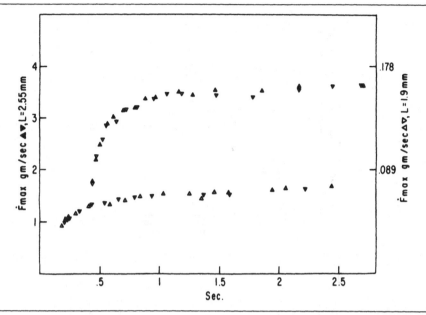

Figure 9–9. Maximum rate of rise of tension, $\dot{F}_{max}$, of test contractions at two muscle lengths plotted as a function of test interval (See figure 9–4 for definitions and pacing protocol). The experiment was performed at two lengths. 2.55mm (solid symbols) and 1.9mm (open symbols). The fixed extra stimulus in the second stage was 0.21 seconds after the fifth regular stimulus. Note the difference in the ordinate scales for the data from the longer length (filled symbols, lefthand ordinate) and from the shorter length (open symbols, righthand ordinate). [Reproduced by permission of the American Heart Association, Inc. from Page A.W. Anderson, Andres Manring, and Edward A. Johnson. 1973. Force-frequency relationship: A basis for a new index of cardiac contractility? *Circulation Research* 33].

isolated heart and in the intact animal [74–76]. For example, in the isolated papillary muscle, after an equilibration period following each change in length, the restitution of contractility, following the contraction at the basic rate, is the same from one preload to another (the maximum rate of increase of force was used (figure 9–9). That is to say, although the values of the maximum rate of force increase in response to the same pattern of stimulation are different at different muscle lengths, the values of the points on the curve of restitution at one muscle length can be scaled to those at another by multiplying them by the same constant. In the isolated heart studied over a range of preloads, restitution could be linearly scaled in a similar manner when the maximum rate of rise of ventricular pressure was used [75, 76] (figure 9–10). Hence, the effects of preload and of the cellular processes which result in the force-interval relationship can be considered as separate functions [75–77]. The force-interval relationship can consequently be studied free of the effects of preload.

By taking the ratio of the post-extrasystolic response to that of the previous regular contraction at the same muscle length or ventricular volume, the constant of proportionality which describes the effect of preload on these

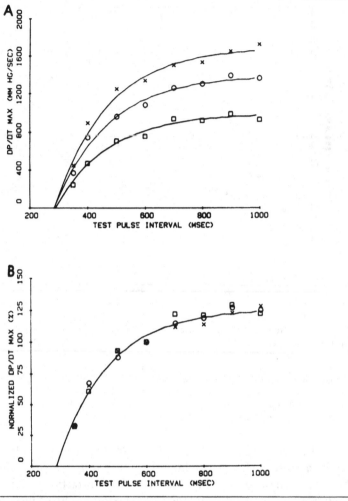

Figure 9–10. Mechanical restitution curves from the left ventricle of an isolated heart, beating isovolumically at volumes of 15 (□), 25 (○), and 35 (×) ml. A pacing protocol, similar, to figure 9–4 was used. A: non-normalized test beat; maximum rate of rise of pressure (dP/dt$_{max}$) values are given. B: responses at each volume normalized by dividing the test responses by the steady-state dP/dt$_{max}$ at that volume. Normalized points were nearly coincident, indicating that volume did not affect either normalized plateau or the time constant of mechanical restitution. [Reproduced from Daniel Burkhoff, David T. Yue, Michael R. Franz, William C. Hunter, and Kiichi Sagawa. 1984. Mechanical Restitution of isolated perfused canine left ventricles. *American Journal of Physiology* 246 (Heart Circ. Physiol. 15), H8–H16.]

responses is eliminated [75–77] (figure 9–11). This permits post-extrasystolic potentiation, for a given pattern of stimulation, to be compared at different times and under different conditions, e.g., during the course of a disease process. It is unnecessary for the studies to be performed at the same point in the length-tension or volume-pressure relationship each time.

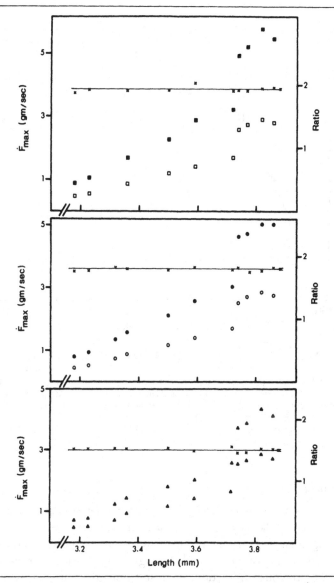

Figure 9–11. The effect of muscle length on the maximum rate of rise of force ($\dot{F}_{max}$) of the post-extrasystole (closed symbols) and the previous contraction at the basic packing rate (closed symbols). Data obtained with the use of pacing protocol described in figure 9–4 from a left ventricular trabecula carnea of an adult dog heart. The force-interval ratio (ratio of $\dot{F}_{max}$ of the potentiated contraction to that of the previous contraction at the basic rate for a given length) describes post-extrasystolic potentiation (crosses). Different extrasystolic intervals were used to obtain the data in panels A, B, and C. The line is drawn through the mean value of the ratios obtained with each extrasystolic interval. [Panel C reproduced with permission of the American Heart Association, Inc., from Page A.W. Anderson, J. Scott Rankin, Carl E. Arentzen, Robert W. Anderson, and Edward A. Johnson. 1976. Evaluation of the force-frequency relationship as a descriptor of the inotropic state of canine left ventricular myocardium. *Circulation Research* 396, 832–839.]

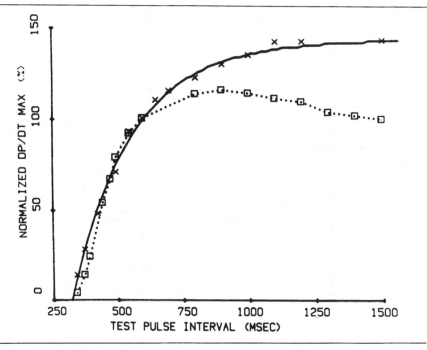

Figure 9–12. Mechanical restitution curves from the left ventricle of an isolated dog heart, at first beating isovolumically (x, solid line) and then allowed to eject (□, dotted line) into a simulated arterial system. The pacing protocol was similar to figure 9–4. The differences between these curves are attributable to effects of changing hemodynamic factors on dP-dt$_{max}$ (the maximum rate of rise of left ventricular pressure). [Reproduced from Daniel Burkhoff, David T. Yue, Michael R. Franz, William C. Hunter, and Kiichi Sagawa. 1984. Mechanical Restitution of isolated perfused canine left ventricles. *American Journal of Physiology* 246 (Heart Circ. Physiol. 15), H8–H16.]

Effect of Afterload

When the effects of afterload on the force-interval relationship were examined, the rising and early-plateau portions of the restitution curve, obtained from the heart ejecting against a varying afterload, were superimposed on those of the isovolumically contracting heart [74]. See figure 9–12. At longer test intervals following the previous contraction, the restitution curve of the isovolumically contracting heart diverged from the auxotonically contracting one and rose above it. At even longer test intervals, the maximum rate of rise of left ventricular pressure in the ejecting heart started to fall (figure 9–12).

These findings demonstrate that the maximum rate of ventricular pressure can be affected if afterload falls sufficiently. However, it does not appear likely that this would occur in the intact patient, given the relatively short test intervals used to evaluate the force-interval relationship. This assumption is supported by experimental observations (figure 9–13). For example, Franz et al. [78] found the plateau of restitution was sustained for over 1000 ms in some

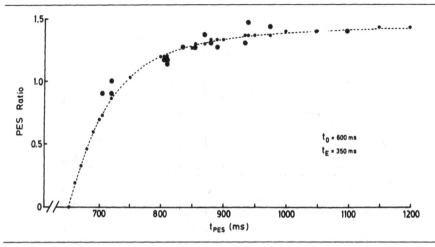

Figure 9–13. The restitution of contractility following an extrasystole. Data obtained from a patient two days following open heart surgery (see figure 9–18 for pacing protocol). The ratio of the maximum rate of rise of left ventricular pressure of the post-extrasystole to the maximum rate of rise of the previous systole at the basic rate (PES ratio) describes the response for each post-extrasystolic interval. The pair of systoles used for each ratio has the same left ventricular end-diastolic dimension. The PES ratio data (large circles) were fitted by an exponential function (dashed line). The basic pacing interval, t_0, was 600 ms and the extrasystolic interval, t_E, was 350 ms. [Reproduced from James D. Sink, Page A.W. Anderson, and Andrew S. Wechsler. 1985. Postoperative Left Ventricular Contractility in the Cardiac Surgical Patient: An Evaluation of the Force-Interval Relationship. *The Annals of Thoracic Surgery* 40:5.]

patients studied during cardiac catheterization. During this period, diastolic pressure would have fallen significantly, yet the maximum rate of rise of pressure appears to have been unaffected. Such measures as post-extrasystolic potentiation should therefore not be significantly affected by afterload in most studies of the in situ heart.

Inotropy

The force-interval relationship was found to be sensitive to alterations in inotropy, e.g., the shapes of the restitution curves and the amount of post-extrasystolic potentiation were altered significantly on exposure to an inotropic agent (sympathomimetic agents, histamine, ouabain, and changes in extracellular calcium) [70, 75, 76]. See figure 9–14.

The effects of inotropic agents on the force-interval relationship provide fascinating examples of how the complex effects of an inotropic agent can be revealed simply by altering the pattern of stimulation. The effects of sympathomimetic agents are the most striking: the restitution curves are changed from monotonic to biphasic or triphasic in the presence of isoproterenol or norepinephrine (figure 9–14).

These results provide strong justification for using the force-interval relationship to assess the effects of the inotropic agent on myocardial function.

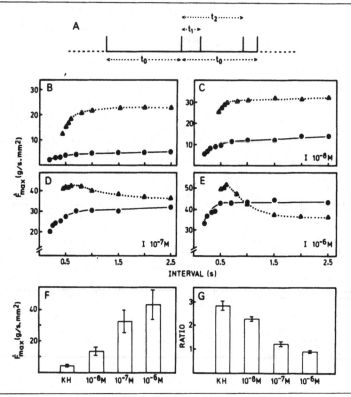

Figure 9–14. Effects of isoproterenol on the force-interval relationship of isolated right ventricular rabbit papillary muscle. A shows the pacing pattern (see figure 9–4 for explanation). The results from the first-stage (circles; solid lines) and the second-stage (triangles; dotted lines, t_1 = 200 ms) experiments are provided for the same muscle before (B) and during exposure to 10^{-8} M (C), 10^{-7} M (D), and 10^{-6} M (E) isoproterenol. $\dot{F}_{max}$ is the maximum rate of rise of force. During exposure to 10^{-7} M and 10^{-6} M isoproterenol, the curves for the second stage of the experiment (dotted lines) were biphasic, i.e., they drooped. Panel F illustrates the increase in $\dot{F}_{max}$ (± se) of the contraction at the basic pacing rate from the control value (KH) to that in isoproterenol (10^{-8}, 10^{-7}, 10^{-6} M). Panel G illustrates the decrease in the force-interval ratio (see figure 9–11 for definition) from the control value (KH) to that in isoproterenol (10^{-8}, 10^{-7}, 10^{-6} M). N = 17. [Reproduced with permission of Pergamon Press Ltd. from Andres Manring, Page A.W. Anderson, Rashid Nassar, and W. Robin Howe, Can sympathomimetic agents be classified by their action on the force-interval relationship? *Life Sciences* 32:4 (1983).]

For example, at a constant rate, all positive inotropic agents will be found to alter the ability of the myocardium to contract, and interventions are consequently required in order to examine the cellular basis of the inotropic change. Varying the pattern of stimulation can provide, by itself, dramatic evidence as to which agent has induced the change in inotropy. As such, it is a potentially valuable tool for testing the underlying mechanisms through which the inotropic agent affects the heart.

Since the force-interval relationship has been shown to fulfill the criteria for an index of contractility, it should be useful in investigating the effects of hypertrophy and heart failure on myocardial function in vivo and in vitro.

Experimental Variability in the Force-Interval Relationship

Before considering how the force-interval relationship may be affected by disease states, we must note that the characteristics of the short-term force-interval relationship, specifically the restitution of contractility, have been found to vary from study to study [23, 24, 73, 75, 76]. A sustained plateau (as seen in figure 9–1) is not always present for instance.

When the peak value of the first derivative of force is used to describe the restitution in the isometrically contracting rabbit papillary muscle, contractility has been shown in some studies to rise from a small initial value to a sustained plateau, but in other studies restitution has been shown to rise and then to fall [23]. If peak force is used, the restitution curve can rise to a plateau value and then fall in a muscle where the peak-first derivative of force provides a sustained plateau [figures 9–8 and 9–9]. The fall in peak force is in contrast to the sustained plateau of aequorin luminescence. Cat myocardium also has been shown to have a biphasic relationship by some investigators [73] but not by others [79, 80].

The differences in the characteristics of restitution may be a consequence of different experimental techniques and species-to-species variations in intrinsic physiologic properties. However, the characteristics of the force-interval relationship within any given system do not change.

The stable and reproducible nature of the responses, which comprise the force-interval relationship, is of great value when searching for changes in myocardial function. When the responses, associated with a disease process or a pharmacologic intervention, differ from those of the control, the differences represent a change in myocardial function. The uniqueness of such changes allows them to be used to examine the course of pathophysiologic changes in the heart, and as a tool for exploring how disease states alter the intrinsic physiological properties of the heart.

CLINICAL FINDINGS: A COMPARISON TO ADRENERGIC STIMULATION

Application of the Force-Interval Relationship to Studies of the Effects of Disease

The ease with which post-extrasystolic potentiation can be used to measure a change in myocardial function allows ready comparison of the function of the normal, the hypertrophied, and the failing heart. Such use of the relationship must be based on an understanding of its basic properties. For example, the timing of the extrasystole has a dynamic effect on the potentiation in the subsequent post-extrasystole. See e.g., figures 9–4, 9–5, and 9–8. The more premature the post-extrasystole, the greater the extent of the potentiation (figures 9–4 and 9–13). Care must be taken to use the same extrasystolic and post-extrasystolic intervals if single observations of post-extrasystolic potentiation in different hearts are to be compared.

If the same extrasystolic interval cannot be used, the function of the heart can still be characterized by using responses induced over a broad range of extrasystolic intervals (figure 9–5). The relationship between extrasytolic interval and post-extrasystolic potentiation can be quantified and used to search for differences in function [84].

Disease States and SR Function

Sarcoplasmic reticular function has been examined in a variety of models of hypertrophy and heart failure. The nature and extent of the effects on SR function appear to be related to the degree and duration of the stress [9, 35–46].

In some forms of hypertrophy, the amount of calcium released may be the same as in normal myocardium, but the rate of calcium uptake and release may be slowed [22]. Indeed, calcium accumulation may be enhanced by mild hypertrophy; but in more severe degrees of hypertrophy, and in heart failure, a progressive decrease is found in the amount of calcium taken up. A decrease in calcium ATPase activity has also been described.

Assessments of alterations in SR function consequent to disease are often performed by reducing a complicated system, the cell, to vesicles. A price is paid for the simplicity: it is no longer possible to explore the ability of the system to modulate activator calcium in the complex manner seen in the intact cell (as evidenced, e.g., by the force-interval relationship). Similarly, attempting to describe the ability of the heart to contract, by observing its response at a single constant rate, fails to bring forth the wide range of responses of which the heart is capable. Descriptions of vesicular function and of steady-state force response ignore much and constitute a very narrow observational window.

In contrast, when the pattern of stimulation is altered, a wide range of contractile responses is elicited, providing a much more nearly complete description of the functional capabilities of the heart. This is a variation on the theme of perturbational analysis. In this respect it is like using exercise to assess the function of a patient's heart. Unlike exercise, however, which induces changes throughout the body, the force-interval relationship can be used to assess myocardial function merely by the introduction of an extrasystole. Examination of the heart can thus be limited to a single functional aspect, e.g., membrane control of cytosolic calcium, without the superimposition of responses from other intra- and extracardiac systems.

In view of the large number of cardiac disease processes and their diverse effects on myocardial structure and function, it should be anticipated that, just as the function of SR vesicles may differ from one form of hypertrophy to another, the force-interval relationship will also be altered in more than one fashion by such diseases.

Hypertrophy: Post-Extrasystolic Potentiation of Isolated Muscle

To study the effects of ventricular hypertrophy on post-extrasystolic potentiation, we compared the responses of papillary muscle from cats which had undergone pulmonary artery banding to sham operated ones [79]. The strength of contraction at the basic pacing rate was found to be unaffected by hypertrophy. This was similar to the findings in several other studies which have compared papillary muscles from hypertrophied and control hearts [48–53]. This state of hypertrophy, called "stable hypertrophy" by Meerson [82], has also been described in the left ventricle of the intact dog, in which no difference in wall stress was found between normal and hypertrophied ventricles, after a recovery period [83].

Post-extrasystolic potentiation, unlike contraction at the basic rate, was affected by hypertrophy, exhibiting greater potentiation (as shown in figure 9–15). Thus, in mild stable hypertrophy, the availability of activator calcium was enhanced in the post-extrasystolic contraction.

In a study of severe hypertrophy, the changes in the relationship between steady-state force and rate suggest that the enhancement in the potentiation found in mild hypertrophy disappears with the acquisition of severe hypertrophy [49].

Hypertrophy: Post-Extrasystolic Potentiation of the in Situ Heart

In a cardiac catheterization study of young patients [54], left ventricular hypertrophy was shown to have an effect on potentiation similar to that which is observed in mild right ventricular hypertrophy in the isolated muscle [79]: that is, hypertrophy did not affect the response at the basic rate. The peak rate of rise of left ventricular pressure in the presence of such lesions as aortic stenosis was the same as in the absence of hypertrophy. However, post-extrasystolic potentiation was greater in the presence of left ventricular hypertrophy. Consequently, although the relationship between potentiation and the extrasystolic interval was qualitatively similar in patients with and without hypertrophy, i.e., the more premature the extrasystole, the greater the subsequent post-extrasystole potentiation. See figure 9–5. The hypertrophied heart demonstrated an ability to modulate activator calcium over a wider range, resulting in a greater potentiation in response to the same stimulus.

This demonstration of an enhancement of post-extrasystolic potentiation in the presence of mild hypertrophy recalls to mind some of the effects of development [84]. The functional and structural similarities suggest that the changes in the cellular processes evoked by development and by mild hypertrophy have similar effects on the control of cytosolic calcium. These relationships will be discussed further.

In view of the variety of the effects of disease on the myocardium, it is not surprising that other effects of hypertrophy on post-extrasystolic potentiation have been found. When post-extrasystolic potentiation was compared among patients with normal and those with abnormal left ventricles, a lack of potentiation was found in patients with extensive coronary artery disease [85, 86]. Patients with cardiomyopathies have been shown to have enhanced post-

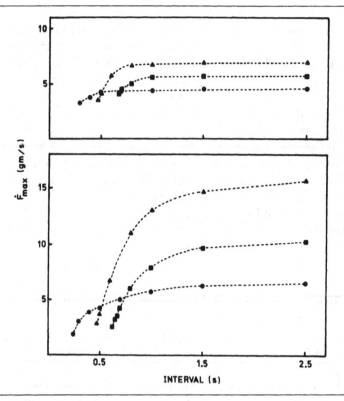

Figure 9–15. Results of a two-stage experiment (see figure 9–4 for pacing protocol and definitions) on the papillary muscle of a cat that had undergone a sham procedure (A) and on a papillary muscle from a cat which had undergone pulmonary artery banding (B). The maximum rate of rise of force ($\dot{F}_{max}$) is plotted against the test stimulus intervals. The circles are the results of the first-stage experiment, the triangles are the results of the second-stage experiment with an extrasystolic interval of 275 ms, and the squares are from the second-stage experiment but with an extrasystolic interval of 400 ms. Basic rate, 20/min. [Reproduced with permission of the American Heart Association, Inc. from Page A.W. Anderson, Andres Manring, Carl E. Arentzen, J. Scott Rankin, and Edward A. Johnson. 1977. Pressure-induced hypertrophy of cat right ventricle: an evaluation with the force-interval relationship. *Circulation Research* 41:4.]

extrasystolic potentiation [87], in comparison to normals or to patients with an atrial septal defect or lessened post-extrasystolic potentiation [88].

Congestive Heart Failure: Post-Extrasystolic Potentiation

When post-extrasystolic potentiation was studied in patients with congestive heart failure, the relationship between potentiation and the timing of the extrasystole was altered quantitatively, and in some instances qualitatively, from that observed in hypertrophied or in normal hearts [54].

In the presence of heart failure, potentiation was absent in some patients. In others, the force-interval relationship became "inverted" in the sense that the stength of the post-extrasystole following the most premature extrasystole

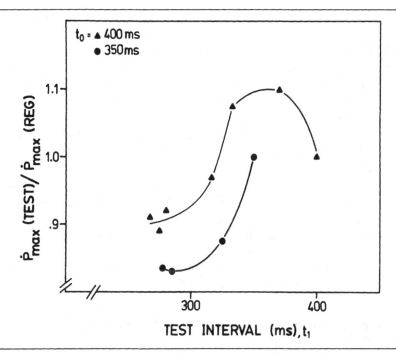

Figure 9–16. The force-interval ratio data from a patient with heart failure (see figure 9–5). The ratio is the maximum rate of rise of left ventricular pressure of the post-extrasystole, $\dot{P}_{max}$ divided by $\dot{P}_{max}$ of the previous systole at the basic rate; end-diastolic dimensions are the same for each pair of systoles). The ratio is plotted as a function of the extrasystolic interval, t_1. Basic pacing intervals were $t_0 = 400$ ms (▲) and $t_0 = 350$ ms (●). Compare the data, in particular the presence of post-extrasystolic depression of this patient with heart failure to the data from a patient with left ventricular hypertrophy shown in figure 9–5. Lines drawn by hand. [Reproduced by permission from Page A. W. Anderson, Andres Manring, Gerald A. Serwer, D. Woodrow Benson, Sam B. Edwards, Brenda E. Armstrong, Richard J. Sterba, and Richard D. Floyd IV. 1979. The force-interval relationship of the left ventricle. *Circulation* 60:2, 334–348.]

was less than the contraction at the basic rate (figure 9–16). This stands in marked contrast to the cases of the normal and the hypertrophied heart, in which the most premature extrasystole elicits the greatest amount of post-extrasystolic potentiation (figure 9–5).

In this group of patients with heart failure, post-extrasytolic depression was present following premature extrasystoles: the maximum rate of rise of left ventricular pressure in the post-extrasystole was less than at the basic rate. When the extrasystolic interval was increased, the strength of the post-extrasystole gradually increased, and, ultimately, post-extrasystolic potentiation occurred. Indeed, potentiation was greater in some of these extrasystolic intervals than it is in the normal and the hypertrophied myocardium. Potentiation disappeared again as the extrasystolic interval approached the basic rate, in a manner similar to that found in the normal heart. In studies of isolated human hearts which have produced heart failure in situ, both post-extrasystolic potentiation and the absence of potentiation have been found [88].

Although our discussion is centered on alterations of myocardial function due to calcium, differences are known to exist in the proteins which make up the contractile apparatus in normal, hypertrophic, and failing hearts. If potentiation were always absent, then alterations in the contractile proteins could explain the absence of potentiation in the failing heart. If the calcium sensitivity of the contractile apparatus were greatly blunted, for instance, the shape of the pCa-force relationship would be so altered that force would change only slightly over a broad range of activator calcium concentrations. A consequence of such a change in myofilament calcium sensitivity would be an uncoupling of the post-extrasystolic potentiation of activator calcium (as shown, e.g., by aequorin luminescence in figures 9–3 and 9–7), and the contractile response. The fact that merely altering the extrasystolic interval can produce post-extrasystolic depression as well as potentiation in the same heart means that the contractile proteins cannot be the primary cause of changes in the force-interval relationship induced by heart failure.

Hypertrophied Myocardium: The Restitution of Contractility in Isolated Muscle

Additional evidence for alterations in membrane function, induced by disease, is provided when we consider the restitution of contractility and how it is altered in the failing heart. The restitution of contractility provides a more complete description of the force-interval relationship than a single measurement of post-extrasystolic potentiation does. It can easily be obtained in the isolated papillary muscle, since restitution can be studied free of changes in muscle length or preload. In both hypertrophied and normal myocardium, restitution is qualitatively the same (figures 9–5 and 9–15). For example, the extrasystole at the shortest extrasystolic interval develops the least force. As the extrasystolic interval is increased, the strength of contraction increases until it reaches a plateau. Similar qualitative characteristics are retained when the restitution of contractility is examined after an extrasystole (figure 9–15).

The Restitution of Contractility in the Presence of an Intact Cardiovascular System

When the restitution of contractility is evaluated in the intact patient, a variety of hemodynamic variables can alter the variables used to derive the relationship. The ventricular end-diastolic volume, for example, is affected by the timing of the extrasystole and the post-extrasystole.

In general, the end-diastolic volume of the extrasystole increases as the extrasystolic interval is increased, until the end-diastolic volume reaches that at the basic rate [54, 76]. Such changes in volume seem to be related directly to the diastolic filling time. Because of the known effects of end-diastolic volume on the maximum rate of rise of pressure, the extrasystolic maximum rate of rise of left ventricular pressure is subject to the combined effects of changes in end-diastolic volume and the intrinsic effect of alterations of the pacing pattern.

In a unique instance, we have been able to describe the restitution of contractility in the intact patient free of the effects of variations in end-diastolic volume [89]. The curve following an extrasystole, shown in figure 9–13, was obtained in a postoperative patient in whom dimension transducers to monitor changes in left ventricular end-diastolic volume and a high fidelity left ventricular pressure manometer to derive changes in the peak first derivative of left ventricular pressure were implanted temporarily at the time of surgery. Because the patient's ventilation was supported by a respirator, large beat-to-beat changes in end-diastolic volume occurred. This allowed us to circumvent the usual relationship between test-interval and end-diastolic volume, namely that left ventricular end-diastolic volume is small at short test intervals. Systoles which began contraction from the same end-diastolic volume were obtained over a wide range of test intervals, allowing us to examine the restitution of contractility at a constant end-diastolic dimension.

The peak rate of rise of left ventricular pressure was smallest at the shortest intervals following the previous contraction. With an increase in the test interval, the maximum value of the derivative of pressure rose to a sustained plateau. These data can be fitted numerically by simple functions, which raises the possibility of describing the restitution of contractility in the intact patient [89]. In the usual case, however, the effects of test intervals on end-diastolic volume alter the peak derivative of left ventricular pressure and the restitution of contractility have precluded the quantitative descripton of the characteristics of restitution among a group of patients.

Congestive Heart Failure and the Restitution of Contractility

The restitution of contractility has been examined in the failing hearts of patients undergoing cardiac catheterization and in diseased hearts removed from patients at the time of cardiac transplantation.

Burkhoff and associates [88] have studied isolated, severely diseased, human hearts. Limitations associated with measurement of the restitution of contractility in the intact patient, such as the effects of varying preload on maximum rate of rise of left ventricular pressure, were avoided by studying the hearts as isolated organs with controlled preload and afterload. Some of them had very slowly rising restitutions of contractility; in others, restitution rose relatively briskly, similar to the normal dog heart.

More complex changes in the restitution of contractility have been found in a few patients with heart failure studied during cardiac catheterization [54].

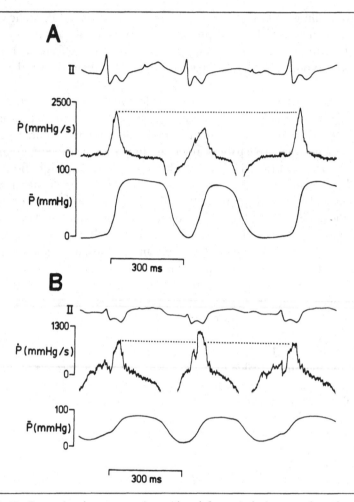

Figure 9–17. Comparison between a patient with no left ventricular hypertrophy and a patient with congestive heart failure. Data obtained during cardiac catheterization. The systoles are, from left, the last systole at the basic rate, the extrasystole, and the post-extrasystole. The end-diastolic dimension was the same for the systoles at the basic rate and the post-extrasystole in each panel; the basic pacing interval was 400 ms for each study. Panel A shows the normal response: compared with the regular systole, the maximum rate of rise of left ventricular pressure of the extrasystole was small and that of the post-extrasystole was large. Panel B shows a response which characterized some patients with heart failure: the extrasystolic maximum rate of rise of left ventricular pressure of the extrasystole was larger than that of the systole at the basic rate, and no post-extrasystolic potentiation was present. II, the electrocardiogram; P, the first derivative of left ventricular pressure; P̄, left ventricular pressure. [Reproduced by permission from Page A.W. Anderson, Andres Manring, Gerald A. Serwer, D. Woodrow Benson, Sam B. Edwards, Brenda E. Armstrong, Richard J. Sterba, and Richard D. Floyd IV. 1979. The force-interval relationship of the left ventricle. *Circulation* 60:2, 334–348.]

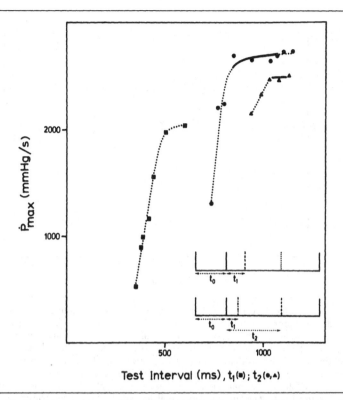

Test Interval (ms), t_1(■); t_2(●,▲)

Figure 9–18. Force-interval curves for a patient with no left ventricular hypertrophy. The insets are schematic representations of the pacing sequence; they include the last two systoles at the basic rate prior to the longer interval, during which an extra systole and a post-extrasystole were introduced (see figure 9–4 for definitions). During the first stage (pacing pattern in upper inset, ■) the timing of the post-extrasystole, t_2, was held constant and the extrasystolic interval, t_1, was varied. During the second stage (lower inset; ●, ▲), t_2 was varied while the extrasystolic interval t_1 was constant at 360 ms (●) or 420 ms (▲). t_0, the basic pacing interval, was 600 ms. Solid lines in the two second stage experiments indicate potentiated systoles with end-diastolic dimension equal to that of systoles at the basic pacing rate. P_{max}, the maximum rate of rise of life ventricule pressure. [Reproduced by permission from Page A.W. Anderson, Andres Manring, Gerald A. Serwer, D. Woodrow Benson, Sam B. Edwards, Brenda E. Armstrong, Richard J. Sterba, and Richard D. Floyd IV. 1979 The force-interval relationship of the left ventricle. *Circulation* 60:2, 334–348.]

Here the force-interval relationship did not rise in a simple way from a small initial value to a sustained plateau. Indeed, the peak first derivative of pressure of the extrasystole was larger, rather than smaller, at the basic rate (figure 9–17). In other words, contractility increased from a small value to one which exceeded the value at the basic pacing rate, and then declined until a lower sustained plateau was achieved (figure 9–19). This should be compared to the monophasic curve exhibited by patients with no left ventricular hypertrophy or with stable left ventricular hypertrophy (figure 9–18).

The biphasic relationship observed in such cases does not appear to be the

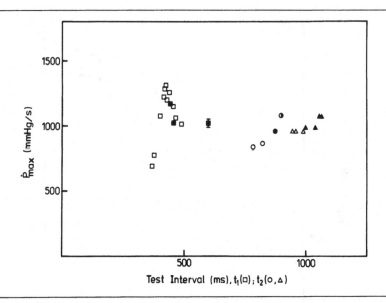

Figure 9–19. Force-interval curves for a patient with heart failure (see figures 9–4 and 9–18 for definitions and pacing protocol). Restitution following a contracting at the basic rate (squares) and following an extrasystole with an extrasystolic interval of 360 ms (circles) and one with an extrasystolic interval of 420 ms (triangles). The symbols denote whether the end-diastolic dimension of the test systole was smaller than (open), equal to (filled), or greater than (half-filled), the end-diastolic dimension of the last regular systole at the basic rate. The first-stage curve (i.e., the restitution curve following a contraction at the basic rate) is biphasic, in contrast to figure 9–18. See also figure 9–20 data from an isolated papillary muscle from a failing heart. [Reproduced by permission from Page A.W. Anderson, Andres Manring, Gerald A. Serwer, D. Woodrow Benson, Sam B. Edwards, Brenda E. Armstrong, Richard J. Sterba, and Richard D. Floyd IV, 1979 The force-interval relationship of the left ventricle. *Circulation* 60:2, 334–348.

result of preload effects. Ventricular volume was monitored with echo-cardiography, and the end-diastolic volumes of extrasystoles with enhanced first derivatives were equal to or less than the volumes of the systoles at the basic rate.

Likewise, decrease in afterload with increasing test interval does not appear to be the cause of such alterations in restitution. In the isolated ejecting heart, the peak first derivative of pressure did not decrease over the range of extrasystolic intervals used in the patients with heart failure (see figure 9–12). In the isolated heart, the peak derivative of pressure did decrease as the test interval was increased. In the patients, however, after the initial rise and fall, the peak rate of rise of pressure remained constant with further increases in the extrasystolic interval.

Changes in the characteristics of restitution observed in patients with a failing heart are reversible. One patient was restudied after repair of his cardiac defect and resolution of his heart failure (the rate of rise of his left ventricular pressure was no longer depressed and his end-diastolic pressure was no longer

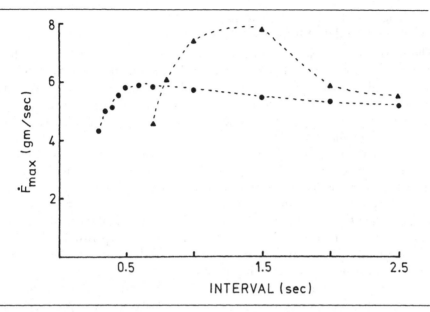

Figure 9–20. The force-interval data from a right ventricular papillary muscle of a cat with heart failure following pulmonary artery banding (see figure 9–4 for pacing protocol and definitions). The restitution following contraction at the basic rate (●) and following an extrasystole (▲) were both biphasic, similar to the restitution described in the patient with heart failure and in marked contrast to data from cats with no hypertrophy or mild right ventricular hypertrophy. See figures 9–15, 9–18, and 9–19 for comparisons. F_{max}, the maximum rate of rise of force.

elevated). The restitution of contractility had become monotonic after his surgery, rising to a sustained plateau. The form of cardiac defect did not appear to be the cause of the abnormal relationship, for other patients, without heart failure but with similar cardiac defects, had the same characteristics of restitution found in patients with a normal heart [54].

The assertion that the changes in restitution associated with heart failure are not caused by alterations in preload and afterload induced by disease is supported by the following evidence: the restitution of contractility of a papillary muscle from a cat in heart failure secondary to pulmonary artery banding (ascites, elevated ventricular end-diastolic pressure and enlarged liver) was biphasic, whether following the contraction at the basic rate or following an extrasystole (figure 9–20). This stood in marked contrast to the monotonic relationships that were obtained for normal or for hypertrophied cat myocardium in that study [79]. See also figure 9–15.

The changes in the force-interval relationship of the isolated muscle associated with heart failure provide support for the supposition that the changes observed in the patient with heart failure were the result of changes in the intrinsic properties of the cell, and were not alterations in preload and afterload.

**Coupling of the Effects of Hypertrophy on the SR
and on the Force-Interval Relationship**

The enhanced potentiation which is found in some forms of hypertrophy indicates that the availability of activator calcium during the post-extrasystole is enhanced. For this to occur, the sarcoplasmic reticulum must have an enhanced ability to release calcium. Alternatively, sarcolemmal function may be altered to allow a greater amount of calcium to enter the cell during the extrasystole or the post-extrasystole.

The hypothesis of greater availability of activator calcium, obtained from the sarcoplasmic reticulum, is supported by morphologic and biochemical observations in the hypertrophied heart. Although a reduction of calcium-binding by the sarcoplasmic reticulum has been found in severe forms of hypertrophy [90], the calcium exchangeable fraction of sarcoplasmic reticulum was found to be higher for hearts in the early stage of hypertrophy than for controls [36]. This suggests that higher intracellular stores are present in hypertrophied hearts. The morphologic evidence for a relative increase in sarcoplasmic reticulum in some forms of hypertrophy [91] also lends weight to the possibility of greater calcium storage capacity in the hypertrophied myocardium.

The hypothesis that greater levels of activator calcium might be available in the hypertrophied heart is reasonable from a teleological standpoint. One might imagine that the patient with a hypertrophied heart has to have a greater reserve of activator calcium in order for his or her heart to respond to the normal daily transient increases in stress. When the patient exercises, for instance, the increased availability of activator calcium would provide a mechanism through which the heart can respond to the increased workload and increase its output.

Evolution from Hypertrophy to Heart Failure

In many congenital and acquired cardiac defects, hypertrophy evolves over time into heart failure. In animal models, the ability of the myocardium to compensate for a time in response to pressure overload, but then to fail, has been demonstrated on many occasions. The range of changes in the force-interval relationship, found in the normal, the hypertrophied, and the failing myocardium, demonstrate that marked changes in membrane function occur with time and with the severity of the cardiovascular defect. However, studies which monitor the simultaneous evolution of membrane function and the associated changes in the characteristics of the force-interval relationship, through the process of hypertrophy to heart failure, have yet to be performed.

Heart Failure and Membrane Function

The presence of post-extrasystolic depression and slowed or biphasic restitutions of contractility in the failing heart indicate that significant changes have occurred in the systems that control calcium movement and its intracellular storages, release, and compartmentalization. In the presence of severe hypertrophy, cardiomyopathy, or congestive heart failure, SR vesicles have a depressed ability to take up calcium and to release it. Such reduction in SR function has been related directly to the severity of the disease process [9].

The depressed ability of SR to take up calcium is consistent with the longer contraction frequently seen in heart failure. By prolonging the time needed to lower cytosolic calcium, the duration of the contraction and the relaxation period are prolonged. The decreased ability of the SR to take up calcium could lead to a greater loss of calcium from the cell, e.g., through sodium-calcium exchange, making other mechanisms more important in the control of cytosolic calcium. The morphologic decrease in the amount of sarcoplasmic reticulum, which has been observed in some failing hearts, will also decrease calcium availability. The depressed ability to take up calcium and the lowered calcium stores will decrease the amount of available activator calcium and produce the weakened force of contraction that is observed in the failing heart.

Changes in sarcolemmal function with disease could also contribute to a decrease in activator calcium. For example, enhanced Na^+-K^+-ATPase has been observed in heart failure. This could lower intracellular sodium concentration, resulting in a reduction in cell stores of calcium as a consequence of the Na-Ca exchange system.

Altered Membrane Function and Changes in Post-Extrasystolic Potentiation and the Restitution of Contractility Induce by Heart Failure

A decrease in the amount of the intracellular calcium which is available with activation could affect the restitution of contractility in several ways. By having less calcium available for release, the cell would not be able to modulate activator calcium over the wide range found in the normal cell. Little difference might then be found between the force of contracting of the extrasystole that closely follows the contraction at the basic rate and the force in that previous contraction.

A more complex derangement of cell calcium control is required to explain the biphasic curve of restitution observed in some failing hearts (figures 9–18 and 9–20). The amount of available activator calcium must increase with time and then fall in order to produce the observed rise and fall in the maximum rate of rise of pressure or force. It has been suggested that such a more complex scheme of activator calcium availability is present in normal myocardium, as in the findings of Edman and Johannsen [23]. Certainly, catecholamine stimulation can induce these effects in the normal myocardium [70, 92]. Refer to figure 9–4.

An increase and a subsequent decline in the availability of activator calcium in heart failure suggests that the myocyte cannot maintain a constant amount of calcium in a releasable form over a physiological interval of time. The loss of calcium from the release site could take place by any of several mechanisms.

Calcium could gradually leak from the release site into the cytosol, could then be extruded across the sarcolemma through sodium-calcium exchange, or be accumulated in an intracellular compartment which does not participate in excitation-contraction coupling from beat to beat (e.g., the mitochondria).

Although the absence of post-extrasystolic potentiation associated with heart failure can be explained by the assumption that there are decreasing intracellular stores of calcium as a result of alterations in uptake and storage, the presence of post-extrasystolic depression and potentiation in the same heart requires the participation of other mechanisms.

Recall that the extent of post-extrasystolic potentiation can be considered to result, in part, from transsarcolemmal influx of calcium during the extrasystole. Using this concept, the following models, which combine a blunting of calcium influx and a depletion of intracellular calcium stores, can explain how the same heart can produce post-extrasystolic depression and potentiation.

The time-dependent recovery of the systems which control transsarcolemmal movement of calcium [1, 2], such as the slow calcium channel, could reduce the availability of calcium during the post-extrasystole. A prolongation of the time required for the recovery of the transsarcolemmal inward movement of calcium following activation would result in a decreased calcium movement into the cell when it is depolarized shortly after the previous action potential. This would cause greater post-extrasystolic potentiation after extrasystoles with relatively longer extrasystolic intervals. However, this model would not account for the enhanced force of contraction observed in the premature extrasystole.

Although a time-dependent recovery of sarcoplasmic reticulum ability to release calcium has been described [32], a time-dependent recovery of the ability of the sarcoplasmic reticulum to pump calcium has not. An exaggeration of such a characteristic, or one induced by disease, could explain the effects of heart failure on the force-interval relationship. Soon after depolarization, the sarcoplasmic reticulum would be least effective in pumping calcium. This would allow calcium, made available transsarcolemmally, to reach the myofilaments and so produce a premature extrasystole which contracts more forcefully than the previous contraction at the basic rate. The decreased ability of the sarcoplasmic reticulum to take up calcium would result in a greater loss of cytosolic calcium to sites other than the sarcoplasmic reticulum, during the most premature extrasystole, producing post-extrasystolic depression. During extrasystoles with longer extrasystolic intervals, the recovery of more effective sarcoplasmic reticulum calcium uptake would allow greater filling of intracellular stores and so post-extrasystolic potentiation.

Models which combine a time-dependent recovery of transsarcolemmal calcium movement and alterations in sarcoplasmic reticulum function can account for the enhanced force of contraction of the extrasystole, post-extrasystolic depression after an extrasystole with a short extrasystolic interval, and post-extrasystolic potentiation after an extrasystole with a longer extrasystolic interval.

Such explanations imply that alterations in the restitution of contractility, induced in disease states, make manifest normal processes which are ordinarily obscured by other systems during the normal function of the heart.

Compensatory Changes During Heart Failure

An alternative exists for interpreting changes in the force-interval relationship induced by disease. Instead of attributing such alterations to abnormalities in membrane function which are central to the fall in myocardial contractility associated with heart failure, the changes in the force-interval relationship could be the consequence of compensatory mechanisms which are induced in response to the overall depression in the ability of the heart to contract and eject blood.

According to this view, the changes in the force-interval relationship in heart failure and in hypertrophy can be considered to be, not the cause of the failure, but byproducts of attempts to compensate for the depression in myocardial function. At first such an interpretation might seem to minimize the changes in function. But in fact it sees them as evidence of the compensatory systems and, as such, of value in exploring the mechanisms used to bolster the function of the failing heart. Such an interpretation is supported by the known effects of sympathomimetic agents on the force-interval relationship of the normal myocardium [70, 92], and the alterations in the sympathetic nervous system which occur with heart failure [14].

Beta Sympathetic Stimulation and the Force-Interval Relationship

When β-agonists such as norepinephrine or isoproterenol are introduced into the bathing medium, the restitution of contractility in the isolated muscle becomes biphasic, and post-extrasystolic potentiation decrease (figure 9–14). Increased concentration of the agent produces post-extrasystolic depression. These changes are similar to those of heart failure. Of course, these sympathomimetic agents markedly enhance the force of contraction, in contrast to the depressed contractile state of the failing myocardium.

A fascinating exception should be noted. Methoxamine is usually considered to be an α-agonist; yet it affects the restitution of contractility in exactly the same manner as isoproterenol or norepinephrine [92]. The rise and fall of the development of force over time after a contraction at the basic rate makes methoxamine a negative inotropic agent (figure 9–21). The difference in the restitution of contractility in the presence and in the absence of methoxamine is analogous to the way in which the biphasic restitution of contractility during heart failure differs from the normal heart.

The effects of such sympathomimetic agents on restitution and post-extrasystolic potentiation are mediated through β-receptors. The effects of

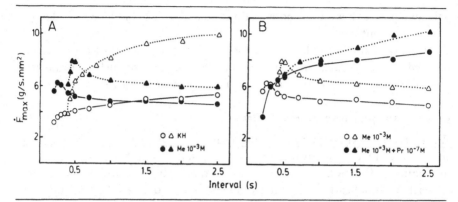

Figure 9–21. Effect of methoxamine on the force-interval relationship of an isolated rabbit right ventricular papillary muscle (see figure 9–4 for pacing protocols and definitions). A: First-stage (circles, solid lines) and second-stage (triangles, dotted lines) curves from muscle prior to (KH; open symbols) and during exposure to 10^{-3} M methoxamine (closed symbols). B: The curves from the muscle during exposure to 10^{-3} M methoxamine (open symbols), and during exposure to both 10^{-3} M methoxamine and 10^{-7} M propranolol (solid symbols). [Reproduced with permission of Pergamon Press Ltd. from Andres Manring, Page A.W. Anderson, Rashid Nassar, and W. Robin Howe. 1983. Can sympathomimetic agents be classified by their action on the force-interval relationship? *Life Sciences* 32:4.]

these agents, including those of methoxamine, are competitively antagonized by propranolol or practolol (figures 9–21 and 9–22).

The changes in the force-interval relationship induced by a β-agonist demonstrate the ability of the normal myocardium to respond in ways which are like those of the failing heart. This suggests that alterations in membrane function, produced by heart failure, are not necessarily pathological, but may be aspects of normal function which are sufficiently amplified to be evident, or by the loss of other normal processes, which otherwise usually obscure these effects. Unlike the changes present in heart failure, however, β-induced ones disappear in normal myocardium within minutes after removal of the β-agonist or are eliminated by a β-antagonist.

Heart Failure and the Response of the Sympathetic Nervous System

The similarity of the effects of sympathomimetic agents on the force-interval relationship to the effects of heart failure suggests that the changes which can be seen in the failing heart may be a result of the chronic stimulation of the myocardium by the sympathetic system.

Changes associated with heart failure in the sympathetic system and its support role have been demonstrated in a large number of studies. During heart failure, the plasma levels of catecholamines and the urinary levels of the byproducts of catecholamine metabolism are markedly increased, while the myocardial concentration of norepinephrine is decreased. The elevated norepinephrine plasma levels have been correlated with the degree of severity

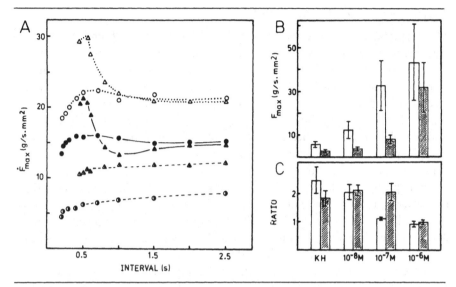

Figure 9–22. Effect of practolol on the isoproterenol-induced changes in the force-interval relationship of isolated rabbit right ventricular papillary muscle (see figure 9–4 for definitions and pacing protocol; P_{max}, the maximum rate of rise of force). Panel A: The first stage (circles) and the second stage (triangles) curves drooped with exposure to 10^{-7} M isoproterenol (open symbols). In the presence of 10^{-6} M practolol and 10^{-7} M isoproterenol, $\dot{F}_{max}$ was less, and post-extrasystolic potentiation was larger and no droop was present (half-filled symbols). Increasing the isoproterenol concentration to 10^{-6} M caused the ratio to fall and the curves to droop (solid symbols), even though practolol was present. Panel B: $\dot{F}_{max}$ of the contraction at the basic rate under control conditions (KH) and in isoproterenol (10^{-8}, 10^{-7}, and 10^{-6}M) are compared in the presence (hatched bars) and the absence (open bars) of 10^{-6} M practolol. Panel C: The force-interval ratio (see figure 9–11 for definition; extrasystolic interval $t_1 = 250$ ms), under control conditions (KH) and in isoproterenol (10^{-8}, 10^{-7}, and 10^{-6} M) are compared in the presence (hatched bars) and the absence (open bars) of 10^{-6} M practolol; N = 6. [Reproduced with permission of Pergamon Press Ltd. from Andres Manring, Page A.W. Anderson, Rashid Nassar, and W. Robin Howe. 1983. Can sympathomimetic agents be classified by their action on the force-interval relationship? *Life Sciences* 32:4 1983.]

of clinical decompensation and to the degree of ventricular depression [14].

An increase in sympathetic activity with heart failure may well be a mechanism for compensation, for norepinephrine has a strong inotropic effect on the myocardium. Although papillary muscles from the failing human heart may have a blunted response to isoproterenol [93, 94], the failing myocardium may be more sensitive to norepinephrine than the normal myocardium [49]. A dependence on extra-cardiac sources of sympathetic stimulation may become greater with worsening heart failure, as shown by the progressive elevation of plasma norepinephrine levels. Such dependence is suggested also by the deleterious effects of beta blockade in some patients with heart failure. In contrast, other investigators have suggested that that β-stimulation is deleterious in itself, and should be blocked in patients with congestive heart failure [15–18].

Norepinephrine Levels in Heart Failure

The surprisingly low myocardial levels of norepinephrine found in patients with heart failure have also been found in many animal models of congestive heart failure [95, 96]. Interestingly, the myocardial content of dopamine is increased in the failing heart [97], while the norepinephrine levels are lower. The depressed tissue levels of norepinephrine can be explained by a reduced cardiac uptake, or by binding. The possibility of enhanced utilization of norepinephrine by the heart is supported by an increase in myocardial norepinephrine turnover rate in the failing heart [98].

In contrast to the low tissue levels, the circulating plasma levels of norepinephrine are elevated [99]. Although the levels might seem to be rather less than would be expected to produce significant pharmacological effects, this is likely not to be the case. Down-regulation of β-receptors has been demonstrated in the failing myocardium of the patient, clearly indicating the presence of elevated β-stimulation [100,101].

Exposure of the failing heart to elevated sympathetic stimulation could be responsible for the changes in the force-interval relationship associated with heart failure, for such changes resemble those produced by β-stimulation in normal myocardium.

Continuous Sympathetic Stimulation and Heart Failure Changes in the Force-Interval Relationship

The heart of the intact patient is obviously exposed to the effects of the sympathetic nervous system. When the isolated papillary muscle is studied, however, the only catecholamines to which it is exposed are those contained within it. Yet the marked alterations in the force-interval relationship remain unchanged after the muscle has been in the tissue bath for hours. Furthermore, exposure of the muscle to propranolol at levels which competitively inhibit the β-effects in the normal myocardium do not affect the alterations in this relationship induced by disease. Although β-stimulation might induce these changes, ongoing sympathetic exposure does not appear to be necessary for their maintenance.

Two alternative hypothese arise from these findings: either

1. the changes in the force-interval relationship induced by disease are due to alterations in cell function which have been caused by symphathetic stimulation and which do not require the continued presence of the agonist for their expression, or
2. the changes in the force-interval relationship associated with heart failure do not result from the altered catecholamine metabolism found in the presence of heart failure but from other mechanisms whose effects are qualitatively similar to those of sympathetic stimulation.

β-agonist Effects on the Cell

β-agonists have a variety of effects on cardiac cells [102–104], among which are the phosphorylation of thin-filament and of membrane-bound proteins (e.g., troponin I and phospholamban, respectively). The phosphorylation of troponin I decreases the affinity of troponin C for calcium and decreases the sensitivity of the myofilaments to calcium [104]. Phosphorylation of the sarcoplasmic-reticulum-bound phospholamban increases the rate of calcium uptake from the cytosol. These effects have been used in suggested explanations for the shortening of the twitch waveform produced by β-stimulation. They do not appear to be a dominant effect in the failing heart, in which the contraction waveform is prolonged.

Although phosphorylation of troponin I and phospholamban has been related to the increase in contractility induced by catecholamines, phosphorylation may not be necessary for the maintenance of the enhancement in contractility. Indeed, in the isolated papillary muscle, the phosphorylation of the contractile proteins is likely to disappear within the time allotted for stabilization of the muscle in the tissue bath [26].

The complex changes induced in the force-interval relationship by catecholamines make alterations in membrane function the most likely cause. It is unlikely that protein phosphorylation would change in such a time-dependent manner, so membrane function would have to have been altered by phosphorylation in such a manner as to acquire this time-dependent characteristic. Calcium availability would first increase, and then fall, after the previous contraction, with transsarcolemmal movement of calcium perhaps depending on time following the previous contraction. In view of the results of studies of isolated muscle preparations, the persistence of such phosphorylation must not be a necessary condition for the presence of the alterations in the force-interval relationship.

With regard to messengers other than calcium that may induce calcium release from intracellular stores, β-agonists could alter the membrane systems so that an increase in the messenger availability or its effectiveness at the release site occurs with time following the previous depolarization. With a further increase in time, these effects would diminish, producing a biphasic restitution of contractility curve.

The Force-Interval Relationship and Dibuteryl Cyclic AMP

Although β-agonists induce changes in cell function through cyclic AMP, this messenger cannot enter the cell from the bathing medium. Dibuteryl cyclic AMP does cross the sarcolemma, and it increases the force of contraction. However, the alterations in the force-interval relationship induced by a β-agonist (figures 9–14, 9–21, and 9–22) are not evoked by this agent. Indeed, post-extrasystolic potentiation is enhanced by dibuteryl cyclic AMP [92].

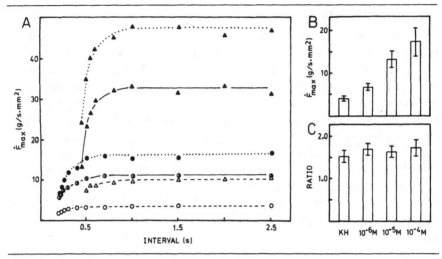

Figure 9–23. Effects of phenylephrine on the force-interval relationship of isolated rabbit right ventricular papillary muscle (see figure 9–4 for pacing protocol and definitions). A: The first-stage (circles) and the second-stage (triangles) curves from a muscle prior to (KH; open symbols, dashed lines) and during exposure to phenylephrine (half-filled symbols, solid lines: 10^{-5} M; filled symbols, dotted lines: 10^{-4} M). B: The maximum rate of rise of force, F_{max}, of the contraction at the basic rate in KH and in phenylephrine (10^{-6}, 10^{-5}, and 10^{-4} M). C: The force-interval ratio (see figure 9–11 for definition; extrasystolic interval $t_1 = 250$ ms) in control conditions and in phenylephrine (N = 9). [Reproduced with permission of Pergamon Press Ltd. from Andres Manring, Page A.W. Anderson, Rashid Nassar, and W. Robin Howe, 1983. Can sympathomimetic agents be classified by their action on the force-interval relationship? *Life Sciences* 32:4.]

These findings suggest that the membrane systems which respond to β stimulation and produce the alterations in the force-interval relationship are being affected by some messenger other than cyclic AMP.

The Force-Interval Relationship and α-Agonists.

Phenylephrine enhances post-extrasystolic potentiation, in contrast to the effects of β-agonists on the force-interval relationship (figure 9–23) [92]. The enhancement of post-extrasystolic potentiation induced by phenylephrine is blocked competitively by phentolamine [92]. Interestingly, α-blockade amplifies the changes in the force-interval relationship, induced by a β-agonist: for example, isoproterenol in the presence of phentolamine produces a greater amount of post-extrasystolic depression and a more prominent biphasic restitution of contractility (figure 9–24).

The enhancement of post-extrasystolic potentiation produced by an α-agonist is similar to the effects of hypertrophy, which also increases post-extrasystolic potentiation. Note that α-agonist stimulation induces cardiac hypertrophy in tissue culture [11–13]. Cell size and protein content increase in response to α-agonist stimulation.

The enhancement in cell growth and the increase in post-extrasystolic

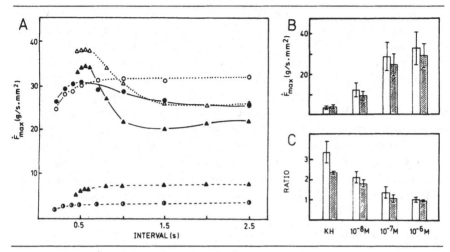

Figure 9–24. Effect of phentolamine on the isoproterenol-induced changes in the force-interval relationship of isolated right ventricular rabbit papillary muscle (see figure 9–4 for definitions and pacing protocol). Panel A: The first-stage curves (circles) and the second-stage curves (triangles) of the same muscle (F_{max}, the maximum rate of rise of force). In 10^{-6} M isoproterenol (open symbols, dotted lines) only the second-stage curve (open triangles) dropped. In 5×10^{-6} M phentolamine and no isoproterenol, the curves (half-filled symbols, dashed line) were monotonic. In the presence of 5×10^{-6} M phentolamine and 10^{-6} M isoproterenol, the first-stage curve (filled circles, solid line) drooped and the droop in the second-stage curve (filled triangles, solid line) was accentuated. Panel B: F_{max} of the contraction at the basic rate under control conditions (KH) and in isoproterenol (10^{-8}, 10^{-7}, and 10^{-6} M) are compared in the presence of (hatched bars) and the absence (open bars) of 5×10^{-6} M phentolamine. Panel C: The force-interval ration (see figure 9–11 for definitions; extrasystolic interval t_1 = 200 ms) under control conditions (KH) and in 10^{-8} 10^{-7}, 10^{-6} M) are compared in the presence (hatched bars) and absence (open bars) of 5×10^{-6} M phentolamine; N = 6. [Reproduced with permission of Pergamon Press Ltd. from Andres Manring, Page A.W. Anderson, Rashid Nassar, and W. Robin Howe. 1983. Can sympathomimetic agents be classified by their action on the force-interval relationship? *Life Sciences* 32:4.]

potentiation induced by α-agonists suggest a corollary hypothesis with regard to the effect of development. During normal growth, cell size increases and post-extrasystolic potentiation is enhanced, as in the case of hypertrophy. With regard to the role of α-agonists in these maturational effects, note that the density of cardiac α-adrenoceptors predominate in the neonatal period and have been shown in the mouse to decline thereafter [105]. This suggests that the mechanisms through which α-agonists affect cell growth and membrane control of cytosolic calcium may be the same as those which the organism uses to produce the cellular response described in the mild hypertrophy of development, and that in response to some disease states.

SUMMARY

The availability of activator calcium is greatly modulated by the cellular processes that give rise to the force-interval relationship of the normal myocardium. Just as vesicular SR function is affected by hypertrophy and heart failure, so qualitative, and sometimes quantitative, changes are induced in the force-interval relationship by disease states. In hypertrophy, the alterations may be a reflection of a stimulus, such as α-agonist stimulation, which induces hypertrophy of the developing heart and which may participate in the process of hypertrophy in response to the stress of a disease process. In heart failure, the alterations (sometimes highly distinctive) in the force-interval relationship may be the result of the chronic β-stimulation which is present in the clinical state of heart failure. Although such stimulation may be necessary to support the failing heart, the alterations in the force-interval relationship found in some patients with heart failure could be used as evidence that β-blockade may be of clinical value in some forms of heart failure.

ACKNOWLEDGEMENTS

The author wishes to thank Dr. Rashid Nassar for his helpful review of the chapter; Chris Brown, Annette Oakeley, and J.H. Johnson for their assistance in illustrating and reviewing the manuscript; and Deborah Hudgins for preparing the manuscript.

REFERENCES

1. Tritthart, H., Kaufmann, R., Volkmer, H-P., Bayer, R., and Krause, H. 1973. Ca-movement controlling myocardial contractility. I. Voltage-, current- and time-independence of mechanical activity under voltage clamp conditions (cat papillary muscles and trabeculae). *Pfluegers Arch.* 338:207–231.
2. Trautwein, W., McDonald, T.F., and Tripathi, O. 1975. Calcium conductance and tension in mammalian ventricular muscle. *Pflugers Arch.* 354:55–74.
3. Fabiato, A., and Fabiato, F. 1977. Calcium release from the sarcoplasmic reticulum. *Circ. Res.* 40:119–129.
4. Morad, M., Goldman, Y.E., and Trentham, D.R. 1983. Rapid photochemical inactivation of Ca^{2+}-antagonists shows that Ca^{2+} entry directly activates contraction in frog heart. *Nature* 304:635–638.
5. Philipson, K.D. 1985. Sodium-calcium exchange in plasma membrane vesicles. *Ann. Rev. Physiol.* 45:561–571.
6. Inesi, G. 1985. Mechanism of calcium transport. *Ann. Rev. Physiol.* 47:573–601.
7. Mechmann, S., and Pott, L. 1986. Identification of Na-Ca Exchange Current in Single Cardiac Myocytes. *Nature* 319:597–599.
8. Kimura, J., Noma, A., and Irisawa, H. 1986. Na-Ca exchange current in mammalian heart cells. *Nature* 319:596–597.
9. Newman, W.H. 1983. Biochemical, structural, and mechanical defects of the failing myocardium. *Pharmacol. Ther.* 22:215–247.
10. Johnson, E.A. 1978. Force-interval relationship of cardiac muscle. In *Handbook of Physiology* section 2, volume 1, Berne, R.M., Sperelakis, N., and Geiger, S.R., eds., pp. 475–496 Bethesda: American Physiological Society.
11. Simpson, P., McGrath, A., and Savion, S. 1982. Myocyte hypertrophy in neonatal rat heart cultures and its regulation by serum and by catecholamines. *Circ. Res.* 51:787–801.
12. Simpson, P. 1983. Norepinephrine-stimulated hypertrophy of cultured rat myocardial cells is an alpha$_1$-adrenergic response. *J. Clin. Invest.* 72:732–738.
13. Simpson, P. 1985. Stimulation of hypertrophy of cultured neonatal rat heart cells through an α_1-adrenergic receptor and induction of beating through and α_1- and β_1-adrenergic receptor interaction. Evidence for independent regulation of growth and beating. *Circ. Res.* 56:884–894.

14. Bristow, M.R., Kantrowitz, N.E., Ginsburg, R., and Fowler, M.B. 1985. -Adrenergic Function in Heart Muscle Disease and Heart Failure. *J. Mol. Cell. Cardiol.* 17(2):41–52.
15. Swedberg, K., Waagstein, F., Hjalmarson, A., and Wallentin, I. 1979. Prolongation of survival in congestive cardiomyopathy by beta-receptor blockade. *Lancet* 1:1374–1376.
16. Swedberg, K., Hjalmarson, A., Waagstein, F., and Wallentin, I. 1980. Beneficial effects of long-term beta blockade in congestive cardiomyopathy. *Br. Heart J.* 44:117–133.
17. Waagstein, F., Hjalmarson, A., Varnauskas, E., and Wallentin, I. 1975. Effect of chronic beta-adrenergic receptor blockade in congestive cardiomyopathy. *Br. Heart J.* 37:1022–1036.
18. Opie, L.H., Walpoth, B., and Barsacchi, R. 1985. Calcium and Catecholamines: Relevance to Cardiomyopathies and Significance in Therapeutic Strategies. *J. Mol. Cell. Cardiol.* 17(2):21–34.
19. Fozzard, H.A. 1977. Heart: excitation-contraction coupling. *Ann. Rev. Physiol.* 39:201–210.
20. Bassingthwaighte, J.B. and Reuter, H. 1972. Calcium movements and excitation-contraction coupling in cardiac cells. In *Electrical Phenomena in the Heart*, De Mello, W.C., ed., pp. 353–395. New York: Academic Press.
21. Morad, M., and Goldman, Y. 1973. Excitation-contraction coupling in heart muscle: membrane control of development of tension. In *Progress in Biophysics and Molecular Biology*, vol. 27, Butler, J.A.V., and Noble, D., eds. pp. 257–313. Oxford: Pergamon Press.
22. Antoni, H. Elementary events in excitation-contraction coupling of the mammalian myocardium. *Basic Res. Cardiol.* 72:140–146.
23. Edman, K.A.P., and Johannsson, M. 1976. The contractile state of rabbit papillary muscle in relation to stimulation frequency. *J. Physiol.* 254:565–581.
24. Wohlfart, B. 1979. Relationships between peak force, action potential duration and stimulus interval in rabbit myocardium. *Acta Physiol. Scand.* 106:395–409.
25. Langer, G.A. 1980. The role of calcium in the control of myocardial contractility: An update. *J. Mol. Cell. Cardiol.* 12:231–239.
26. Mensing, H.J., and Hilgemann, D.W. 1981. Inotropic effects of activation and pharmacological mechanisms in cardiac muscle. *Trends Pharmac. Sci.* 2:303–307.
27. Yue, D.T., Burkhoff, D., Franz, M.R., Hunter, W.C., and Sagawa, K. 1985. Post-extrasystolic potentiation of the isolated canine left ventricle. Relationship to mechanical restitution. *Circ Res.* 56:340–350.
28. Burkhoff, D., Yue, D.T., Franz, M.R., Hunter, W.C., Sunagawa, K., Maughan, W.L., and Sagawa, K. Quantitative comparison of the force-interval relationships of the canine right and left ventricles. *Circ. Res.* 54:468–473.
29. Sutko, J.L., Ito, K., and Kenyon, J.L. 1985. Ryanodine: a modifier of sarcoplasmic reticulum calcium release in striated muslce. *Fed. Proc.* 44:2984–2988.
30. Wier, W.G., Yue, D.T., and Marban, E. 1985. Effects of ryanodine on intracellular Ca^{2+} transients in mammalian cardiac muscle. *Fed. Proc.* 44:2989–2993.
31. Wier, W.G., and Yue, D.T. 1986. Intracellular, calcium, transients underlying the short-term force-interval relationship in ferret ventricular myocardium. *J. Physiol.* (in press)
32. Fabiato, A. and Baumgarten, C.M. 1984. Methods for detecting calcium release from the sarcoplasmic reticulum of skinning cardiac cells and the relationships between calculated transsarcolemmal calcium movements and calcium release. In *Physiology and Pathophysiology of the Heart*, Sperelakis, N., ed., pp. 215–254. Boston: Martinus Nijhoff Publishing.
33. Morgan, J.P. 1985. The effects of digitalis on intracellular calcium transients in mammalian working myocardium as detected with aequorin. *J. Mol. Cell. Cardiol.* 17:1065–1075.
34. Fabiato, A. 1986. Inositol^{1,4,5} trisophosphate-induced release of Ca^{2+} from the sarcoplasmic reticulum of skinning cardiac cells. *Biophys. J.* 49:190a.
35. Lamers, J.M.J., Stinis, J.T., Kort, W.J., and Huelsmann, W.C. 1978. Biochemical studies on the sarcolemmal function in the hypertrophied rabbit heart. *J. Mol. Cell. Cardiol.* 10:235–248.
36. Villani, F.P., Pelosi, G., Agliati, G., Piccinini, F., and Pensa, P. 1976. Calcium exchangeable fraction of sarcoplasmic reticulum in hypertrophic dog heart. *Pharmacology* 14:140–147.
37. Wyse, R.K.H., and Welham, K.C., Jones, M., Silove, E.D., and de Leval, M.R. 1983. Hemodynamics, regional myocardial blood flow, and sarcoplasmic reticulum calcium uptake in right ventricular hypertrophy and failure. In *Advances in Myocardiology*, vol. 4, Chazov, E., Saks, V., and Rona, G., eds., pp. 97–105. New York: Plenum Medical Book Co.
38. Lamers, J.M.J., and Stinis, J.T. 1979. Defective calcium pump in the sarcoplasmic reticulum

of the hypertrophied rabbit heart. *Life Sci.* 34:2313–2320.

39. Dhalla, N.S., Das, P.K., and Sharma, G.P. 1978. Subcellular basis of cardiac contractile failure. *J. Mol. Cell. Cardiol.* 10:363–385.
40. Lentz, R.M. Harrison, Jr. C.E., Dewey, J.D., Barnhorst, D.A., Danielson, G.K., and Pluth, J.R. 1978. Functional evaluation of cardiac sarcoplasmic reticulum and mitochondria in human pathologic states. *J. Mol. Cell. Cardiol.* 10:3–30.
41. Prasad, K., Khatter, J.C., and Bharadwaj, B. 1979. Intra- and extracellular electrolytes and sarcolemmal ATPase in the failing heart due to pressure overload in dogs. *Cardiovasc. Res.* 13:95–104.
42. Limas, C.J. and Cohn, J.N. 1977. Defective calcium transport by cardiac sarcoplasmic reticulum in spontaneously hypertensive rats. *Circ. Res.* 40:I, 62–69.
43. Gwathmey, J.K. and Morgan, J.P. 1985. Altered calcium handling in experimental pressure-overload hypertrophy in the ferret. *Circ. Res.* 57:836–843.
44. Ito, Y., Suko, J., and Chidsey, C.A. 1974. Intracellular calcium and myocardial contractility v. calcium uptake of sarcoplasmic reticulum fractions in hypertrophied and failing rabbit hearts. *J. Mol. Cell. Cardiol.* 6:237–247.
45. Mead, R.J., Peterson, M.B., and Welty, J.D., 1971. Sarcolemmal and sarcoplasmic reticular ATPase activities in the failing canine heart. *Circ. Res.* 29:14–20.
46. Gertz, E.W., Stam, Jr. A., Bajusz, E., and Sonnenblick, E.H. 1972. A biochemical defect in the function of the sarcoplasmic reticulum in the hereditary cardiomyopathy of the Syrian hamster. In *Recent Advances in Studies on Cardiac Structure and Metabolism*, vol. 1, Bajusz, E. and Rona, G., eds., pp. 243–250. Baltimore: University Park Press.
47. Anderson, P.A.W., Manring, A., Arentzen, C.E., Rankin, J.S., and Johnson, E.A. 1977. Pressure-induced hypertrophy of cat right ventricle. An evaluation with the force-interval relationship. *Circ. Res.* 41:582–588.
48. Pannier, J.L. 1971. Contractile state of papillary muscles obtained from cats with moderate right ventricular hypertrophy. *Arch. Int. Physiol. Biochim.* 79:743–752.
49. Spann, Jr. J.F., Buccino, R.A., Sonnenblick, E.H., and Braunwald E. 1967. Contractile state of cardiac muscle obtained from cats with experimentally produced ventricular hypertrophy and heart failure. *Circ. Res.* 21:341–354.
50. Grimm, A.F., Kubota, R., and Whitehorn, W.V. 1963. Properties of myocardium in cardiomegaly. *Circ. Res.* 12:118–124.
51. Fisher, V.J. Kavaler, F. 1971. Maximal force development by hypertrophied right ventricular papillary muscles remaining in situ. In *Cardiac Hypertrophy*, Alpert, N.R., ed., pp. 371–385. New York: Academic Press.
52. Bing, O.H.L., Matsushita, S., Fanburg, B.L., Levine, H.J. 1971. Mechanical properties of rat cardiac muscle during experimental hypertrophy. *Circ. Res.* 28:234–245.
53. Kerr, A.R., Winterberger, A.R., and Giambattista, M. 1961. Tension developed by papillary muscles from hypertrophied rat hearts. *Circ. Res.* 9:103–105.
54. Anderson, P.A.W., Manring, A., Serwer, G.A., Benson, D.W., Edwards, S.B., Armstrong, B.E., Sterba, R.J., and Floyd IV, R.D. The force-interval relationship of the left ventricle. *Circulation* 60:334–348.
55. Anderson, P.A.W., Manring, A. Johns, P., Gilbert, P.P., and Johnson, E.A. 1977. Force-interval relationship in the intact heart. *Circulation* 56(2):231.
56. Braveny, P, and Kruta, V. 1958. Dissociation de deux facteurs: restitution et potentiation dans l'action de l'intervalle sur l'amplitude de la contraction du myocarde. *Arch. Int. Physiol. Biochim.* 66:633–652.
57. Anderson, P.A.W., Manring, A., Sommer, J.R., and Johnson, E.A. 1976. Cardiac muscle: An attempt to relate structure to function. *J. Mol. Cell. Cardiol.* 8:123–143.
58. Nassar, R., Reedy, M.C., and Anderson, P.A.W. 1983. Isolated ventricular myocytes: Electron microscopic and contractile characteristics. *Fed. Proc.* 43:819.
59. Nassar, R., Anderson, P.A.W., and Reedy, M.C. 1984. Sarcomere dynamics in the isolated myocyte: the interaction of calcium and the pattern of stimulation. *Biophys. J.* 45:158a.
60. Anderson, P.A.W., Reedy, M.C., and Nassar, R. 1986. Structure-function comparisons in cardiac myocytes from adult and three-week-old rabbits. *Biophys. J.* 49:81a.
61. Bassett, A.L. and Gelband, H. 1973. Chronic partial occlusion of the pulmonary artery in cats change in ventricular action potential configuration during early hypertrophy. *Circ. Res.* 32:15–26.
62. Kaufmann, R.L., Homburger, H., and Wirth, H. 1971. Disorder in excitation-contraction

coupling of cardiac muscle from cats with experimentally produced right ventricular hypertrophy. *Circ. Res.* 28:346–357.

63. Konishi, T. 1965. Electrophysiological study on hypertrophied cardiac muscle experimentally produced in the rabbit. *Jap. Circ. J.* 29:491–503.

64. Yue, D.T. 1986. Interrelations between intracellular calcium, strength of contraction, and stimulus interval in the mammalian heart. (Ph.D. dissertation, Johns Hopkins University, Baltimore, 1986).

65. Sommer, J.R. and Johnson, E.A. 1979. Ultrastructure of cardiac muscle. In *Handbook of Physiology*, section 2, volume 1, Berne, R.M. Sperelakis, N., and Geiger, S.R. eds., pp.113–186. Bethesda, American Physiological Society.

66. Jorgensen, A.O., Shen, A. C-Y, and Campbell, K.P. 1985. Ultrastructural localization of calsequestrin in adult rat atrial and ventricular muscle cells. *J. Cell Biol.* 101:257–268.

67. Fabiato, A. 1983. Calcium-induced release of calcium from the cardiac sarcoplasmic reticulum. *Am. J. Physiol.* 245:C1–C14.

68. Allen, D.G., Jewell, B.R., and Wood, E.H., 1976. Studies of the contractility of mammalian myocardium at low rates of stimulation. *J. Physiol.* 254:1–17.

69. Hiraoka, M. and Sano, T. 1976. Role of slow inward current in the genesis of ventricular arrhythmia. *Jap. Circ. J.* 40:1419–1427.

70. Anderson, P.A.W., Manring, A., and Johnson, E.A. 1977. The force of contraction of isolated papillary muscle: a study of the interaction of its determining factors. *J. Mol. Cell. Cardiol.* 9:131–150.

71. Bers, D.M. 1983. Early transient depletion of extracellular Ca during individual cardiac muscle contraction. *Am. J. Physiol.* 244:H462–H468.

72. Fabiato, A. and Fabiato, F. 1978. Calcium-induced release of calcium from the sarcoplasmic reticulum of skinned cells from adult human, dog, cat, rabbit, rat, and frog hearts and from fetal and new born rat ventricles. *Ann. N.Y. Acad. Sci.* 307:491–522.

73. Pidgeon, J., Lab, M., Seed, A., Elzinga, G., Papadoyannis, D., and Noble, M.I.M. 1980. The contractile state of cat and dog heart in relation to the interval between beats. *Circ. Res.* 47:559–567.

74. Burkhoff, D., Yue, D.T., Franz, M.R., Hunter, W.C., and Sagawa, K. 1984. Mechanical restitution of isolated perfused canine left ventricles. *Am. J. Physiol.* 246:H8–H16.

75. Anderson, P.A.W., Manring, A., and Johnson, E.A. 1973. Force-frequency relationship: a basis for a new index of cardiac contractility? *Circ. Res.* 33:665–671.

76. Anderson, P.A.W., Rankin, J.S., Arentzen, C.E., Anderson, R.W., and Johnson, E.A. 1976. Evaluation of the force-frequency relationship as a descriptor of the inotropic state of canine left ventricular myocardium. *Circ. Res.* 39:832–839.

77. Manring, A. and Anderson, P.A.W. 1980. The contractility of cardiac muscle. *CRC Crit. Rev. Bioeng.* 4:165–201.

78. Franz, M.R., Schaefer, J., Schoettler, M., Seed, W.A., and Noble, M.I.M. 1983. Electrical and mechanical restitution of the human heart at different rates of stimulation. *Circ. Res.* 53:815–822.

79. Anderson, P.A.W., Manring, A., Arentzen, C.E., Rankin, J.S., and Johnson, E.A. 1957. Pressure-induced hypertrophy of cat right ventricle. An evaluation with the force-interval relationship. *Circ. Res.* 41:582–588.

80. Maylie, J.G. 1982. Excitation-contraction coupling in neonatal and adult myocardium of cat. *Am. J. Physiol.* 242:H834–H843.

81. Gwathmey, J.K. and Morgan, J.P. 1985. Altered calcium handling in experimental pressure-overload hypertrophy in the ferret. *Circ. Res.* 57:836–843.

82. Meerson, F.Z. and Kapelko, VI. 1972. The contractile function of the myocardium in two types of cardiac adaptation to a chronic load. *Cardiology* 57:183–199.

83. Sasayama, S., Ross, Jr. J., Franklin, D., Bloor, C.M., Bishop, S., and Dilley, R.B. Adaptations of the left ventricle to chronic pressure overload. *Circ. Res.* 38:172–178.

84. Anderson, P.A.W., Glick, K.L., Manring, A., and Crenshaw, C., Jr. 1984. Developmental changes in cardiac contractility in fetal and postnatal sheep: in vitro and in vivo. *Am. J. Physiol.* 247:H371–H379.

85. Schwarz, F., Thormann, J. and Winkler, B. 1975. Frequency potentiation and post-extrasystolic potentiation in patients with and without coronary arterial disease. *Br. Heart J.* 37:514–519.

86. Van Der Werf, T., Van Poelgeest, R., Herbschleb, H.H., Meijler, F.L. 1976. Post-

extrasystolic potentiation in man. *Eur. J. Cardiol.* 4; 131–141.

87. Kvasnicka, J., Liander, B., Broman, H., and Varnauskas, E. 1975. Quantitative evaluation of post-ectopic beats in the normal and failing human heart using indices derived from catheter-tip manometer readings. *Cardiovasc. Res.* 9:336–341.

88. Burkhoff, D., Yue, D.T., Oikawa, R., Flaherty, J.T., Herskowitz, A., Franz M.R., Stewart, S., Baumgartner, W.A., Schaefer, J., Reitz, B.A., Sagawa, K. 1984. Insights into the pathophysiology of cardiomyopathy from studies of isolated supported human hearts. *Circulation* 70(2):46

89. Sink, J.D., Anderson, P.A.W., and Wechsler, A.S. 1985. Postoperative left ventricular contractility in the cardiac surgical patient. An evaluation of the force-interval relationship. *Ann. Thor. Surg.* 40:475–482.

90. Ito, Y., Suko, J., and Chidsey, C.A. 1974. Intracellular calcium and myocardial contractility. V. Calcium uptake of sarcoplasmic reticulum fractions in hypertrophied and failing rabbit hearts. *J. Mol. Cell. Cardiol.* 6:237–247.

91. Singh, S., White, F.C., and Bloor, C.M. 1982. Effect of acute exercise stress in cardiac hypertrophy II. Quantitative ultrastructural changes in the myocardial cell. *Virchows Arch.* 39:293–303.

92. Manring, A., Anderson, P.A.W., Nassar, R., and Howe, W.R. 1983. Can sympathomimetic agents be classified by their action on the force-interval relationship? *Life Sci.* 32:329–336.

93. Ginsburg, R., Bristow, M.R., Billingham, M.E., Stinson, E.B., Schroeder, J.S., and Harrison, D.C. 1983. Study of the normal and failing isolated human heart: Decreased response of failing heart to isoproterenol. *Am. Heart J.* 106:535–540.

94. Ginsburg, R., Esserman, L.J., and Bristow, M.R. 1983. Myocardial performance and extracellular ionized calcium in a severely failing human heart. *Ann. Intern. Med.* 98:603–606.

95. Chidsey, C., Kaiser, G.A., Sonnenblick, E.H., Spann, J.F., and Braunwald, E. 1964. Cardiac norepinephrine stores in experimental heart failure in the dog. *J. Clin. Invest.* 43:2386–2393.

96. Chidsey, C., Braunwald, E., Morrow, A.G., and Mason, D.T. 1963. Myocardial norepinephrine concentration in man. Effects of reserpine and of congestive heart failure. *New Eng. J. Med.* 269:653–658.

97. Sole, M.J., Helke, C.J., and Jacobowitz, D.M. 1982. Increased dopamine in the failing hamster heart: transvesicular transport of dopamine limits the rate of norepinephrine synthesis. *Am. J. Cardiol.* 49:1682–1690.

98. Sole, M.J., Lo, C-M., Laird, C.W., Sonnenblick, E.H., and Wurtman, R.J. 1975. Norepinephrine turnover in the heart and spleen of the cardiomyocpathic Syrian hamster. *Circ. Res.* 37:855–862.

99. Thomas, J.A., and Marks, B.H. 1978. Plasma norepinephrine in congestive heart failure. *Am. J. Cardiol.* 41:233–243.

100. Bristow, M.R., Ginsburg, R., Minobe, W., Cubicciotti, R.S., Sageman, W.S., Lurie, K., Billingham, M.E., Harrison, D.C., and Stinson, E.B. 1982. Decreased catecholamine sensitivity and -adrenergic-receptor density in failing human hearts. *New Eng. J. Med.* 307:205–211.

101. Bristow, M.R. 1984. Myocardial -adrenergic receptor downregulation in heart failure. *Int. J. Cardiol.* 5:648–652.

102. Stull, J.T., Manning, D.R., High, C.W., and Blumenthal, D.K. 1980. Phosphorylation of contractile proteins in heart and skeletal muscle. *Fed. Proc.* 39:1552–1557.

103. Kranias, E.G. and Solaro, R.J. 1983. Coordination of cardiac sarcoplasmic reticulum and myofibrillar function by protein phosphorylation. *Fed. Proc.* 42:33–38.

104. Winegrad, S., McClellan, G., Horowits, R., Tucker, M., Lin, L-E., and Weisberg, A. 1983. Regulation of cardiac contractile proteins by phosophorylation. *Fed. Proc.* 42:39–44.

105. Yamada, S., Yamamura, H.I., and Roeske, W.R. 1980. Ontogeny of mammalian cardiac α_1-adrenergic receptors. *Eur. J. Pharmac.* 68:217–221.

10. RIGHT ATRIAL ULTRASTRUCTURE IN CORONARY ARTERY DISEASE: CHARACTERIZATION OF CHRONIC ISCHEMIA

JOHN J. FENOGLIO, JR. AND TUAN DUC PHAM

Cardiac disease causes changes in cardiac structure that may have functional consequences. For example, an increase in connective tissue may decrease ventricular compliance, alterations in myocardial cell structure may affect contractility, and changes in intercellular junctions may influence impulse initiation and conduction. There have been numerous detailed studies on the ultrastructural changes of ventricular myocardium in both congenital and acquired disease; however, there has been little focus on the changes in atrial ultrastructure in either congenital or acquired disease [1–12]. One of the long-term interests of our laboratory has been atrial ultrastructure and its relationship to cardiac function. In addition to studies in animal models we have studied the atria of patients with both congenital and acquired disease. [13–15].

In congenital heart disease, the atrial myocardium is not primarily affected by a disease process. Changes in atrial ultrastructure are therefore probably related to hemodynamic alterations, such as atrial pressure and/or volume overload, secondary to the congenital anomaly. To determine whether such structural changes occur and whether they are related to hemodynamic alterations, we compared the ultrastructure of atrial tissue from patients with

This study was supported by U.S. Public Health Service Grant HL-12738, HL-30557 and HL-26588 from the National Heart, Lung and Blood Institute, Bethesda, Maryland.

219

ventricular septal defects and normal atrial hemodynamics, patients with atrial septal defects and increased right atrial volume, and patients with endocardial defects and significantly elevated right atrial pressure and volume [4, 5]. The atria of patients with ventricular septal and atrial septal defects were ultrastructurally normal. In contrast, the atria of patients with endocardial cushion defects demonstrated numerous ultrastructural changes. The cells were hypertrophied, measuring up to 24μ in diameter; the nuclei were lobulated; the intercalated discs were focally widened; there was an increase in interstitial connective tissue, and there were scattered degenerating cells, characterized by loss of myofilaments and accumulation of dilated segments of sarcoplasmic reticulum. The results of these studies suggest that changes in right atrial ultrastructure in congenital heart disease are related to alterations in right atrial pressure.

In a companion study, we characterized right atrial ultrastructure in patients with acquired valvular heart disease, including chronic rheumatic heart disease [12]. The structural changes in the patients with chronic rheumatic heart disease were distinctive. These changes included extensive interstitial fibrosis: severe degenerative changes in 10–50% of cells examined and marked cellular hypertrophy with mean cell diameters of 12–21μ. In contrast, the right atria of patients with isolated aortic stenosis and floppy mitral valve demonstrated cellular hypertrophy, with mean cell diameters of 11–19μ but only minimal increases in interstitial connective tissue and rare degenerative changes (less than 2% of cells examined in 2 of 6 patients studied). The mean right atrial pressures were slightly elevated but similar in both groups of patients. These studies suggest that changes in right atrial ultrasturcture are dependent not only on elevations of atrial pressure but also on the underlying disease process.

The conclusions of these structural studies are strengthened by the multivariate analysis of the structural clinical and electrophysiologic data in a large series of patients [16]. These studies suggest that atrial pressure is best correlated with electrophysiologic and ultrastructural alterations in the right atrial and the occurence of atrium fibrillation.

None of these studies, however, has considered whether the structural and ultrastructural changes described are secondary to ischemia, nor have structural and ultrastructural changes associated with chronic ischemia been well characterized in human atrium. The purpose of the present study was to characterize the structural and ultrastructural changes in the human atrium that are associated with chronic ischemia. Right atrial specimens from fourteen patients with multivessel coronary artery disease were studied. In each of these patients, there was significant disease of the right coronary artery. The structural and ultrastructural changes in the atria of these patients are different from the structural and ultrastructural changes described in patients with valvular heart disease [9, 12] or congenital heart disease [4, 5]. It seems likely that these changes are related to chronic ischemia.

MATERIALS AND METHODS

Patients Studied

Fourteen patients with multiple vessel coronary artery disease, documented by arteriography, were included in this study (table 10–1). Each patient had occulsive lesions (greater than 75% luminal narrowing) in at least two coronary arteries, including the right coronary artery. Twelve patients had a history of a previous myocardial infarct, and two patients (1 and 2) had ECG evidence of ischemic damage to the myocardium but no documented history of a previous myocardial infarct. All patients had a history of angina, and three patients (3, 6 and 11) had ventricular premature beats. The patients ranged in age from 38 to 57 years; their average age was 50 years. Four patients underwent right heart catheterization (patients 1, 2, 4 and 6) and, in each patient, the right atrial mean pressures were normal (less than 5mm Hg). At the time of surgery, the right atrium was mildly dilated in patient 3, but of normal size in the other 13 patients.

Tissue Preparation

The atrial tissue was obtained adjacent to the atriotomy site on the anterior wall of the right atrium in all patients. In ten patients, the tissue was fixed in phosphate-buffered (pH 7.3) 2.5% glutaraldehyde after electrophysiologic study as previously described [17]. In four patients (2, 4, 9 and 14) the tissue was divided into 1×1 mm blocks and fixed in the operating room for morphometric analysis. All tissue was fixed overnight and then postfixed for one hour in 1 percent osmium tetroxide in 0.1 molar phosphate buffer (pH 7.3). The tissue was rinsed in phosphate buffer, dehydrated in graded acetones, and embedded in Durcupan ACM. Flat silicone embedding molds were used to facilitate orientation of muscle fibres to the endocardium [8]. Thick sections (0.5 to 1μ) were cut with glass knives on a Sorvall MT-2 ultramicrotome from all tissue blocks and stained with 1 percent toluidine blue. Ultrathin section (60–80 nm) were cut with a diamond knife on a Sorvall MT-2 ultramicrotome, stained with uranyl acetate and lead citrate and examined with a Philips EM 300 electron microscope at 80 kV.

Cell size and the degree of interstitial fibrosis were evaluated from thick sections. Cell size was determined by measuring cell diameters at the nuclear level of longitudinally sectioned cells with a calibrated eyepiece. The degree of interstitial fibrosis was graded on a 0 to 3+ scale as follows: 0 = no increase, 1+ = diffuse increase of collagen in all fields, 2+ = separation of bundles of myofibers by dense collagen, and 3+ = separation of individual cells within bundles of myofibers by dense collagen. The incidence of ultrastructural changes in the right atrium was evaluated from low power (×3,500) electron micrographs. At least 4 blocks and about 600 cells were studied in each patient. The cells with ultrastructural changes were counted and an approximate incidence of each change calculated. The incidence of Z-band and intercalated

Table 10-1. Clinical and Structural Findings

	Clinical Findings			Structural Findings**				
Patient	Age (yrs) & Sex	Diagnosis*	Cell Size† (μ)	Z Band	Disc	Glycogen	Fibrosis
CAD Patients							
1	38 M	LAD, RC	12	0	0	1+	0
2	42 M	LAD, RC	13	1%	5%	3+	1+
3	46 M	LAD, LC, RC	12	0	1%	2+	1+
4	48 F	LAD, LM, RC	13	0	3%	3+	1+
5	48 M	LAD, LC, RC	13	1%	0	1+	1+
6	48 M	LAD, RC	11	5%	1%	2+	1+
7	50 M	LAD, LM, RC	13	1%	1%	3+	1+
8	50 F	LAD, RC	14	0	0	3+	1+
9	51 M	LAD, RC	12	1%	0	3+	1+
10	52 M	LAD, LC, RC	11	0	0	1+	1+
11	54 M	LAD, LC, RC	12	1%	0	1+	0
12	54 F	LAD, RC	13	0	0	1+	0
13	56 M	LM, RC	13	1%	1%	2+	1+
14	57 M	LAD, RC	12	5%	1%	3+	1+
AS Patients							
1	45 M	AS	10	1%	0	0	0
2	53 F	AS	10	1%	0	0	0

* Site of major coronary artery lesion determined by coronary arteriography prior to coronary by-pass surgery, or pathologic diagnosis.
† Average cell diameter measured at the nuclear level.
** STRUCTURAL FINDINGS:
 Z band and Disc: Percentage of cells and discs examined with changes (see text).
 Glycogen: Grading of increased glycogen (see text):
  1+ = confined to perinuclear region;
  2+ = expanded to intercalated disc;
  3+ = extended to subsarcolemmal region.
 Fibrosis: Extent of fibrosis as assessed by light microscopy:
  1+ = increased interstitial and perivascular fibrous tissue;
  2+ = separation of group of myocytes;
  3+ = separation of individual myocytes.

AS = Aortic Stenosis; CAD = Coronary Artery Disease; Disc = widened, irregular intercalated discs; F = female; M = male; LAD = left anterior descending coronary artery; LC = left circumflex coronary artery; RC = right coronary artery; Z band = accumulation of Z-band-like material.

disc changes are expressed as the percent of the total cell population studied in table 10-1. Glycogen accumulation was variable but present in all cells studied. The extent of glycogen accumulation was graded on a 0 to 3+ scale as follows: 0 = no inclusion, 1+ = small inclusion confined to the perinuclear region, 2+ = moderate inclusion at both perinuclear and between myofibrils, and 3+ = extensive inclusion extending to subsarcolemmal regions.

Morphometric Study

Five blocks of tissue that contained longitudinally oriented myocardial cells were selected from each of the four patients in whom atrial tissue was fixed in the operating room for morphometric study. Ultrathin 60 nm sections were cut from these blocks and mounted on formvar-coated 100 mesh grids. Each grid was systematically scanned and longitudinally sectioned cardiac cells with centrally located nuclei and distinct intercalated discs at both ends of the cells were photographed. A total of five cells were photographed from each block and a total of 25 cells from each patient were analyzed. The electron microscope was calibrated daily using a diffraction grating replica and the electron micrographs photographically enlarged to a final magnification of 9,000x. The electron micrographs were overlaid with a transparent plastic sheet with a test lattice which has 10 mm spacings. The lattice was placed on the electron micrographs in order that the horizontal lines of the lattice formed 19° angles with the longitudinal axis of the myofibrils [18, 19]. Intersections of the lines were used as points, and the points over different components of cardiac cells were counted. Volume fractions of myofibrils, mitochondria, glycogen inclusions, and others (nucleus, Golgi apparatus, lipofuscin, lipid droplets, and "clear" sarcoplasm) were calculated according to standard point-counting techniques [20].

Control Patients

Our unpublished studies have indicated that the right atrial cells of patients with aortic valvular disease are "normal" if the right atrial pressure is not elevated, and the atrium is not dilated. Atrial tissue of two patients with aortic stenosis and normal right atrial pressure (less than 5 mm Hg) was immediately fixed in the operating room and processed as described above for both routine electron microscopic study and morphometric analysis. The patients were included in this study only after the routine electron microscopic study confirmed that the atrial cells were not hypertrophied, and severely degenerative changes were not present. The clinical and structural findings in these patients are included in table 10-1.

RESULTS

Cell Size and Interstitium:

The majority of the right atrial cells were slightly enlarged in all patients. The diameters of these cells ranged from 6 to 16u, with a mean value of 12µ.

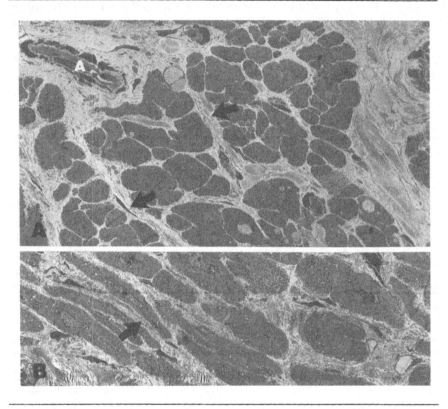

Figure 10-1. At low magnification (Panel A), the increased connective tissue was most prominent around blood vessels (A) and between muscle bundles (arrows). Focally (Panel B), there was increase connective tissue between individual myocytes and with slight separation of myocytes (arrow).

Panel A × 1,000
Panel B × 1,125

Eleven of the fourteen patients had increased amounts of connective tissue around blood vessels and between muscle bundles (figure 10-1, panel A) or between individual cardiac cells (figure 10-1, panel B). The interstitial connective tissue consisted of normal appearing bundles of collagen fibers, elastic materials and scattered fibroblasts.

Cell Structure

Myofibrils were arranged orderly and did not increase in number even in enlarged atrial cells. In general, two to six myofibrils could be seen across the width of the cells. The sarcomeres were normal with distinct A, I, and Z bands. Focal widening of Z bands was found in eight patients (table 10-1) but in less than 5 percent of the cells examined.

Prominent inclusions of glycogen particles were present in most atrial cells

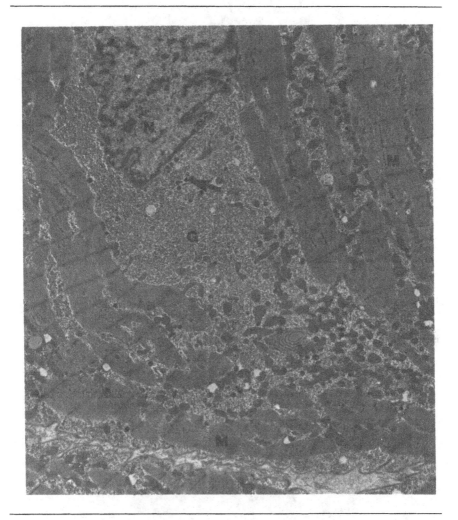

Figure 10–2. The amount of glycogen appeared increased in all atrial cells. In this cell, the increased glycogen (G) was most prominent at the perinuclear region and displaced the myofibrils (M) to the periphery of the cell. Atrial-specific granules (arrows) were numerous. The nucleus (N) appeared normal.

× 6,500

of patients with coronary artery disease. The extent of glycogen accumulation was graded on a scale of 0 to 3+ (table 10–1). In two patients (4 and 14) glycogen inclusions were associated with large aggregates of lipofuscin. In the majority of the atrial cells, glycogen inclusions were most prominent (figure 10–2) but were limited to the perinuclear regions (Grade 1). In other cells (figure 10–3), glycogen inclusions expanded from the perinuclear regions to the intercalated discs (Grade 2). In the most severely affected cells (figure 10–4), glycogen inclusions extended to the periphery of the cells (Grade 3).

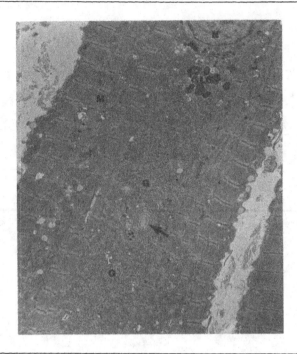

Figure 10–3. In cells with separated myofibrils, accumulations of glycogen (G) extended beyond the perinuclear region and were interspersed between individual myofibrils (M). The central region of the cells was filled with glycogen inclusions which often extended to the intercalated discs. N = nucleus; Arrow = Golgi apparatus; LG = lipofuscin granules.

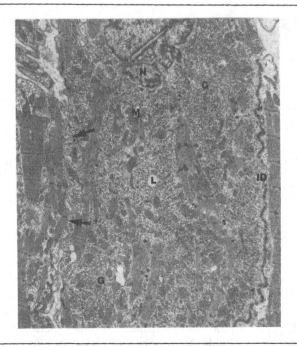

Figure 10–4. In severely affected cells, the accumulation of glycogen (G) extended to the intercalated disc (ID) as well as to the sarcolemma (arrows). The myofibrils were in disarray. N = nucleus; L = lipid.

× 7,000

Accumulation of dilated segments of sarcoplasmic reticulum was not observed in areas of glycogen accumulation. In table 10–1, the numbers represent the amount of glycogen accumulation present in the majority of the atrial cells examined.

Mitochondria were variable in size and shape, but giant forms were not seen. Large mitochondria often showed electron lucent areas with focal disintegration of cristae (figure 10–5). The majority of small mitochondria were slim, elongated projections of the large ones. These small mitochondria had one or two cristae and a dense matrix. Both types of mitochondria were found in the perinuclear regions and between myofibrils and glycogen inclusions. A Golgi apparatus and numerous atrial specific granules were often found in the perinuclear regions. Lipid droplets were abundant in some atrial cells and were either juxtaposed to mitochondria or in areas of glycogen inclusions (figure 10–6). An elliptical nucleus, often with prominent nucleoli, was situated at the center of the atrial cells.

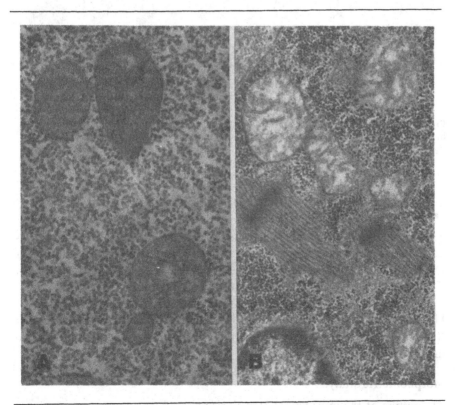

Figure 10–5. Electron-lucent central areas (Panel A) and focal crista degeneration (Panel B) were present in scattered mitochondria. The majority of mitochondria, however, appeared normal with regular cristae.

Panels A & B: × 32,800

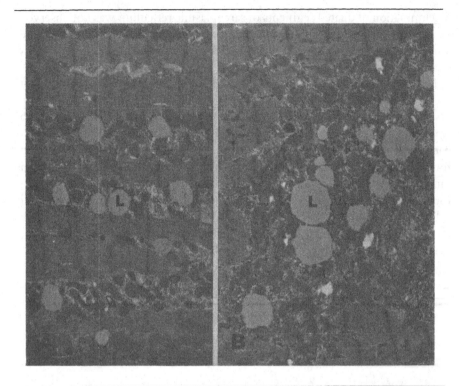

Figure 10-6. In some atrial cells, lipid droplets (L) were numerous and were present both between myofibrils (Panel A) and in areas with accumulation of glycogen and mitochondria (Panel B).

Panels A & B: × 9,900

Sarcolemma and Cell Junctions

The sarcolemma of the atrial cells was normal and the basement lamina was not thickened. Irregular invaginations of the sarcolemma to form T-tubules were found in less than 1% of the atrial cells examined in two patients. T-tubules were not found in the atrial cells of the other 14 patients.

The majority of intercalated discs were normal (figure 10-7 panel A). However, about 5 percent of intercalated discs were widened and irregular (figure 10-7, panel B) in five patients. Both side-to-side and end-to-end intercalated discs were present.

Morphometric Study:

The results of the morphometric analysis in the four patients with coronary artery disease and in the two patients with aortic stenosis are summarized in table 2. The volume fractions of myofibrils and mitochondria were significantly decreased in the atrial cells of patients with coronary artery

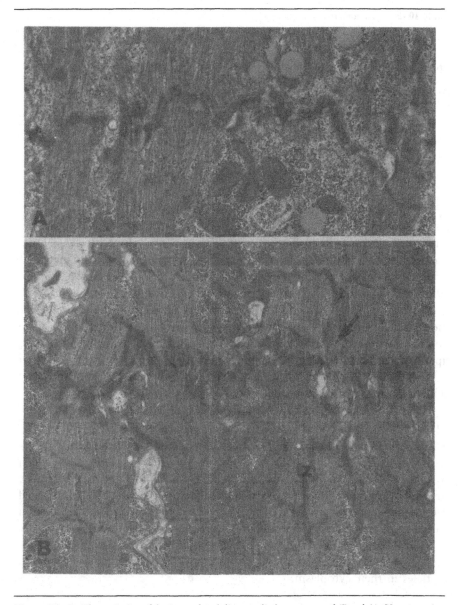

Figure 10–7. The majority of the intercalated discs studied were normal (Panel A). However, in seven patients, about 5% of the intercalated discs were widened and irregular (Panel B). These abnormal discs were associated with accumulation of Z-band (Z) and fibrillar material (arrow).

Panel A: × 20,400

Panel B: × 16,500

Table 10–2. Morphometric Analysis

Group	N	Diameter*	Volume Fraction				
			Myofibrils	Mitochondria	Glycogen	Sarcoplasm	Others[†]
AS	50	10.0 μ	50.3±7.1%	26.5±4.6%	2.1±1.3%	14.8±8.3%	6.06%
CAD	100	12.5 μ	36.9±5.3%	12.5±3.2%	11.4±6.3%	29.7±7.3%	8.98%

AS = aortic stenosis; CAD = coronary artery disease; N = number of cells measured in each group of patients;
* mean cell diameter measured at the level of the nucleus; + AS = mean value of the following structures: nucleus
(5.10±4.25%), Golgi apparatus (0.25±0.21%), lipofuscin (0.31±0.31%), lipid droplets (0.16±0.26%), atrial-specific granules (0.24±0.24%). † CAD = nucleus (6.78±5.24%), Golgi apparatus (0.29±0.39%), lipofuscin (1.42±1.25%), lipid droplets (0.18±0.32%), atrial-specific granules (0.31±0.55%).

disease (36.9 ± gp 5.3% and 12.5 ± gp 3.2%) as compared to those of patients with aortic stenosis (50.3 ± 7.1% and 26.5 ± 4.6%). In contrast, volume fractions of glycogen inclusions and *clear* sarcoplasm were markedly increased in the atrial cells of patients with coronary artery disease (11.4 ± 6.3% and 29.7 ± 7.3%) as compared to those of patients with aortic stenosis (2.3 ± 1.3% and 14.8 ± gp 8.3%). The *clear* sarcoplasm was arbitrarily defined as areas of the atrial cells occupied by scattered glycogen particles or empty spaces. The volume fractions of other cell organelles such as the nucleus, Golgi apparatus, lipid droplets and atrial specific granules, were approximately 9% in the atrial cells of patients with coronary artery disease as compared to 6% in the atrial cells of patients with aortic stenosis.

DISCUSSION

The most striking ultrastructural changes in the right atrial cells of the patients with coronary artery disease were extensive accumulation of glycogen particles and abnormal reduction of myofibrils and mitochondria. Moreover, myofibrils and mitochondria were displaced toward the periphery of enlarged cells by glycogen inclusions. Although the extent of glycogen accumulation varied from cell to cell and from patient to patient, it was present in virtually every atrial cell examined and in all patients with coronary artery disease. Thus the hallmark of ischemic atrial cells is the abnormal accumulation of glycogen particles in their cytoplasm.

Hypertrophy

The ultrastructural criteria of hypertrophy [4, 9, 21] are:

1. increased numbers of myofilaments and mitochondria
2. large lobulated nuclei
3. abnormal accumulations of Z band-like material
4. focal widening of Z bands
5. increased amounts of rough endoplasmic reticulum

6. irregular invaginations of the sarcolemma and
7. widened convoluted intercalated discs.

The majority of the atrial cells of the patients with coronary artery disease were hypertrophied by size but only minor changes of the Z bands and intercalated discs were present. Other criteria were not found in enlarged atrial cells. Moreover, based on morphometric analysis, there was a significant decrease in the volume fractions of myofibrils and mitochondria and an abnormal increase in the volume fractions of glycogen inclusions and *clear sarcoplasm*. These changes indicated that the enlarged atrial cells were in the process of degeneration.

Degeneration

The ultrastructural changes in the atrial cells of the patients with coronary artery disease are slightly different from the severely degenerative changes previously reported in the atrial cells of patients with congenital heart disease [4] and valvular heart disease [9, 12]. In these studies, severely degenerative changes were characterized by:

1. loss of myofilaments with preferential loss of thick filaments,
2. aggregation of glycogen and mitochondria in areas of myofilament loss,
3. proliferation of sarcoplasmic reticulum in areas of myofilament loss,
4. aggregation of Z-band-like material and cytoskeletal filaments,
5. abnormal mitochondrial size, shape and configuration and,
6. accumulation of myelin figures and electron dense residual bodies.

In the present study, aggregates of dilated segments of sarcoplasmic reticulum, cytoskeletal filaments, myelin figures and electron dense residual bodies were not found in the atrial cells of patients with coronary artery disease. The absence of these changes indicated the moderate degree of degeneration in these cells.

Effects of Chronic Ischemia

Increases in glycogen accumulation have been reported in ventricular myocardial cells following chronic hypoxia and ischemia in experimental animal models [18, 19]. Similar changes have also been reported in the left ventricular myocardial cells of patients with coronary artery disease [20, 21]. In patients with stable angina (chronic coronary insufficiency) there was a loss of mitochondrial cristae and increased amounts of glycogen particles in ventricular myocardial cells. In patients with acute coronary insufficiency, there was a loss of mitochondrial mass in addition to increased amounts of glycogen particles. Similar changes have also been reported in the atrial cells of patients with atherosclerotic heart disease and fixed intra-atrial block [7].

Increased glycogen in myocardial cells was presumed to be secondary to ischemia, especially chronic ischemia [7, 20].

Degenerative changes, especially loss of myofilaments, have been reported in the left ventricular myocardial cells of patients with coronary artery disease but these changes were not extensive unless there was at least 90% coronary artery stenosis [21]. In patients with less than 80% stenosis, there was no loss of myofilaments but there was increased interstitial connective tissue. Increases in interstitial connective tissue were present in patients with 50% stenosis and grew proportionally to the degree of coronary artery stenosis. Similar increases in interstitial connective tissue were reported in so-called ischemic cardiomyopathy [22].

There was significant coronary narrowing with greater than 75% stenosis in all patients in this study. The blood supply of the right atrium, with the exception of the sinus and atrioventricular nodes and the atrial septum which have a dual blood supply, is usually derived from the right coronary artery [23]. Since the right coronary artery was diseased, we have presumed that the blood supply to the right atrium was compromised in these patients. The structural changes in the atria of the patients in this study — increased cell size, accumulation of glycogen particles, focal mitochondrial degeneration and interstitial fibrosis — are similar to structural changes reported in chronic ischemia and are presumably secondary to stenosis of the right coronary artery. The absence of severely degenerative changes may reflect less severe coronary artery disease in our patients or differences in susceptibility of atrial and ventricular myocardial cells to the effects of chronic ischemia.

This study has defined the structural and ultrastructural changes associated with chronic ischemia in the right atrium. These changes include:

1. increase in interstitial and perivascular connective tissue,
2. decrease in volume fractions of myofibrils and mitochondria,
3. increase in volume fractions of glycogen inclusions and "clear" sarcoplasm,
4. increase in lipofuscin and lipid droplets and,
5. degeneration of mitochondrial cristae.

REFERENCES

1. Lannigan, R.A., and Zaki, S.A. 1966. Ultrastructure of the myocardium of the atrial appendage. Br. Heart J. 28:796–807.
2. Roy, P.E., and Morin, P.J. 1971. Variations of the Z band in human auricular appendages. Lab. Invest. 25:422–426.
3. Tomisawa, M., Onouchi, Z., Gloto, M., et al. 1975. Congenital left atrial enlargement. A case report with special reference to myocardial fine structure. Jpn. Circ. J. 39:417–424.
4. Pham, T.D., Wit, A.L., Hordof, A.J., Malm, J.R., and Fenoglio, J.J. Jr. 1978. Right atrial ultrastructure in congenital heart disease. I. Comparison of ventricular septal defect and endocardial cushion defect. Am. J. Cardiol. 42:973–982.
5. Fenoglio, J.J. Jr., Pham, T.D., Hordof, A., Edie, R.N., and Wit, A.L. 1979. Right atrial ultrastructure in congenital heart disease. II. Atrial septal defect: effects of volume overload. Am. J. Cardiol. 43:820–827.

6. Legato, M.J. 1973. Ultrastructure of the atrial, ventricular and Purkinje cell, with special reference to the genesis of arrhythmias. *Circulation* 47:178–189.
7. Legato, M.J., Bull, M.B., and Ferrer, M.I. 1974. Atrial ultrastructure in patients with fixed intra-atrial block. *Chest* 65:252–261.
8. Thiedemann, K-U., and Ferrans, V.J. 1976. Ultrastructure of sarcoplasmic reticulum in atrial myocardium of patients with mitral valvular disease. *Am. J. Path.* 83:1–38.
9. Thiedemann, K-U., and Ferrans, V.J. 1977. Left atrial ultrastructure in mitral valvular disease. *Am. J. Path.* 89:575–604.
10. Thiedemann, K-U., and Ferrans, V.J. 1978. Ultrastructure of left atrial myocardium in patients with mitral valvular disease. In Cardiomyopathy and Myocardial Biopsy, Kaltenbach M, Loogen F, and Olsen EGJ, eds. pp.141–156. New York: Springer-Verlag.
11. Fenoglio, J.J. Jr. and Wagner, B.M. 1973. Studies in rheumatic fever. VI. Ultrastructure of chronic rheumatic heart disease. *Am. J. Path.* 73:623–640.
12. Pham, T.D., and Fenoglio, J.J. Jr. 1982. Right atrial ultrastructure in chronic rheumatic heart disease. *Int. J. Cardiol.* 1:289–304.
13. Friedman, P.L., Fenoglio, J.J. Jr., and Wit, A.L. 1975. Time course for the reversal of electrophysiological and ultrastructural abnormalities in subendocardial Purkinje fibers surviving extensive myocardial infarction in dogs. *Circ. Res.* 36:127–144.
14. Eisenberg, B.R., Kuda, A.M., and Peter, J.B. 1974. Stereological analysis of mammalian skeletal muscle. I. Soleus muscle of the adult guinea pig. *J. Cell Biol.* 60:732–744.
15. Loud, A.V., Barany, W.C., and Pack, B.A. 1965. Quantitative evaluation of cytoplasmic structures in electron micrographs. *Lab. Invest.* 14:966–1008.
16. Weibel, E.R. 1972. Stereological techniques for electron microscopic morphometry. In Principles and Techniques of Electron Microscopy: Biological Applications, Hayat, M.A., ed., pp. 237–296. New York: Van Nostrand Rheinhold Company.
17. Jones, M., Ferrans, V.J., Morrow, A.G., and Roberts, W.C., 1975. Ultrastructure of crista supraventricular is muscle in patients with congenital heart diseases associated with right ventricular outflow tract obstruction. *Circulation* 51:39–67.
18. Ferrans, V.J., and Roberts, W.C., 1971. Myocardial ultrastructure in acute and chronic hypoxia. *Cardiology* 56:144–160.
19. Schwartz, A., Wood, J.M., Allen, J.C., et al. 1973. Biochemical and morphological correlates of cardiac ischemia. I. Membrane systems. *Am. J. Cardiol.* 32:46–61.
20. Laguens, R.P., Weinschelbaum, R., and Favaloro, R. 1979. Ultrastructural and morphometric study of the human heart muscle cell in acute coronary insufficiency. *Human Pathol.* 10:695–705.
21. Schwarz, F., Flameng, W., Thiedemann, K-U., Schaper, W., and Schlepper, M. 1978. Effects of coronary stenosis of myocardial function, ultrastructure and aortocoronary bypass graft hemodynamics. *Am. J. Cardiol.* 42:193–201.
22. Boucher, C.A., Fallon, J.T., Johnson, R.A., and Yurchak, P.M. 1979. Cardiomyopathic syndrome caused by coronary artery disease. III: Prospective clinicopathological study of its prevalence among patients with clinically unexplained chronic heart failure. *Br. Heart J.* 41:613–620.
23. Baroldi, G., and Scomazzoni, G. 1965. *Coronary circulation in the normal and the pathologic heart.* Washington, D.C.: Armed Forces Institute of Pathology.

11. CONNECTIVE TISSUE IN THE NORMAL
AND HYPERTROPHIED HEART

THOMAS F. ROBINSON

A complete analysis of the dynamic, three-dimensional shape changes that occur in the heart during the cardiac cycle must include consideration of the structural and mechanical integration of the large population of variously oriented muscle cells of the myocardium. From this viewpoint, the study of hypertrophied myocardium is not only a vehicle for pathophysiological investigation, but represents an opportunity to examine adaptation to extreme functional demands that can increase our understanding of basic physiological mechanisms.

Structural integration of myocytes involves the branching and nonuniform orientation of the long axes of myocytes, the connective tissue, and specialized membrane junctions, most notably the intercalated discs. This chapter focuses on changes that occur in connective tissue of heart muscle during hypertrophy and their implications in cardiac physiology and pathophysiology. A synopsis of the structure of connective tissue in normal myocardium is presented, followed by a selective review of studies related to connective tissue in several types of hypertrophy.

CONNECTIVE TISSUE IN NORMAL MYOCARDIUM

After being virtually ignored for several decades, the connective tissue of the myocardium has recently been intensively studied. A landmark paper [1] in a series by Caulfield and Borg [1–4] demonstrated the advantages of modern microscopical techniques, most notably scanning electron microscopy, to increasing our understanding of the disposition of collagen fibers relative to myocytes, and called attention to several classic histological studies from the early part of this century. Robinson and co-workers [5–10] have studied the dispositions of collagen, elastin, microfibrils, and the collagen fibril-micro-thread-granule lattice (CML), and changes in those dispositions in correlation with mechanical state. They used a variety of fixation, staining, and microscopical techniques, including light microscopy, standard and high-voltage transmission, and scanning electron microscopy.

Historical Background

Holmgren, in a paper published in German in 1907 [11], used light microscopy of tissue sections stained with silver or other histological compounds to study striated skeletal and heart muscles from various vertebrates and crustacea. His interpretations regarding tracheal function were incorrect, but in some of his 105 figures, he clearly demonstrates that extracellular fibers interconnect muscle fibers and capillaries. His drawings of membrane systems and cellular organelles are also of interest as a complement to modern ultrastructural studies.

Nagel used stretched sarcolemmas and silver-stained sections to study mechanical characteristics of internal perimysium and sarcolemma. Unfortunately, these beautiful experiments were confined to skeletal muscle [12], but his studies of the mechanical properties of capillary coat and its relation to connective tissue [13] included diagrams of connective tissue in heart as well as skeletal muscle.

Bairati, in his 1937 paper [14], studied the correlation of resistance to stretch and the conformation of extracellular fibers associated with the sarcolemmas of extracted skeletal muscles using microdissection needles and light microscopy, including darkfield or polarization, and silver-stained sections in brightfield. He proposed a "cargo net" type of model for the sarcolemma of skeletal muscle, whereby the woven network of inextensible collagen fibers can be reversibly deformed up to lengths at which the woven fibers become aligned. One limitation of these elegant experiments is that work with isolated sarcolemmas does not permit any estimate of the relevant sarcomere lengths at which the wrapped, woven, extracellular fibers pinch in upon the included volume of muscle and thereby preclude further changes in length. Bairati also observed that the fibrillar reticulum of the sarcolemma is embedded in a dense colloidal interfibrillar cement analogous to the basal membranes of epithelial cells.

Studies of elastic tissue in cross-striated muscles are few and most are published in German. Benninghoff, in the 1930 *Handbuch der mikroskopischen Anatomie des Menschen* [15] reviewed the previous decades of histologic work on elastic fibers in blood vessels and heart. In addition to reporting the results of localization studies of elastin, he reviewed several important and provocative theories regarding the function of elastic fibers, including plasticity of the tissue in hypertrophy, the higher concentrations of elastic fibers in apex and atria than in ventricular midwall, the probable role of elastic fibers in storing energy during systole to promote return to diastolic configuration, and the hypertrophy of the elastic fiber system with aging and with arteriosclerosis. Feneis, in his 1935 paper [16], studied the angles of collagen and forces relative to muscle axes in skeletal muscle, as well as the histological localization of elastic fibers. Nagel, in 1945, published a paper [17] on the importance of the elastic-muscle systems for the development of shoulder alignment.

The 1965 paper of Puff and Langer [18] is the only recent major study (found by this author) that specifically addresses the subject of elastic tissue in the heart. The paper is entitled, in translation, "The problem of diastolic development of the heart chamber: an understanding of the elastic web in myocardium." The authors, based on their histological studies, concluded that the elastic fibers in the right ventricular heart muscle of man occur in two major configurations: as low-angle spirals wrapped around myocytes and as intercellular reticular networks.

Benninghoff [15] was aware of the problems involved in classifying fine networks of extracellular fibers based on histological silver stain. In 1979, Puchtler and Meloan [19] reinvestigated Unna's concept (1894) regarding the limitations of specificity of histochemical staining of elastic fibers. They concluded that although orcein and resorcin-fuchsin had similar staining properties, their specificity for elastic tissue was uncertain for embryonic, experimentally or pathologically altered collagens, and meshworks of fine fibers. Thus "collastin" or "pseudo-elastica" cannot be conclusively identified by these histological methods. Highly resolved localization of small elastic and other types of fibers thus awaited the development and utilization of modern ultrastructural and antibody labeling techniques.

Current Understanding

The various components of myocardial connective tissue can be systematically catalogued as epimysium, perimysium, and endomysium. Epimysium, the sheath of connective tissue surrounding an entire muscle, has been studied in cardiac papillary muscles and atrial trabeculae.

Robinson, et al. [7–10] have shown that the epimysium of atrial trabeculae of rat and hamster hearts is comprised predominantly of collagen and elastin fibers, on the order of one micron in diameter, that are larger than other extracellular fibers in the muscle (figure 11–1). The elastic fibers are associated with microfibrils that are about 15 nm. in diameter. The intervening extracellular space is filled with a *collagen* fibril-*microthread*-granule *lattice* (CML) whose preservation is enhanced by the inclusion of cationic dyes in the fixation medium and is probably the dense colloid that Bairati described from his light microscopic studies [14]. The collagen fibrils of the CML are 30–70 nm. in diameter and are linked by the microthreads, approximately 3 nm. in diameter (figure 11–2). Granules, 10–40 nm. in diameter, usually occur at the inter-

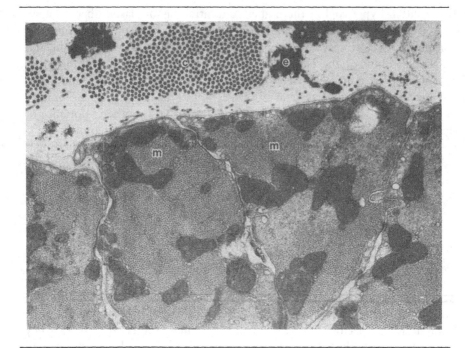

Figure 11–1. Transmission electron micrograph of a transverse section through a normal rat atrial trabecula. Note the close association of collagen fibers (c), comprised of collagen fibrils, and elastic (e) fibers in the epimysial sheath that surrounds the myocytes (m).

sections of microthreads with collagen fibrils, cell coats, or other microthreads. Fine filaments between cells had been mentioned in cardiac muscle of dog by Bahr and Jennings [20]. Cationic dyes had been effectively employed by Sommer and Johnson [21] to demonstrate that the extracellular "space" is really an extracellular lattice filled with cationic-positive material.

Robinson, et al, [8–10] have studied the orientations of the epimysial sheath of collagen fibers in isolated papillary muscles from rat heart. Using electron microscopy and silver stain for light microscopy, they found that epimysial fibers are more highly aligned with the long axes of stretched muscles than those analyzed at slack length. They invoked a "cargo net" hypothesis, similar to that used by Bairati for skeletal muscle sarcolemma [14], whereby the collagen fibers exert little resistance to stretch until they are aligned and taut. A more complete model that accounts for the combined tensile strengths of the slightly thinner but numerous longitudinal collagen fibers that occur throughout the thickness of the muscle is being developed.

The CML is found throughout the extracellular compartment of heart muscle; that is, in the perimysium and endomysium, as well as the epimysium. Elastic and collagen fibers in the endomysium are relatively small, and large perimysial collagen fibers, common in the ventricle, are rare in atrial muscles.

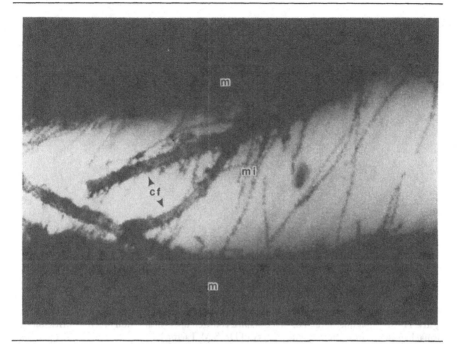

Figure 11-2. High voltage transmission electron micrograph of a ¼ μm-thick section of rat papillary muscle that was fixed in a solution containing the cationic dye, ruthenium red, in order to preserve the CML (collagen fibril-microthread-granule lattice). Microthreads, (mi) 3–6 nm. in diameter, inter-connect cell coats of adjacent myocytes (m) and collagen fibrils (cf) to cell coat.

The preservation and imaging of the CML is improved by the use of cationic dyes. The CML has been observed, however, in specimens fixed with glutaraldehyde alone, or glutaraldehyde with ruthenium red, alcian blue, safranin-O, cetylpyridium chloride, or tannic acid. Recently, Frank and Beydler [22] have demonstrated the CML in unfixed tissue. They obtained striking-transmission electron micrographs of the lattice with the techniques of rapid freezing, deep etching, and rotary shadowing of rabbit papillary muscles. Ahumada and Saffitz [23] have recently labeled microthreads that connect collagen fibrils to the cell coats of myocytes and to other collagen fibrils with antibody to fibronectin. More work will be needed to determine whether microthreads are comprised only of fibronectin or if some micro-threads do not contain fibronectin. Glycosaminoglycans and proteoglycans are present in the cardiac interstitium [24] and the CML resembles proteoglycan networks according to criteria of structure and positive reaction with cationic dyes [25]. Since proteoglycans are a major constituent of the CML, their water-binding properties, and hence, their effect on interstitial viscosity, should be of major importance in lubricating the extracellular regions between the continually moving cardiac myocytes.

Caulfield and Borg used scanning-electron microscopy to beautifully

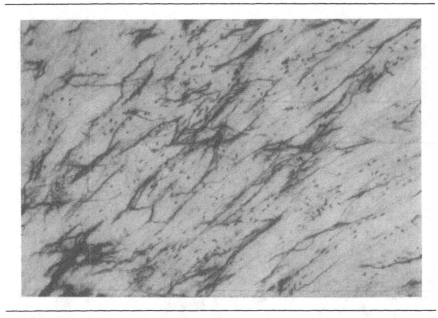

Figure 11-3. Light micrograph of silver-stained collagen fibers in a section of left ventricle of normal hamster heart. (Micrograph courtesy of Dr. S.M. Factor.)

demonstrate the disposition of collagen fibers relative to the surfaces of myocytes and capillaries in papillary muscle and ventricular wall [1]. They defined "struts" as the collagen fibers, 120–150 nm. in diameter in rodents, that interconnect the lateral surfaces of myocytes and capillaries. Their ultrastructural techniques undoubtedly reveal strands smaller than those seen using histologic stain. Recent studies have shown that collagen types I and III are principal components of struts [26, 27]. Caulfield and Borg [1] also described "weaves" of collagen fibers that envelop groups of myocytes and are interconnected by collagen fibers. Figures 11–3 and 11–4 show collagen waves in heart. The first reference found by this author for the application of scanning electron microscopy to the study of collagen fibers relative to myocyte surfaces was published in a short paper on skeletal muscle by Khoroshkov in 1976 [28], but no correspondence or subsequent publications have come from his laboratory.

Robinson, et al. [5–10], and recently Frank and Beydler [22] demonstrated that some collagen fibrils are very closely apposed to the outside of the cardiac myocyte sarcolemma. This strong looking "husk" portion of the sarcolemma had been described in skeletal muscle by Bairati [14] in 1937, using the light microscope, and in 1961 by Mauro and Adams [29], using the transmission electron microscope. Schmalbruch [30] performed experiments correlating the disposition of sarcolemmal collagen fibrils in skeletal muscle as a function of sarcomere length. Using a shadowed replica technique, he found that the collagen fibrils became straight and nearly co-aligned with the long axis of the

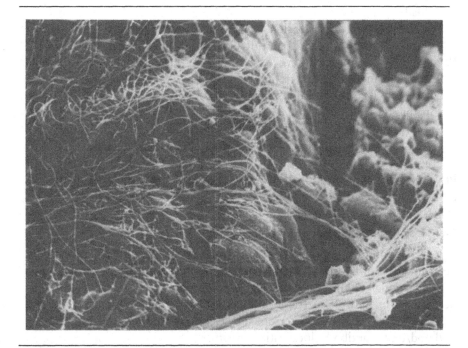

Figure 11–4. Scanning electron micrograph of a collagen weave that surrounds myocytes in a papillary muscle from normal rat heart. Sarcolemmal contours of underlying mitochondria and Z bands are evident.

myocyte at sarcomere lengths of 3 μm. At that sarcomere length resistance to stretch increases sharply, and Dulhunty and Franzini-Armstrong [31] have shown that the caveolae (sarcolemmal inpouchings) open and become co-planar with the rest of the lateral surface of the sarcolemma.

Microfibrils, usually associated with elastin, were defined and named by Battig and Low [32] in their ultrastructural study of human cardiac muscle and its associated tissue space. Hanak and Böck [33] postulated an adhesion and shock absorbing role for microfibrils in the tendon-muscle junction of papillary muscle.

Fine filaments between the cell coat and the trilamellar membrane portions of the sarcolemma have been reported by Robinson, et al. [6–8], and Frank and Beydler [22]. Orenstein, Hogan, and Bloom [34] have described "surface cables" that connect longitudinally adjacent regions of the sarcolemma that lie over M bands. The biochemical identities and the inter-relationships of these structures are unknown.

CONNECTIVE TISSUE IN HYPERTROPHIED MYOCARDIUM
Types of Hypertrophy

The etiology of hypertrophy has been categorized by Sonnenblick, et al. [35] as follows:

Overloads:

Systolic pressure: hypertension, aortic stenosis

Volume: aortic and mitral regurgitation, atrial septal defect, A-V shunt

Reactive (loss of myocardium):

Segmental: myocardial infarction

Diffuse: myocarditis, cardiomyopathy

Myopathies:

Primary: idiopathic.

Secondary: Decreased contractility, leading to increased load, leading to increased mass.

Physiological and hormonal: exercise, normal growth, catecholamines, thyroid excess or hypertryroidism

Methods of Analyzing Connective Tissue

1. Total amounts of collagen in heart tissue are estimated biochemically by determination of hydroxyproline content [36] or by amino acid analysis [37].

2. Fractional volume or fractional area occupied by connective tissue is determined by morphometric techniques [38].

3. Types of collagen are determined by electrophoresis of extracted collagen [39] and/or by antibody localization in situ.

4. Size, distribution, and characterization of connective tissue fibers are determined by histological and ultrastructural methods [1, 8].

5. Functional role of connective tissue is deduced by correlation of mechanical properties with quantitative estimation of connective tissue [40].

6. Functional role of connective tissue is more directly deduced by correlation of mechanical properties of muscle with optically determined disposition and assessment of type of connective tissue fibers [10, 41].

Myocardial Connective Tissue in Hypertrophy

Robinson, et al. have found enlarged collagen fibers (figure 11–5) in papillary muscles of rats whose hearts had hypertrophied with age. Resting tension was also significantly elevated compared to that in papillary muscles of younger animals with smaller fibers. In the genetically cardiomyopathic Syrian hamster, four stages occur in the myocardium during progression of the disease: myocyte necrosis, fibrosis secondary to the loss of myocytes, subsequent reactive hypertrophy of remaining myocytes due to the need to sustain the increased load, and ultimately a decrease in myocardial function and heart failure. Figure 11–6 shows a focal calcified lesion in hamster myocardium during the stage of reactive hypertrophy. Abnormally large collagen fibers emanate from the lesion to apparently normal tissue and may amplify the region of dysfunction to surrounding myocardium.

Caulfield [42] used scanning electron microscopy to examine hypertensive human hearts. His criteria for selection included heart weight of 550–650 g,

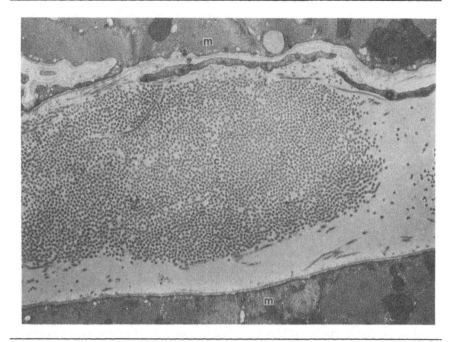

Figure 11–5. Transmission electron micrograph of a cross-section of papillary muscle from hypertrophied heart of a 25-month-old (aged) rat (specimen courtesy of Dr. J.M. Capasso). The collagen fiber (c) between two myocytes (m) is very large relative to those of non-hypertrophied heart muscle and is commonly found in hypertrophy associated with aging.

coronary artery occlusion of 60% or less, and an absence of focal scars. He found two types of alterations of the collagen struts and collagen weaves in those hearts: first, an increase in diameters of struts from the normal values of 180–200 nm to 250–300 nm and an increase in diameters of weave fibers to a maximum of 230 nm; and second, in three of the hearts studied, the weave network was replaced by broad bands and sheets of collagen that could make the ventricle less compliant. Weber and co-workers [43] have observed a thickened weave and thickened collagen fibers connecting weaves in hypertrophied primate hearts.

Bing and co-workers [40] studied experimental hypertrophy, as evidenced by increased left ventricle-to-body weight ratios, in the hearts of rats subjected to aortic arch constriction for up to four weeks. In comparing hypertrophied to normal hearts, they observed elevated hydroxyproline content, as well as elevated resting tension. They explained an observed depression in muscle shortening velocity as either an increased stiffness in parallel elastic components or an altered contractile state. In subsequent studies [44] they administered an inhibitor of collagen cross-linking, BAPN (beta amino proprionitrile), to experimental rats and found that both the increase in left ventricular collagen content and the increase in resting tension were inhibited,

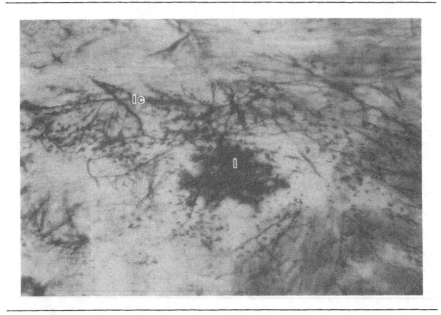

Figure 11-6. Light micrograph of silver-stained collagen fibers in a hypertrophied section of left ventricle of cardiomyopathic hamster heart. Focal calcified lesion (l) is bordered laterally by a clear region that lacks stained fibers, and longitudinally by long, abnormally large fibers (lc). (Micrograph courtesy of Dr. S.M. Factor.)

but the decrease in maximum velocity of shortening persisted. They concluded that decrease in shortening speed was independent of collagen content, whereas the elevated resting tensions appeared to depend upon increased collagen content.

Lund, et al. [45] studied the changes in cardiac muscle fiber diameters and collagen content (hydroxyproline method) in 16-week-old rats with spontaneous hypertension, aortic constriction, and hypoxia. They also studied spontaneously hypertensive and aortic constricted groups exposed to six weeks of hypobaric hypoxia (simulated altitude of 6100 m). Lund et al. noted that even though blood pressure was enhanced to the same magnitude after aortic constriction and spontaneous hypertension, an increase in hydroxyproline concentration was found only in the aortic constricted animals in both the stressed and nonstressed ventricles. The connective tissue response in the left ventricle of the spontaneously hypertensive rat lags behind fiber hypertrophy, but is readily activated by exposure to hypoxia. The authors concluded that connective tissue response produced by aortic constriction is significantly different from the response produced by essential hypertension, and they suggested that the factors governing muscle fiber hypertrophy might be independent from those governing connective tissue proliferation.

Wendt-Gallitelli and Jacob [46] and Wendt-Gallitelli et al. [47] studied the time course of ultrastructural alterations in hypertrophied myocardium of

Goldblatt type II rats (induction of left ventricular pressure hypertrophy by coarctation of one renal artery). Although they limited their study to the period of compensatory hypertrophy in order to emphasize alterations in the myocardial cell itself, they found considerable increases in connective tissue near blood vessels and in diffuse scar tissue after six months of coarctation. Increase in total connective tissue was determined by the hydroxyproline method and morphometry. They attributed impairment of rate of development of tension as well as unloaded shortening velocity to the increase of connective tissue. They also found a correlation between the presence of diffuse scar tissue and most evident impairment of mechanical performance. The decrease in relaxation velocity after four to eight weeks, where an increase in connective tissue is not yet observed, has been attributed to impairment of calcium ion pumping by the sarcoplasmic reticulum. This implies an, as yet, unproved concept of subcontracture of the hypertrophied myocardium. Such questions demonstrate the importance of testing more than the correlation between function and total amount of connective tissue in hypertropy; i.e., the type of connective tissue, as well as its disposition relative to the muscle cells, should be determined for more rigorous testing of its functional importance.

The physiological properties of papillary muscles have been used as a measure of functional states of the myocardium, whereas most of the extensive morphometric investigations of the effects of hypertrophy have been performed in the ventricular wall. Anversa et al. [48], however, performed experiments important to providing a basis for structure-function correlations in hearts made hypertrophic by pressure overload (aortic constriction). They directly studied papillary muscles of rat by morphometric techniques. Although their study was performed on the tissue, cellular, and subcellular levels, this discussion will be focused on changes in connective tissue. They found that their experimental papillary muscles hypertrophied by an average of 51%, almost entirely in lateral expansion of the muscle, and that alterations in most of the domains were proportional. Disproportionate alterations, however, were observed in the volumes of endothelium (100%) and of connective tissue cells (121%), which included fibroblasts, pericytes, macrophages, and round cells. In these interstitial cell populations, both cellular hyperplasia, evaluated by an increased number of nuclei, and cellular hypertrophy, measured by the increase of mean cell volume, were found to coexist at statistically significant levels. In both normal and hypertrophied papillary muscle, connective tissue cells and extracellular space together comprise 9.4% of the volume. Fibroblasts constitute approximately 80% of the volume of these cellular components. Rough endoplasmic reticulum in fibroblasts increased by 150% in eight days, but no significant addition of collagen was detected until one to two weeks following the onset of muscle hypertrophy. Overall structural comparisons indicate that the magnitude of alterations in papillary muscle are less than those in the left ventricular wall; as a consequence, prediction of the magnitude of physiological changes in the ventricle, by extrapolation of results from the papillary muscle, could lead to significant underestimation of the alterations due to hypertrophy.

Medugorac [49], in studies of the hearts of spontaneously hypertensive rats, obtained results parallel to those of Anversa for aortic constriction in the rat. Both found that the hydroxyproline concentration in hypertrophied left ventricular papillary muscles was lower than the average hydroxyproline concentration in the hypertrophied left ventricle as a whole. Medugoric cautioned that in using hydroxyproline measurements for the quantitative determination of collagen content, the presence of other hypdroxyproline-containing proteins such as elastin, as well as the occurrence of different proportions of various collagens with different hydroxyproline content, must be taken into account. He further emphasized that the concentration of collagen varies as a function of age and region of the heart in normal as well as hypertrophied myocardium, and therefore advised caution in categorizing any given region from pathophysiological studies of another region. He found that, in normal and hypertrophied hearts from rats aged 10 and 16 months, the hydroxyproline content was predictably lower in the left ventricular free wall than in the right ventricle and septum. In normal left ventricle, the hydroxyproline level was approximately the same in endomyocardial, epicardial, and papillary muscle. Hydroxproline concentration was elevated in all regions of the myocardium in the 16-month-old relative to 10-month-old normal rats, and was increased in all parts of the hypertrophied myocardium in the spontaneously hypertensive rats. The increase in the hydroxyproline concentration was greatest in endomyocardial areas of the left ventricular wall, in agreement with changes reported for left ventricle after aortic stenosis in the rat [40] and in the right ventricle after coarctation of the pulmonary artery in the cat [50]. The difference in the increase in hydroxproline concentration, between epimyocardial and endomyocardial areas, was greater in the 10-month-old than in the 16-month-old hypertensives. He suggested that diminished blood flow in the endocardium, relative to the epicardium in hypertrophy, might lead to necrosis and subsequently elevated levels of collagen synthesis.

In subsequent studies, Medugorac and Jacob [51] characterized collagen types I and III in the left ventricles of normal rats at ages four weeks, four months, and 24 months, as well as rats subjected to various types of hypertrophy (induced by aortic stenosis, Goldblatt hypertension, swimming training, and spontaneous hypertension). Extraction of collagen from left ventricles was accomplished with dilute-acid solutions (0.3–0.6% of total collagen), neutral salt solutions (lower yield), and pepsin digestion (50–65% of total collagen). The distribution of various types of collagen molecules was analysed in pepsinsolubilised collagen, with the aid of electrophoresis in polyacrylamide gels. The proportion of type I collagen was significantly larger than type III collagen in all samples, but varied with growth, aging, and hypertrophy. The connective tissue of the hearts of young rats contains a higher proportion of collagen type III than those of adult rats; those of old rats reveal only traces of type III. The proportion of type III is also higher in ventricles of the hypertrophied hearts.

The limited yields obtained in these extractions further demonstrates the need for data regarding the localization of collagen types relative to myocytes in order to ascribe physiological significance to varying ratios of types of collagen in different regions of the heart under various conditions. The markedly different biochemical, structural, and mechanical properties of type I and type III collagens underscore the need to localize the usually large fibers of collagen type I, the more compliant fine reticular network of type III, and fibers of mixed type.

The question of whether the enhanced synthesis of collagen type III in hypertrophied endocardium is due to scarring subsequent to ischemia in that region, or whether ventricular growth during these types of hypertrophy partly reverts to an embryonic pattern of sythesis, is raised in the Medugorac and Jacob study [51] and answered in their subsequent paper [52], in which connective tissue content and myocardial stiffness are measured in pressure-overload hypertrophy (spontaneous hypertensive and Goldblatt rats) in a combined study of morphologic, morphometric, biochemical, and mechanical parameters. They observed that these types of hypertrophy are accompanied by myocardial fibrosis, and an increase in stiffness that is better reflected in morphometric data than in chemical analysis.

Dawson et al. [53] used changes in solubility and phenotype composition to study collagen composition of total hearts in which hypertrophy was induced by copper deficiency. In copper-supplemented animals, 35–45% of the collagen could be extracted with pepsin, but in the hypertrophied copper-deficient hearts, up to 74% could be extracted. The increase in solubility was attributed to either an inhibition or a decreased synthesis of the copper-containing enzyme lysyl oxidase, which is involved in the cross-linking process. Electrophoretic analysis of the extracts showed that the type III/type I ratio increased threefold (to a maximum of 2.3) between two and six weeks, the period of most rapid growth, then returned to the initial level at eight weeks. In the hypertrophied copper-deficient hearts, however, the type III/type I ratio increased almost twice as much from two to six weeks and remained significantly higher at eight weeks. The authors note that this is consistent with the fact that collagen type III binds more strongly to fibronectin than does type I, and that these observations could indicate that one of the functions of type III collagen is to provide a network attached to the basement membranes that then acts as a scaffold for deposition of collagen type I. They also present evidence of an increase in collagen type V in copper-deficient hearts that is as yet unexplained.

CONCLUSIONS

Collagen comprises a few percent and elastin less than one percent of the dry weight of the heart, but they are widely distributed in a complex manner.

Collagen is the more completely studied. Based on its distribution, its known properties, and the correlation of its disposition with physiological state, collagen is expected to play a significant role in myocardial dynamics. Furthermore, some aspects of pathophysiological performance have been attributed to increased amounts and altered configurations of collagen in hypertrophy. Two recent and especially dramatic correlations have indicated the profound functional effect of collagen and the importance of applying structural as well as biochemical analysis to such problems. Factor et al. [54] have noted the complete absence of collagen fibers in regions of ventricular rupture in autopsied human myocardium, and Caulfield et al. [55] have observed a dramatic loss of myocardial stiffness and the disappearance of collagen fibers within hours of experimentally induced coronary artery occlusion in dog heart.

Despite such intriguing findings, the role of connective tissue is difficult to assess beyond the level of simple correlations of function with content of collagen. A more complete assessment of the role of connective tissue in myocardial function is dependent upon an extensive knowledge of basic structure, identity, and base-line regional variations. As further studies are performed, therefore, it will be vital to determine several variables.

1. The total amount of collagen and elastin should be known, preferably as a function of region of the heart. Small differences in the amount of collagen present have potentially large effects on respective tensile strength and elastic properties.

2. The types of collagen should be determined in view of their differences in elastic moduli.

3. The size of fibers is a critical parameter since the cross-sectional area, and hence the tensile strength of the fibers, varies as the square of the diameter of the fiber. Caulfield [42] has calculated that a fiber undergoing an increase in diameter from 200 to 300 nm can support an increase in stress of over 100%.

4. The determination of the orientations of fibers, relative to the myocytes and relative to inter-myocyte and myocyte-capillary directions of stress, is vital to an evaluation of their function. For example, Robinson et al. [8] have shown a dramatic correlation among the orientation of epimysial collagen fibers, resistance to stretch, and sarcomere lengths for optimal myofilament cross-bridge overlap in normal papillary muscles from rat heart.

Extending studies from model systems, such as the papillary muscle, to the determination of convolutions (waviness) of extracellular fibers and their changes in angle as a function of contractile state in the geometrically complicated wall of the ventricle will be especially difficult, but extremely important to a complete understanding of the anatomical basis of the mechanical properties of the myocardium of normal and hypertrophied hearts.

ACKNOWLEDGEMENTS

I thank Drs. M.J. Legato, J.M. Capasso, S.M. Factor, E.H. Sonnenblick, O.O. Blumenfeld, S. Seifter, and C. Dickson for helpful discussion and encouragement; Mrs. L. Cohen-Gould for excellent technical assistance and discussion, Mrss. K. Cohen, M. Abercrombie, and Ms. L. DiDia for translations of articles; Ms. J. Fant and Mr. F. Macaluso for use of the Analytical Ultrastructure Center facilities; Dr. K. R. Porter, Dr. M. Fotino, Mr. F. Wray, and Mr. F. Charlie of the High Voltage EM Laboratory of the University of Colorado, Boulder; and Miss D. Ditizio for expert help with preparation of the manuscript. Work supported in part by NIH research grants HL-24336, HL-18824, AG-05554, NIH Research Career Development Award HL-00568, and a N.Y Heart Association Grant-in-Aid.

REFERENCES

1. Caulfield, J.B., and Borg, T.K. 1979. The collagen network of the heart. *Lab. Invest.* 40: 364–372.
2. Borg, T.K., and Caulfield, J.B. 1979. Collagen in the heart. *Texas Rep. Biol. Med.* 39: 321–333.
3. Borg, T.K., and Caulfield, J.B. 1981. The collagen matrix of the heart. *Fed. Proc. Fed. Am. Soc. Exp. Biol.* 40:2037–2041.
4. Borg, T.K., Ranson, W.F., Moslehy, F.A., and Caulfield, J.B. 1981. Structural basis of ventricular stiffness. *Lab. Invest.* 44:49–54.
5. Winegrad, S., and Robinson, T.F. 1978. Force generation among cells in the relaxing heart. *Eur. J. Cardiol.* 7 (Suppl.): 63–70.
6. Robinson, T.F. 1980. Lateral connections between heart muscle cells as revealed by conventional and high voltage transmission electron microscopy. *Cell Tissue Res.* 211: 353–359.
7. Robinson, T.F., and Winegrad, S. 1981. A variety of intercellular connections in heart muscle. *J. Mol. Cell. Cardiol.* 13:185–195.
8. Robinson, T.F., Cohen-Gould L., and Factor, S.M. 1983. The skeletal framework of mammalian heart muscle: Arrangement of inter-and pericellular connective tissue structures. *Lab. Invest.* 49:482–498.
9. Robinson, T.F., 1983. The physiological relationship between connective tissue and contractile filaments in heart muscle. *Einstein Q. J. Biol. Med.* 1(3):121–127.
10. Robinson, T.F., 1985. Cohen-Gould, L., Remily, R.M. Capasso, J.M., Factor, S.M. Extracellular Structures in Heart Muscle. In *Advances in Myocardiology*, Vol. 5, Harris, P., and Poole-Wilson, P.A., eds. pp. 243–255. New York: Plenum Publishing Corporation.
11. Holmgren, E. 1907. Uber die Trophospongien der quergestreiften Muskelfasern, nebst Bemerkungen uber den allgemeinen Bau dieser Fasern. *Arch. Mikrosk. Anat.* 71:165–247.
12. Nagel, A. 1935. Die mechanischen Eigenschaften von Perimysium internum und Sarkolemm bei der quergestreiften Muskelfaster. *Z. Zellforsch.* 22:695–706.
13. Nagel, A. 1934. Die mechanischen Eigenschaften der Kapillarwand und ihre Beziehungen zum Bindegewebslager. *Z. Zellforsch.* 21:376–387.
14. Bairati, A. 1937. Struttura e proprieta fisiche del sarcolemma della fibra muscolare striata. *Z. Zellforsch.* 27:100–124.
15. Benninghoff, A. 1930. Das perimysium internum. *Handbuch der mikrosk. Anatomie von v. Mollendorf.* 6:192–196.
16. Feneis, H. 1935. Uber die Anordnung und die Bedeutung des Bindegewebes fur die Mechanik der Skelettmuskculatur. *Gegenhaurs Morphol. J.* 76:161–202.
17. Nagel, A. 1945. Die Bedeutung elastische-muskuloser Systems fur die Ausbildung von Schutzeinrichtengen. *Nova Acta Leopold. N.F.* 14 (102): 9–31.
18. Puff, A., and Langer, H. 1965. Das Problem der diastolischen Entfaltung der herzkammer

(Eine Untersuchung uber das elastische Gewebe im Myocard). *Gegenhaurs Morphol. J.* 7: 184–212.

19. Puchtler, H., and Meloan, S.N. 1979. Orcein, collastin, and pseudoelastica: a re-investigation of Unna's concepts. *Histochem.* 64:119–130.
20. Bahr, G.F., and Jennings, R.B. 1961. Ultrastructure of normal and asphyxic myocardium of the dog. *Lab. Invest.* 10:548–571.
21. Sommer, J., and Johnson, T. 1979. Ultrastructure of Cardiac Muscle. In: *Handbook of Physiology: The Cardiovascular System I*, pp. 113–186.
22. Frank, J., and Beydler, S. 1985. Intercellular connections in rabbit heart as revealed by quick-frozen, deep-etched, and rotary-replicated papillary muscle. *J. Ultrastruc. Res.* 90:183–193.
23. Ahumada, G.G., and Saffitz, J.E. 1984. Fibronectin in rat heart: a link between cardiac myocytes and collagen. *J. Histochem. Cytochem.* 32:383–388.
24. Manasek, F.J. 1976. Macromolecules of the extracellular compartment of embryonic and mature hearts. *Circ. Res.* 38:331–337.
25. Myers, D.B., Highton, T.C., and Rayns, D.G. 1973. Ruthenium red-positive filaments interconnecting collagen fibrils. *J. Ultrastruct. Res.* 42:87–92.
26. Robinson, T.F., Factor, S.M., Capasso, J.M., Wittenberg, B.A., Blumenfeld, O.O., and Seifter, S. 1986. Morphology, composition, and function of struts between cardiac myocytes of rat and hamster, *Cell Tiss. Res.* (In Press).
27. Borg, T.K., Buggy, J., Sullivan, T., Laks, J., and Terracio, L. 1986. Morphological and biochemical characteristics of the connective tissue network during normal development and hypertrophy. *J. Molec. Cell. Cardiol.* 18 (Suppl. 1):247.
28. Khoroshkov, Y.A. 1976. (Title in Russian) The structure of the collagenous framework of skeletal muscle. *Arkhiv. Anatomii Gistologii* 71:97–100.
29. Mauro, A., and Adams, W.R. 1961. The structure of the sarcolemma of the frog skeletal muscle fiber. *J. Biophys. Biochem. Cytol.* 10:177–186.
30. Schmalbruch, H. 1974. The sarcolemma of skeletal muscle fibers as demonstrated by a replica technique. *Cell Tiss. Res.* 150:377–387.
31. Dulhunty, A.F., and Franzini-Armstrong, C. 1975. The relative contributions of the folds and caveolae to the surface membrane of frog skeletal muscle fibres at different sarcomere lengths. *J. Physiol.* 250:513–539.
32. Battig, C.G., and Low, F.N. 1961. The ultrastructure of human cardiac muscle and its associated tissue space. *Am. J. Anat.* 108:199–252.
33. Hanak, H., and Böck, P. 1971. Die Feinstruktur der Muskel-Sehnenverbindung von Skelettund Herzmuskel. *J. Ultrastrct. Res.* 36:68–85.
34. Orenstein, J. Hogan, D., and Bloom, S. 1980. Surface cables of cardiac myocytes. *J. Molec. Cell. Cardiol.* 12:771–780.
35. Sonnenblick, E.H., Strobeck, J.E., Capasso, J.M. and Factor, S.M. 1983. Ventricular hypertrophy: models and methods. In *Perspectives in Cardiovascular Research,* Vol. 8, Tarazi, R.C., and Dunbar, J.B., 1983 eds., pp. 13–20. New York: Raven Press.
36. Prockup, O.J., and Udenfriend, S. 1960. Specific method for the analysis of hydroxyproline in tissues and urine. *Anal. Biochem.* 1:228–239.
37. Blumenfeld, O. 1985. Personal Communication.
38. Page, and E., McCallister, L.P. 1973. Quantitative electron microscopic description of heart muscle cells: application to normal, hypertrophied, and thyroxin-stimulated hearts. *Am. J. Cardiol.* 31:172–181.
39. Light, N.D. 1982. Estimation of types I and III collagens in whole tissues by quantitation of CNBr peptides on SDS-polyacrylamide gels. *Biochem. Biophys. Acta* 702:30–36.
40. Bing, O.H.L., Matsushita, S., Fanburg, B.L., and Levine, H.J. 1971. Mechanical properties of rat cardiac muscle during experimental hypertrophy. *Circ. Res.* Vol. XXVIII, pp. 234–245.
41. Broom, N.D. 1978. Simultaneous morphological and stress-strain studies of the fibrous components in wet heart valve leaflet tissue. *Connect. Tiss. Res.* 6:37–50.
42. Caulfield, J.B. 1983. Alterations in Cardiac Collagen with Hypertrophy. In *Perspectives in Cardiovascular Research,* Vol. 8, Tarazi, R.C., and Dunbar, J.B., eds., pp. 49–57. New York: Raven Press, 1983.
43. Weber, K. et al. (Personel Communication, 1985).
44. Bing, O.H.L., Fanburg, B.L., Brooks, W.W., and Matsushita, S. 1978. The effect of the lathyrogen β-amino proprionitrile (BAPN) on the mechanical properties of experimentally

hypertrophied rat cardiac muscle. *Circ. Res.* Vol. 43(4), pp. 632–637.

45. Lund, D.D., Twietmeyer, T.A., Schmid, P.G., and Tomanek, R.J. 1979. Independent changes in cardiac muscle fibers and connective tissue in rats with spontaneous hypertension, aortic constriction, and hypoxia. *Cardiovasc. Res.* 13:39–44.

46. Wendt-Gallitelli, M.F., and Jacob, R. 1977. Time course of electron microscopic alterations in the hypertrophied myocardium of Goldblatt rats. *Basic Res. Cardiol.* 72:209–213.

47. Wendt-Gallitelli, M.F., Ebrecht, G., and Jacob, R. 1979. Morphological alterations and their functional interpretation in the hypertrophied myocardium of Goldblatt hypertensive rats. *J. Molec. Cell. Cardiol.* 11:275–287.

48. Anversa, P., Olivetti, G., Melissari, M., and Loud, A.V. 1980. Stereological measurement of cellular and subcellular hypertrophy and hyperplasia in the papillary muscle of adult rat. *J. Molec. Cell. Cardiol.* 12:781–795.

49. Medugorac, I. 1980. Collagen content in different areas of normal and hypertrophied rat myocardium. Cardiovasc. Res. 14:551–554.

50. Buccino, R.A., Harris, E., Spann, J.F. Jr., and Sonnenblick, E.H. 1969. Response of myocardial connective tissue of development of experimental hypertrophy. *Am. J. Physiol.* 216:425–428.

51. Medugorac, I., and Jacob, R. 1983. Characterization of left ventricular collagen in the rat. Cardiovasc. Res. 17:15–21.

52. Thiedemann, K.U., Holubarsch, C.H., Medugorac, I., and Jacob, R. 1983. Connective tissue content and myocardial stiffness in pressure overload hypertrophy. A combined study of morphologic, morphometric, biochemical and mechanical parameters. *Basic Res. Cardiol.* 78:140–155.

53. Dawson, R., Milne, G., and Williams, R.B. 1982. Changes in the collagen of rat heart in copper-deficient-induced cardiac hypertrophy. *Cardiov. Res.* 16:559–565.

54. Factor, S.M. Robinson, T.F., and Cho, S.H. 1985. Alterations of the myocardial skeletal framework in acute myocardial infarction with and without ventricular rupture. *Amer. J. Cardiovasc. Pathol.* (In press).

55. Caulfield, J.B., Xuan, J.C., and Ranson, W. 1985. Morphology and ventricular strain rates with infarction. *Proc. 38th Annu. Conf. Engineering in Med. & Biol.* 198.

12. MYOCARDIAL HYPERTROPHY AND CARDIAC FAILURE: A COMPLEX INTERRELATIONSHIP

BARRY M. MASSIE

The interrelationship between myocardial hypertrophy and cardiac function is complex and controversial [1-5]. This relationship is often viewed as a dynamic continuum, with hypertrophy developing as an adaptive response to excessive loading conditions but ultimately becoming associated with myocardial dysfunction and, in the intact organism, cardiac failure.

Figure 12-1 illustrates the interdependance of myocardial hyertrophy and cardiac failure. The initiating stimulus is usually an increase in the load faced by the left or right ventricle. In the most physiologic forms of hypertrophy, such as normal growth and aerobic exercise training, the heart enlarges to keep pace with requirements for increasing cardiac output [6, 7]. Valvular insufficiency, left-to-right shunting, and a variety of other stimuli, produce more abnormal forms of volume overload. Left ventricular pressure overload is most commonly encountered in man as aortic stenosis or systemic hypertension. Despite the different underlying pathophysiologies, each of these processes increases left ventricular systolic or diastolic circumferential wall stress which, as defined by the Laplace equation shown below, is a product of intracavitary pressure (P) times the chamber radius (R) divided by the myocardial wall thickness (h) [3, 6, 7].

This work was supported in part by grant no: HL-28146 from the National Institute of Health and by the Veterans Administration Research Service. This manuscript was published in part in the American Journal of Medicine 75 (Suppl 3A):67, 1983.

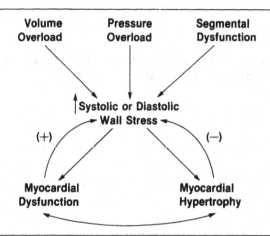

Figure 12–1. The complex interrelationship between myocardial hypertrophy and cardiac dysfunction is shown schematically. See text for details. Reproduced with permission from reference 1.

$$\text{Stress} = \frac{PR}{2h}$$

Similarly, wall stress of the residual healthy myocardium increases when segmental dysfunction results in chamber dilatation and increased diastolic volume and pressure. Finally, in the congestive cardiomyopathies, wall stress is increased as a result of left ventricular dilatation.

A number of regulatory mechanisms are available by which wall stress can be reduced despite increased external load. However, when myocardial contractile reserve is impaired, wall stress will remain elevated and lead to further depression of cardiac performance. Myocardial hypertrophy provides one mechanism by which the heart may adapt to a chronically excessive load. As wall thickness increases, systolic and/or diastolic stress return toward normal levels [3, 7, 8]. This unloads the heart and improves cardiac performance.

A major unresolved question is whether, in some situations, the function of the hypertrophied myocardium is abnormal or becomes so over time and, therefore, eventually results in worsening cardiac performance [1–5]. This uncertainty provides the basis for two potentially divergent views of the hypertrophy process. Some workers consider hypertrophy to be entirely a compensatory adaptation to excessive loading conditions and view the onset of cardiac failure as the result of an insufficient degree of hypertrophy. Other investigators hypothesize that in pressure- and volume-overload situations, hypertrophy may be a pathologic process, either from its initiation or as the result of evolving biochemical, energetic, or contractile abnormalities.

As is often the case when conflicting interpretations arise, there is experimental and clinical evidence supporting both points of view. Central to both hypotheses is the mechanism of transition between compensated hypertrophy and heart failure. Thus far, identification and characterization of such a transitional phase has remained an elusive goal, and, more than likely, no single transitional process is characteristic of all clinical conditions or experimental models.

Much of the work that has provided our present understanding of the hypertrophy process and its interrelationship with myocardial function is experimental. Although this review will consider some of this information, it will focus primarily on the more clinical aspects of the problem.

EVOLUTION OF CARDIAC HYPERTROPHY

As mentioned above, the stimulus to hypertrophy in most experimental models and disease states is a hemodynamic one [1, 3, 7, 8]. It is also apparent that other factors may initiate hypertrophy. Thyrotoxicosis has long been known to stimulate cardiac growth. Laks and his co-workers have produced left ventricular hypertrophy (LVH) with long-term sub-hypertensive infusions of norephinephrine [9]. This and other inferential evidence indicates that the sympathetic nervous system plays a role in the pathogenesis of LVH [10].

The mechanisms by which the stimulus for hypertrophy is translated into sarcomerogenesis remain speculative. Meerson hypothesized that the increased engergy requirements, resulting from supranormal workloads, deplete high energy phosphate stores and that this in turn stimulates nuclear and mitochondrial protein synthesis [11]. Others have postulated a role for cyclic AMP and for changes or compartmental shifts in calcium ion concentration [12]. Although further substantiation for these hypotheses is required, the biochemical sequence of events leading to hypertrophy is better documented [13]. In the stressed heart, messenger RNA synthesis increases within minutes. In a period of 1–3 hours, ribosomal RNA concentration increases. New contractile protein synthesis can be demonstrated within a few hours, and mitochondrial protein and DNA synthesis soon follow.

Since myocardial cell division does not occur in adult mammals, cardiac hypertrophy results from an increase in the volume of existing myocytes [7, 14]. Newly formed sarcomeres may be added in series or in parallel. Data from human subjects suggest that in the volume-overloaded heart, with cardiac dilatation and a normal or increased chamber radius/wall thickness ratio ("eccentric" hypertrophy), sarcomeres are added in series. In contrast, pressure-overloaded states produce "concentric" hypertrophy, characterized by a lower than normal chamber radius/wall thickness ratio and the parallel addition of sarcomeres. In either case, as hypertrophy proceeds, there is an accompanying deposition of fibrous tissue and hyperplasia of stromal elements, including capillaries, although not always in proportion to the degree of myocyte enlargement [14–16]. Ultrastructural changes in myocardial hypertrophy have been reviewed recently [17] and are discussed elsewhere in this volume.

HYPERTROPHY AS A COMPENSATORY PROCESS

Experimental Models

Ontologically, it is attractive to view myocardial hypertrophy as a compensatory process [1, 3, 6, 7, 14]. Ample experimental and clinical evidence suggests that this is usually the case. This adaptational role is most obvious in the hypertrophy which occurs with normal growth or in response to athletic training. Hypertrophy is also seen in the adaptation to increased metabolic demand, such as thyrotoxicosis. These forms of hypertrophy have been termed "physiologic" [2, 4, 6, 14]. Physiological hypertrophy is characterized by normal indices of systolic contraction, diastolic relaxation, myocardial oxygen utilization, and coronary blood flow [2, 4]. Cardiac myosin ATPase activity has been used to distinguish physiologic from pathologic hypertrophy; this is increased, or remains normal, in the former, but diminished in the latter [2, 18]. In addition physiologic forms of hypertrophy appear to be fully reversibe without residual functional or structural changes [4].

In many animal models, hypertrophy also serves to normalize, or at least minimize, the impairment of cardiac-pump performance. In most volume-overload models, cardiac performance remains normal [19–22]. The situation is more complex in pressure-overloaded models [5, 23]. Initially, particularly when the load is applied acutely to the right ventricle and when small mammals are studied, function is reduced [24–27]. However, a compensatory role for hypertrophy has been demonstrated in a number of more chronic studies [28–33]. For instance, while indices of contractility are depressed and chamber dilation is present for several days following aortic contriction in the dog, after several weeks LVH develops, and pump function indices return toward baseline levels as the chamber radius/wall thickness ratio normalizes. (figure 12–2) [29]. Normal function after an initial depression has also been reported after pulmonary artery banding in the rabbit [31], and during chronic pressure overload applied to the right ventricle in the rat [32] and to the left ventricle in the pig [33].

Further evidence for the compensatory nature of hypertrophy is available from studies of left ventricular function in experimental hypertension. In the spontaneously hypertensive rat, global indices of function, such as peak-stroke volume during fluid loading and maximal developed pressure during aortic occlusion, are normal during the early phases of the disease [34–36]. During this time period, despite markedly increased systemic arterial pressure, peak-systolic stress is maintained within normal limits as a result of progressive hypertrophy. Significant left ventricular dysfunction in the intact animal occurs only at a later stage, when LVH does not keep pace with the work load [35].

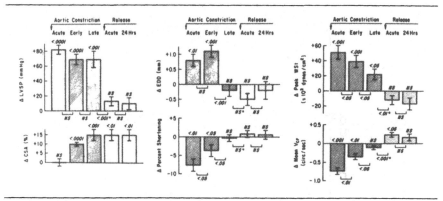

Figure 12-2. The six panels exhibit the average changes (Δ) from control of left ventricular systolic pressure (LVSP), cross-sectional area (CSA), internal end diastolic diameter (EDD), percent internal diameter shortening, peak wall stress (WST), and normalized mean circumferential fiber shortening (VCF). Measurements immediately after aortic constriction (acute), after 9 days (early), after 2½ weeks (late), immediately after release (acute) and 24 hours after release are shown. Probability values above the bars indicate significance of changes from control. Note that with time LV CSA rises, and concomitantly, EDD and measurements of LV function return to baseline. Reproduced with permission from reference 29.

However, studies evaluating contractile function in isolated muscle preparations and perfused hearts have often not confirmed these findings [23]. Cooper et al. demonstrated depressed contractile function in papillary muscles from cats with chronic pressure overload of the right ventricle even though these same animals exhibited normal pump function [27]. Other workers have shown depressed contractility in the chronic phase of renovascular hypertension in rats [37, 38]. These results will be discussed below in the section on pathologic aspects of hypertrophy.

Hypertrophy in Human Pressure and Volume Overload States

It has long been recognized that hypertrophy serves a compensatory function in human subjects as well [3, 4, 6–8]. Grossman and his associates have investigated the role of LVH in patients with aortic stenosis [39, 40]. They found that when hypertrophy was adequate to maintain wall stress within the normal range, despite markedly increased intracavity pressures, left ventricular systolic function was preserved. Systolic dysfunction and signs of congestive heart failure were associated with elevated wall stress [41]. Nonetheless, even in the majority of these subjects, the same linear relation between wall stress and systolic function was maintained, as in the case of normal subjects, indicating that cardiac failure resulted from excessive afterload rather than impaired contractility (figure 12–3). This finding, together with improvement in left ventricular function observed after valve replacement, suggests that LVH is compensatory and physiologic in these individuals. Strauer and others have reported similar findings [42].

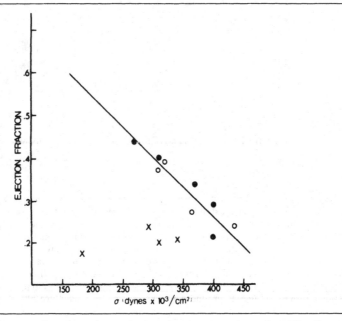

Figure 12-3. Left ventricular ejection fraction is plotted against mean circumferential wall stress in patients with aortic stenosis and congestive heart failure. The patients shown by circles exhibited a postoperative rise in ejection fraction and clinical improvement; in contrast, those shown by x experienced pump failure perioperatively or failed to improve. The authors hypothesize that the preoperative ventricular dysfunction in the first group was due to afterload mismatch with inadequate hypertrophy, whereas in the second group a primary disorder of contractility was present. Reproduced with permission from Reference 41.

In the volume-overloaded setting of aortic insufficiency, hypertrophy appears to play a similar compensatory role [8, 39]. As can be seen in figure 12-4, despite an increase in chamber diameter, systolic wall stress remains normal by virtue of increased wall thickness in compensated patients. However, in an important subset of volume-overloaded patients, systolic dysfunction develops; many of these manifest an elevated chamber radius/wall thickness ratio, suggesting inadequate hypertrophy [8, 43]. However, in contrast to patients with aortic stenosis in whom left ventricular function usually returns to normal postoperatively, patients with aortic insufficiency often continue to exhibit left ventricular dysfunction [4, 43, 44]. Persistent postoperative dysfunction is most pronounced in patients with the greatest degree of cellular hypertrophy on preoperative biopsies [44]. Krayenbuehl has interpreted these findings as indicating that LVH secondary to aortic valve disease is not solely a physiological adaptation [4].

Hypertrophy in Congestive Cardiomyopathy

LVH is a consistent finding in the chronic congestive cardiomyopathies, whether they are primary or result from ischemic heart disease. Again, LVH appears to play a compensatory role. A number of authors have noted fewer

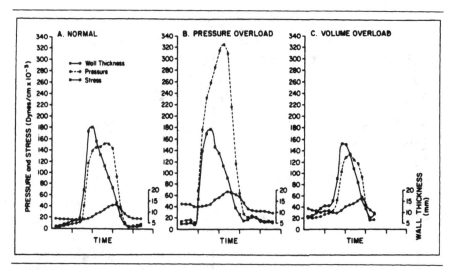

Figure 12-4. The 3 panels show plots of intraventricular pressure, wall thickness and calculated wall stress during the cardiac cycle in a normal subject (A) and compensated patients with pressure overload due to aortic stenosis (B) and volume overload due to aortic insufficiency (C). Systolic stress is maintained in the normal range despite the excessive pressure and volume. Reproduced with permission from reference 39.

symptoms and a better prognosis in patients with dilated cardiomuyopathy who have more advanced hypertrophy [45–47]. Feild and his co-workers performed quantitative angiography in 36 patients with primary cardiomyopathy [46]. Patients with a left ventricular mass/volume ratio above 0.9 g/ml had better survival; this measurement provided additional prognostic information even when the patients were subdivided by ejection fraction (figure 12–5).

These findings were corroborated in a postmortem study evaluating the role of hypertrophy in congestive cardiomyopathy [47]. Patients with a greater left ventricular wall thickness/chamber diameter ratio had a more prolonged clinical course, and this measurement was of greater predictive value than either chamber size for left ventricular mass alone. These findings, again, support the hypothesis that hypertrophy, by preventing excessive wall stress, is an important adaptation to left ventricular dysfunction.

LVH is also a frequent finding in patients with coronary heart disease following myocardial infarction. Theoretically, this may also be an adaptive response to compensate for loss of myocardium, but whether it is ultimately beneficial, particularly in the setting of a compromised coronary circulation, is uncertain [48].

PATHOLOGIC NATURE OF CARDIAC HYPERTROPHY

While the concept that myocardial hypertrophy is primarily an adaptive response is ontologically satisfying, the view that hypertrophy is a pathologic

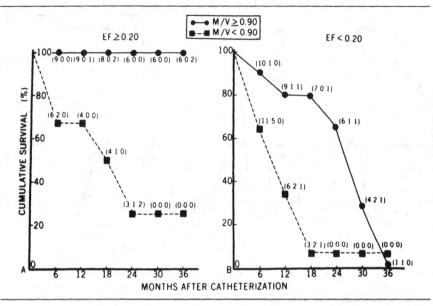

Figure 12–5. Survival curves of patients with congestive cardiomyopathy based upon their left ventricular mass (M) to volume (V) ratio are shown. Whether the ejection fraction was above or below 0.20, the M/V ratio indicated discriminated high and low risk groups. Reproduced with permission from reference 46.

process in many disease states is also supported by compelling evidence. The Framingham study has demonstrated dramatically that LVH is associated with a poor prognosis [49]. There is a strong relation between electrocardiographic and radiographic evidence of LVH and the subsequent appearance of congestive heart failure. Furthermore, electrocardiographic LVH was associated with an eightfold increase in cardiovascular mortality. Belying the argument that hypertrophy plays a solely compensatory role in patients with severe hypertension is the finding that at any level of blood pressure, mortality was twice as high in patients with diagnostic criteria for LVH. In fact, a considerable body of predominantly experimental and pathologic data indicates that significant abnormalities exist in hypertrophied myocardium.

Experimental Models

The literature on the pathologic aspects of myocardial hypertrophy is both extensive and contradictory [1–3]. Much of the confusion results from the fact that many findings are not reproducible in different experimental models, so that the species studied, the severity and acuteness of the stimulus to hypertrophy applied, the ventricle subjected to overload, and the timing of subsequent observations, are all critical in determining the results [2]. Various investigators have documented biochemical and structural abnormalities in hypertrophy and have found associated disorders of contractility, myocardial blood flow, and myocardial metabolism. These abnormalities are easier to demonstrate in models in which the stimulus to hypertrophy is abrupt and severe, when it involves a pressure overload to the right ventricle and when smaller animals are studied.

Many workers have demonstrated decreased indices of contractility in isolated cardiac muscle from hearts subjected to pressure overload of either the right or left ventricle [23–27, 37]. The most consistent abnormality is a depression of the velocity-related contractility indices in isolated muscle taken from the overloaded ventricle. This decrease in shortening velocity (V_{max}) is associated with a reduction in myosin ATPase activity. Of note is that this abnormality precedes any depression in isometric indices of contraction and can be observed at a time when pump function in vivo and in the perfused heart are normal [27, 31, 50]. The depression in V_{max} has been interpreted as being an early sign of myocardial dysfunction and, together with the depressed myosin ATPase activity, considered to be a marker for pathologic hypertrophy [2, 23, 37].

Another interpretation is possible, as has been recently presented by Swynghedauw et al. [5]. In the pressure-overloaded heart, the reduction in shortening velocity produces a more energy-efficient contraction, thus permitting additional external work to be performed with relatively less energy utilization [36, 51]. The finding that these indices are less abnormal when hypertrophy develops gradually and may return to normal in a more chronic compensated phase supports the argument that these changes are adaptive [28, 31–33]. Similarly, a number of workers have found that depression in V_{max} is completely reversible when the stimulus to hypertrophy is removed [52–54], even at a time when hypertrophy persists [55]. This suggests that the changes in contractility are more closely related to the excessive load than to the hypertrophy process itself and again supports the concept that they may be playing an adaptive role.

Thus, controversy persists about the degree, chronicity, and implications of contractile dysfunction in the overloaded heart. Nonetheless, several careful studies have shown that in some models, chronic pressure overload is associated with impaired myocardial function either from the outset or during the course of follow-up [23]. Thus, Cooper was able to show that in kittens a gradually progressive pressure overload resulting from an initially nonconstricting pulmonary artery band demonstrated abnormalities of isotonic shortening and isometric tension development at 25 and 60 weeks after banding [27]. Coulsen studied two groups of cats, one having moderate pulmonary stenosis and the second having severe obstruction [56]. Ejection-phase indices were abnormal in both and reversed with relief of the obstruction. The severe-stenosis group developed signs of congestive heart failure and also exhibited depressed tension development that did not reverse when the pressure overload was removed. This was interpreted as demonstrating that, with increasing loads, initially reversible dysfunction progresses to an irreversible stage of failure.

Pfeffer et al. have studied cardiac function in the spontaneously hypertensive rat longitudinally. At six months of age, significant LVH is present, but contractile indices are normal or even supranormal [34]. Similar observations have been made in our laboratory in isovolumically contracting perfused hearts [36]. Of note is that this compensation is achieved with lower energy requirements, indicating a successful adaptation. After 18 months, LVH has progressed, but the pump performance of the heart becomes depressed. A similar evolution has been observed in the renal hypertensive rat [57].

These data support the hypothesis, most elegantly put forth by Meersen, that in pressure overload there is a continuum from normal to impaired contractile function [11]. Meerson proposed three stages of cardiac hypertrophy. The first is characterized by progressive hypertrophy and supernormal function. In the second stage, hypertrophy is stable and cardiac function remains normal; in the final stage, there is "exhaustion" of the heart, high energy substrate depletion, and progressive dysfunction.

Cardiac Function During Hypertrophy in Humans

The compensatory nature of LVH in patient with aortic valve disease has been discussed previously [40, 41, 42]. However, although most patients with aortic stenosis exhibit normal indices of contractility when examined in relation to load, virtually every study includes a smaller group with depressed function [41, 42, 44]. Of note is that those with impaired contractility generally have greater degrees of LVH, suggesting that there may be an element of pathologic dysfunction in advanced hypertrophy [4, 44].

LVH and Hypertension

Chronic hypertension is the most frequent cause of LVH [49]. With the availability of echocardiography, it is now clear that hypertrophy often occurs earlier in the clinical course of hypertension than was previously appreciated [58, 59]. Surprisingly, the correlation between the level of blood pressure and the degree of LVH is poor [10, 60]. Since hypertension is a major etiological factor in many patients with congestive heart failure [61], the question of whether hypertrophy plays a compensatory or pathologic role is of obvious importance.

The evolution of hypertrophy and heart failure in animal models has been discussed previously. Progression of cardiac involvement in hypertensive human subjects appears to parallel that in the spontaneously hypertensive rat [62–64). See table 12–1. Hypertrophy may precede the appearance of "fixed" hypertension. Early in the course of hypertension, many patients exhibit a hyperkinetic picture, characterized by increased blood volume and cardiac output, together with supernormal indices of contractility. During the phase of chronic, stable hypertension, LVH progresses and left ventricular performance generally remains normal, although investigators have demonstrated reduced systolic function with exercise [64, 65].

Table 12–1. Evolution of hypertensive heart disease

	Early Hypertension	Hypertension	Congestive Heart Failure
Blood pressure	increased	increased	increased or unchanged
Cardiac output	increased or unchanged	unchanged	decreased
Left ventricular mass	unchanged or increased	increased	increased
Left ventricular volume	unchanged or decreased	unchanged	increased
Contractility	increased	unchanged or decreased	decreased
Ejection fraction	unchanged or increased	unchanged	decreased

Table 12–2. Left ventricular functional reserve in hypertension

	Normals	Hypertension	Hypertension with LVH	Hypertension with LVH and abnormal EF
N	13	40	23	7
Rest EF (%)	67 ± 8	62 ± 7	67 ± 7	55 ± 10*#@
Rest PSP/ESV (mmHg/ml/m²)	3.0 ± 1.2	3.8 ± 1.6	4.2 ± 1.7	3.3 ± 1.0
Rest ESS (10^3 × dyn/m²)	54 ± 15	55 ± 14	64 ± 6	83 ± 11*#@
Δ EF (%)	+15	+11	+8*	+4*#@
Δ PSP/ESV (mmHg/ml/m²)	+5.5	+3.5	+2.3*	+0.5*#@
Maximum workload (kpm/min)	1130 ± 180	853 ± 200	680 ± 220*	670 ± 220*#

* $p < .01$ vs. normal, # $p < .05$ vs. hypertensives, @ $p < 0.5$ vs. hypertensives with LVH.

Abbreviations:
EF = ejection fraction;
ESS = end-systolic stress;
PSP/ESV = peak systolic pressure to end-systolic volume ratio.

In our experience, patients with uncomplicated hypertension generally exhibit normal cardiac reserve, as estimated by their ejection fraction response to exercise [66]. However, a continuum of responses was apparent [67]. See table 12–2. All patients without LVH exhibited a normal exercise ejection fraction response. Approximately 25% of patients with LVH had an abnormal resting ejection fraction or a subnormal increase during exercise. The remaining patients exhibited a normal ejection fraction response but exhibited a smaller increase in their peak systolic pressure/end-systolic pressure ratio with exercise. Interestingly, end-systolic stress was normal in the hypertensives without LVH, elevated in those with impaired ejection fraction response, and intermediate in those with LVH and a normal ejection fraction response.

These findings again raise the question of whether the hypertrophied myocardium is functioning normally, or whether the degree of hypertrophy is inadequate for the load to the heart. As noted previously, it has been argued that hypertrophy, by maintaining relatively low systolic wall stress in the face of increased systolic pressures, reduces and prevents decompensation. However, it is difficult to ignore the consistent finding that in clinical pressure overload states, it is the subjects with the most advanced hypertrophy that show overt signs of heart failure or more subtle abnormalities of contractile function [4]. Furthermore, as discussed above, LVH itself appears to be a poor prognostic sign.

Diastolic Function in LVH

Until recently, most studies of the relation between myocardial hypertrophy and cardiac function have concentrated on left ventricular systolic performance. It has now become obvious that LVH is frequently accompanied by diastolic dysfunction, and that this often precedes measurable impairment of contractility [66, 68, 69]. Increased chamber stiffness or reduced left ventricular distensibility is an early finding in most experimental models of hypertrophy [35, 70]. This is likely to be a result of the increased wall thickness, and disappears when hypertrophy is reversed. However, at a later stage, myocardial wall stiffness or muscle stiffness also becomes abnormal. These changes may not be reversible and appear to be related to collagen deposition and myocardial fibrosis [70–72]. Abnormalities in left ventricular relaxation and increased myocardial stiffness have been detected in patients with aortic valve disease in the presence of normal contractile function [73, 74]. When these findings are correlated with myocardial biopsies, they appear to be more closely related to the fibrous tissue content of the heart, rather than to myocardial cell diameter.

The literature on diastolic function and essential hypertension is growing rapidly. While the status of systolic function in this entity remains controversial, diastolic abnormalities are found consistently. In a study of 39 patients with mild and moderate essential hypertension, selected by virtue of their normal left ventricular ejection fraction at rest and during exercise, we found diastolic abnormalities in 84% of patients [66] (figure 12–6). When the correlation between these abnormalities and the degree of LVH was examined, the relation was only modest. However, when a group of previously untreated patients was examined the relation was significantly tighter [75]. Shapiro examined isovolumic relaxation times as well as the rate of wall thinning in a group of previously untreated hypertensive subjects and again found a close relationship with left ventricular mass [68]. Interestingly, he found no such changes in a group of athletes who had comparable degrees of LVH, supporting the concept that there are physiological differences between forms of hypertrophy. We have recently noted that diastolic filling rates improve

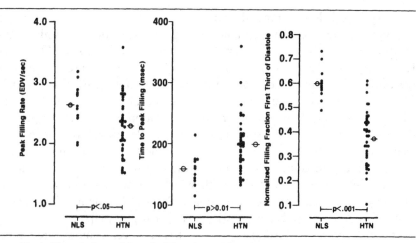

Figure 12-6. Three indices of diastolic filling derived from blood pool scintigrams are shown. Each was abnormal in hypertensive subjects compared to age-matched controls. Reproduced with permission from reference 66.

when LVH is reversed by antihypertensive therapy [76]. This would suggest that at least some of the changes relate to increased chamber stiffness, although a component of increased myocardial wall stiffness cannot be excluded.

These findings concerning diastolic function in hypertension have raised the possibility that such measurements may facilitate the detection of the previously elusive transitional stage between compensated myocardial function and left ventricular failure. However, in animal models diastolic and systolic function are more closely related, and the preponderance of data suggests that the observed changes may be more related to ventricular geometry and changes in nonmyocardial components, rather than to an alteration in the function of heart muscle itself. Most important will be longitudinal examinations in man which will demonstrate whether patients with subtle diastolic dysfunction will proceed to left ventricular failure.

Whatever the pathophysiologic implications of these diastolic changes, they appear to have important clinical implications. Impaired diastolic function probably explains the early appearance of left atrial enlargement in patients with hypertension [77]. It probably is also a common cause for the symptoms of dyspnea on exertion and orthopnea, which some hypertensive patients experience at a time when measurements of systolic function are normal. Prior to the ready availability of noninvasive measurements of cardiac function, these symptoms were often attributed to incipient congestive heart failure and led to inappropriate medical therapy with digitalis.

Coronary Blood Flow and Ischemia in LVH

The physiology and anatomy of the coronary circulation in experimental LVH has been extensively studied [78–84]. There is general agreement that resting coronary blood flow is normal, but that coronary reserve, as measured by minimal coronary vascular resistance during pharmacological vasodilation or situations of increased oxygen demand, is reduced. These changes have been described in both large and small mammals. This diminished reserve has been ascribed to alterations in coronary vasomotor regulation, external compression of blood vessels, particularly in the sub-endocardial region, and anatomic changes. Some workers have observed a correlation between the impairment of coronary reserve and the severity of LVH, while others have not and have even noted a reversal of the abnormalities while hypertrophy progresses. In any case, the pathologic significance of these findings in some situations is indicated by the work of Bache et al. which has demonstrated lactate production and adenosine release correlating with the reduction in subendocardial blood flow in dogs with left ventricular hypertrophy [85].

Abnormal coronary vasodilator reserve has also been demonstrated in man in the setting of aortic stenosis and, more importantly, in essential hypertension [86–91]. In the former condition, the changes again correlate with clinical and metabolic evidence of ischemia. Decreased coronary reserve has been observed in patients with chest pain and normal coronary arteries in the presence of LVH [90, 91]. In a recent study, the coronary blood flow abnormalities were correlated with scintigraphic evidence of myocardial ischemia [91]. It is tempting to speculate that some of the electrocardiographic repolarization abnormalities of severe LVH may also reflect changes in coronary blood flow, but confirmation for this is not yet available. Also of potential clinical importance is the finding of Marcus and his co-workers that dogs with LVH tolerate coronary occlusion less well [92, 93]. They observed an increase in the size of myocardial infarction relative to the area at risk and a higher mortality during experimental myocardial infarction. Along these same lines, Strauer has observed that the reduction in coronary reserve is greater in patients with hypertension and accompanying coronary disease than in those with similar degrees of LVH and normal coronary arteries [87]. Taken together, these experimental and clinical observations may help explain why hypertension is a prominent risk factor for coronary disease as well as the high proportion of deaths due to ischemic heart disease in the hypertensive population.

Perhaps related to the changes in coronary blood flow is evidence that the hypertrophied myocardium may suffer from an inadequate energy supply. The biochemical, ultrastructural and anatomic observations that support this view are presented in depth elsewhere in this volume. However, it is important to observe that decreases in capillary density within the myocardium, increases in interstitial elements such as collagen, and the reduction in cell surface/cell volume ratio, which necessarily accompanies concentric hypertrophy, all may impair the transfer of substrates and metabolites in and out of the cell [14–16]. Metabolic changes in the hypertrophied heart at the cellular level consistent with the presence of ischemia have been detected

[94–95]. Ischemia could well explain the presence of cell necrosis and fibrosis which are usually present in both experimental and clinical hypertrophy. It was noted previously the increase in collagen content of the hypertrophied myocardium is the likely explanation for the increase in muscle stiffness and reduced diastolic compliance noted in many hypertrophic states. Furthermore, Bing et al. have demonstrated that the progressive systolic dysfunction with aging in the spontaneously hypertensive rat is primarily a function of increasing fibrosis [72]. Taken together, these findings raise the possibility that the transition from myocardial hypertrophy to cardiac failure is mediated predominantly by the effects of ischemia rather than a primary change at the cellular level.

REGRESSION OF MYOCARDIAL HYPERTROPHY

Regression of LVH has been demonstrated in animal models and in man, and this subject has been reviewed extensively [96–99]. The ability to reverse LVH raises a number of important issues. If LVH carries a poor prognosis, it is natural to speculate that morbidity and nortality will be diminished with its reversal. Whether such an improvement is more beneficial than that expected from successful treatment of the underlying pathology alone is speculative. More appropriate to the current discussion is the potential for understanding the pathophysiology of hypertrophy, which the capability to reverse the disorder provides. In pressure-overload hypertrophy models involving right or left ventricular outflow tract obstruction, myocardial hypertrophy can be reversed with removal of the stenosis. In most studies, contractile dysfunction reverses as myocardial hypertrophy diminishes [52–55]. This is associated with a return to the pre-overload pattern of isomyosin distribution. In both the renal and spontaneously hypertensive rat, the evolution of LVH may be prevented and established LVH may be reversed with therapy [96, 97]. Again, the changes in systolic and diastolic function are also prevented or reversed. One interesting observation from these experimental studies is the occasional dissociation between hypertrophy regression and blood pressure control, suggesting that nonhemodynamic factors may play a role in the reversal, and, by implication, in the development of LVH. However, after LVH regression, an abnormal amount of collagen may remain [100]. This has been associated with a permanent reduction in left ventricular compliance.

In humans, regression of LVH has been frequently demonstrated after surgical treatment of aortic and pulmonary valve disease. This is usually associated with the normalization of contractile indices and coronary blood flow reserve, but some patients, particularly those with the most severe preoperative hypertrophy and myocardial dysfunction, do not demonstrate reversal of dysfunction [4]. In these, excessive fibrosis has been shown to persist. LVH reversal has been demonstrated during the course of antihypertensive therapy with many agents [98, 99]. While some have argued that agents with an anti-sympathetic nervous system mechanism of action are more effective in reversing LVH, a growing body of information suggests that most medications which effectively lower blood pressure have a potential to regress LVH. Nonetheless, there is marked heterogeneity in responses of individual patients. It is not yet possible to generalize about the functional consequences of LVH reversal, secondary to antihypertensive therapy. The limited information available suggests that systolic function is at least maintained and that diastolic function may improve [76].

SUMMARY

In man, LVH carries a poor prognosis, being associated with a markedly increased risk of developing congestive heart failure and an excessive mortality. This knowledge has led to intensive investigation of the changes in myocardial function during experimentally induced hypertrophy. In some models, the expected evolution from normal function to a phase of depressed contractility, to an eventual stage of overt cardiac failure, has been demonstrated. In other models, the detection of this transition has been elusive. Similarly, in humans, the demonstration of depressed systolic function prior to the appearance of overt failure, has not been clear-cut. More commonly, in both the clinical setting and the laboratory, groups with normal contractility and those with definite dysfunction have been detected, but an intermediate group has been less apparent.

During the course of these investigations, it has also become obvious that hypertrophy plays an adaptive role. The increased myocardial mass permits the maintenance of normal pump function in the presence of excessive load. Some workers believe that myocardial dysfunction supervenes only when hypertrophy is inadequate. Indeed, the depression in ejection phase indices such as V_{max}, the changes in isomyosin composition, and the associated decrease in myosin ATPase activity may also be adaptive by increasing the efficiency of cardiac performance.

Perhaps these two views of the relation between myocardial hypertrophy and function can best be reconciled by viewing the transition from the compensatory stage of hypertrophy to a dysfunctional one as being the result of an ischemic process. In this regard, a growing body of data suggests that the hypertrphied heart is more susceptible to ischemia, and that many of the functional abnormalities at the late stages of hypertrophy result from myocardial fibrosis, which may be the result of ischemia. This view would fit with the clinical picture of the evolution of hypertensive heart disease, where the juxtaposition of hypertrophy and coronary artery disease is the cause of most mortalities.

REFERENCES

1. Massie, B.M. 1983. Myocardial hypertrophy and cardiac failure: A complex interrelationship. *Am. J. Med.* 75, Suppl. 3A:67–74.

2. Wikman-Coffelt, Parmley, W.W., and Mason, D.T. 1979. The cardiac hypertrophy process: Analyses of factors determining pathological vs. physiological development. *Circ. Res.* 45:697–707.

3. Grossman, W. 1980. Cardiac hypertrophy: useful adaptation or pathologic process? *Am. J. Med.* 69:576–584.

4. Krayenbuehl, H.P., Hess, O.M., Schneider, J., and Turina, M. 1983. Physiologic or pathologic hypertrophy. *Eur. Heart. J.* 4:29–34.

5. Swynghedauw, B., Schwartz, K., and Apstein, C.S. 1984. Decreased contractility after myocardial hypertrophy: Cardiac failure or successful adaptation? *Am. J. Cardiol.* 54: 437–440.

6. Badeer, H.S. 1964. Editorial, Biological significance of cardiac hypertrophy. *Am. J. Cardiol.* 14:133–138.

7. Ford, L.E. 1976. Heart size. *Circ. Res.* 39:297–303.

8. Gaasch, W.H. 1979. Left ventricular radius to wall thickness ratio. *Am. J. Cardiol.* 43:1189–1194.

9. Laks, M.M., Morady, F., and Swan, H.J.C. 1973. Myocardial hypertrophy produced by chronic subhypertensive doses of norephinephrine in the dog. *Chest* 64:75–80.

10. Frohlich, E.D., and Tarazi, R.C. 1979. Is arterial pressure the sole factor responsible for hypertensive cardiac hypertrophy? *Am. J. Cardiol.* 44:959–963.

11. Meerson, F.Z., and Breger, A.M. 1977. The common mechanism of the heart's adaptation and deadaptation: hypertrophy and atrophy of the heart muscle. *Basic Res. Cardiol.* 72: 228–234.

12. Rasmussen, H., and Goodman, D.B.P. 1977. Relationship between calcium and cyclic nucleotides in cell activation. *Physiol. Rev.* 57:421–509.

13. Rabnowitz, M., and Zak, R. 1972. Biochemical and cellular changes in cardiac hypertrophy. *Ann. Rev. Med.* 23:245–262.

14. Linzbach, A.J. 1960. Heart failure from the point of view of quantitative anatomy. *Am. J. Cardiol.* 5:370–382.

15. Buccino, R.A., Harris, E., Spann, J.F., and Sonnenblick, E.H. 1969. Response of myocardial connective tissue to development of experimental hypertrophy. *Am. J. Physiol.* 216: 425–428.

16. Gerdes, A.M., Callas, G., and Rasten, F.H. 1979. Differences in regional capillary distribution and myocyte sizes in normal and hypertrophic rat hearts. *Am. J. Anat.* 156:523–532.

17. Bishop, S.P. 1983. Ultrastructure of the myocardium in physiology and pathologic hypertrophy in experimental animals. In *Myocardial Hypertrophy and Failure*, N.R. Alpert, ed., pp. 127–147. New York: Raven Press.

18. Scheuer, J., and Bhan, A.K. 1979. Cardiac contractile proteins. *Circ. Res.* 45:1–12.

19. Taylor, R., Covell, J.W., and Ross, J. Jr. 1968. Left ventricular function in experimental aorto-canal fistula with circulatory congestion and fluid retention. *J. Clin. Invest.* 47: 1333–42.

20. Turina, M., Bussmann, W.D., and Krayenbuehl, H.P. 1969. Contractility of the hypertrophied canine heart in chronic volume overload. *Cardiovasc. Res.* 3:486–495.

21. Cooper, G., Puga, F.J., Aujko, K.J., Harrison, E.C., and Coleman, H-N. 1973. Normal myocardial function and energetics in volume-overload hypertrophy in the cat. *Circ. Res.* 32:140–148.

22. Carey, R.A., Natarajan, G., Bove, A.A., Coulson, R.L., Spann, J. F. 1979. Myosin adenosine triphosphatase activity in the volume-overloaded hypertrophied feline right ventricle. *Circ. Res.* 45:81–87.

23. Spann, J.F. 1983. Contractile and pump function of the pressure-overloaded heart. In *Myocardial Hypertrophy and Failure*, N.R. Alpert, ed. pp. 19–38. New York: Raven Press.

24. Spann, J.F., Buccino, R.A., Sonnenblick, E.H., and Braunwald, E. 1967. Contractile state of cardiac muscle obtained from cats with experimentally produced ventricular hypertrophy and failure. *Circ. Res.* 21:341–54.

25. Bing, O.H.L., Matsushita, S., Fanburg, B.L., and Levine, H.J. 1971. Mechanical properties of rat cardiac muscle during experimental hypertrophy. *Circ. Res.* 28:234–45.

26. Cooper, G., Satava, R.M. Jr., Harrison, C.E., and Coleman, H.N. 1973. Mechanism for the abnormal energetics of pressure-induced hypertrophy of cat myocardium. *Circ. Res.* 33:313–23.

27. Cooper IV, G., Tomanek, R.J., Ehrhardt, J.C., and Marcus, M.L. 1981. Chronic

progressive pressure overload of the cat right ventricle. *Circ. Res.* 48:488–97.

28. Williams, J.F. Jr., and Potter, R.D. 1974. Normal contractile state of hypertrophied myocardium after pulmonary artery construction in the cat. *J. Clin. Invest.* 54:1266–72.

29. Sasayama, S., Ross, J., Franklin, D., Bloor, C.M., Bishop, S., and Dilley, R.B. 1976. Adaptations of the left ventricle to chronic pressure overload. *Circ. Res.* 38:172–78.

30. Carabello, R.A., Mee, R., Collins, J.J. Jr., Kloner, R.A., and Levin, D., Grossman, W. 1981. Contractile function in chronic gradually developing subcoronary aortic stenosis. *Am. J. Physiol.* 240:1180–86.

31. Hoffman, H., and Covell, J.W. 1984. Relationship between ejection phase indices of performance and myocardial functions during the development of pressure-overload hypertrophy. *Am. Heart J.* 107:738–44.

32. Julian, F.J., Morgan, D.L., Moss, R.L., Gonzalez, M., and Dwivedi, P. 1981. Myocyte growth without physiological impairment in gradually induced rat cardiac hypertrophy. *Circ. Res.* 49:1300–10.

33. Wisenbaugh, T., Allen, P., Cooper IV, G., Holzegrefe, H., Beller, G., and Carabello, B. 1983. Contractile function, myosin ATPase activity and isozymes in the hypertrophied pig left ventricle after a chronic progressive pressure overload. *Circ. Res.* 53:332–41.

34. Pfeffer, J.M., Pfeffer, M.A., Fishbein, M.C., and Frohlich, E.D. 1979. Cardiac function and morphology with aging in the spontaneously hypertensive rat. *Am. J. Physiol.* 237: H461–68.

35. Burger, S.B., and Strauer, B.E. 1981. Left ventricular hypertrophy in chronic pressure load due to spontaneous essential hypertension. I Left ventricular function, left ventricular geometry and wall stress. In *The Heart in Hypertension*, B.E. Strauer, ed., pp. 13–35. Berlin: Springer-Verlag.

36. Tubau, J.F., Wikman-Coffelt, J., Sievers, R., Parmley, W.W., and Massie, B.M. 1984. Improved myocardial efficiency in the isolated perfused heart of hypertensive rats. *Clin. Res.* 32:340A.

37. Capasso, J.M., Strobeck, J.E., and Sonnenblick, H. 1981. Myocardial mechanical alterations during gradual onset long-term hypertension in rats. *Am. J. Physiol.* 241:H435–41.

38. Alfaro, A., Schaible, T.F., Malhotra, A., Yipintsoi, T., Scheuer, J. 1983. Impaired coronary flow and ventricular function in hearts of hypertensive rates. *Cardiovasc. Res.* 17:553–561.

39. Grossman, W., Jones, D., and McLaurin, L.P. 1975. Wall stress and patterns of hypertrophy in the human left ventricle. *J. Clin. Invest.* 56:56–64.

40. Gunther, S., and Grossman, W. 1979. Determinants of ventricular function in pressure-overload hypertrophy in man. *Circulation* 59:679–688.

41. Carabello, B.A., Green, L.H., Grossman, W., Cohn, L.W., Koster, J.K., and Collins, J.J. 1980. Hemodynamic determinants of prognosis of aortic valve replacement in critical aortic stenosis and advanced congestive heart failure. *Circulation* 62:42–48.

42. Strauer, B.E. 1981. Performance, wall dynamics, and coronary function of the left ventricle in hypertensive heart disease. In *The Heart in Hypertension*, B.E. Strauer, ed., pp. 251–84. Berlin: Springer-Verlag.

43. Gaasch, W.H., Andrios, C.W., and Levine, H.W. 1978. Chronic aortic regurgitation: the effect of aortic valve replacement on left ventricular volume, mass, and function. *Circulation* 58:825–36.

44. Schwartz, F., Flameng, W., Schaper, J., Langebartels, F., Sesto, M., Hehrlein, F., and Schlepper, M. 1978. Myocardial structure and function in patients with aortic valve disease and their relation to postoperative results. *Am. J. Cardiol.* 41:661–69.

45. Goodwin, J.F. 1970. Congestive and hypertrophic cardiomyopathies. *Lancet:*731–39.

46. Feild, B.J., Baxley, W.A., Russell, R.O. Jr., Hood, W.P., Holt, J.H., Dowling, J.T., and Rackley, C.E. 1973. Left ventricular function and hypertrophy in cardiomyopathy with depressed ejection fraction. *Circulation* 47:1022–31.

47. Benjamin, I.J., Schuster, E.H., and Bulkley, B.H. 1981. Cardiac hypertrophy in idiopathic dilated congestive cordiomyopathy: A clinicopathologic study. *Circulation* 64:442–47.

48. 1974. The Coronary Drug Project Research Group: Left ventricular hypertrophy and prognosis. Experience postinfarction in the coronary drug project. *Circulation* 49:862–69.

49. Kannell, W.B., Gordon, T., and Offutt, D. 1969. Left ventricular hypertrophy by electrocardiogram. Prevalence, incidence, and mortality in the Framingham Study. *Ann. Intern. Med.* 71:89–101.

50. Hammell, B.B., Alpert, N.R. 1977. The mechanical characteristics of hypertrophied rabbit cardiac muscle in the absence of congestive heart failure. *Circ. Res.* 40:20–25, 1977.
51. Alpert, N.R., and Muller, L.A. 1982. Increased myothermal economy of isometric force generation in compensated cardiac hypertrophy, induced by pulmonary artery constriction in the rabbit. *Circ. Res.* 50:491–500.
52. Cooper, G., Satava, R.M., Hamson, C.E., and Coleman, H.N. 1974. Normal myocardial function and energetics after reversing pressure-overload hypertrophy. *Am.J. Physiol.* 226:1158–65.
53. Carey, R., Bove, A.A., Coulson, R.L., and Spann, J.R. 1958. Recovery of myosin ATPase after relief of pressure-overload hypertrophy. *Am. J. Physiol.* 234:H711–17.
54. Capasso, J.M., Strobeck, J.E., Malhotra, A., Scheuer, J., and Sonnenblick, E.H. 1982. Contractile behavior of rat myocardium after reversal of hypertensive hypertrophy. *Am. J. Physiol.* 242:H882–89.
55. Wisenbaugh, Allen, P., Cooper IV, G., O'Connor, W.N., Mezaros, L., Streter, F., Bahinski, A., Houser, S., and Spann, J.F. 1984. Hypertrophy without contractile dysfunction after reversal of pressure overload in the cat. *Am. J. Physiol.* 247:H146–54.
56. Coulson, R.L., Yazdanfar, S., Rubio, E., Bore, A.A., Lemote, G.M., and Spann, J.F. 1977. Recuperative potential of cardiac muscle following relief of pressure-overload hypertrophy and right ventricular failure in the cat. *Circ. Res.* 40:41–49.
57. Jacob, R., and Kissling, G. 1981. Left ventricular dynamics and myocardial function in Goldblatt hypertension of the rat. In *The Heart in Hypertension*, B.E. Strauer, ed., Berlin: Springer-Verlag.
58. Savage, D.D., Drayer, J.I.M., Henry, W.L., Mathews, E.C., Ware, J.H., Gardin, J.M., Cohen, E.R., Epstein, G.E., and Laragh, J.H. 1979. Echocardiographic assessment of cardiac anatomy and function in hypertensive subjects. *Circulation* 59:623–32.
59. Scheiken, R.M., Clarke, W.R., and Lauer, R.M. 1981. Left ventricular hypertrophy in children with blood pressure in the upper quantile of the distribution. The Muscatine Study. *Hypertension* 3:669–75.
60. Devereux, R.B., Savage, D.D., Sachs, L., and Laragh, J.H. 1983. Relation of Hemodynamic load to left ventricular hypertrophy and performance in hypertension. *Am. J. Cardiol.* 51:171–76.
61. Kannell, W.B., Castelli, W.P., Mellumara, A.M., McKee, P.H., and Fernleib, M. 1972. Role of blood pressure in the development of congestive heart failure. *N. Engl. J. Med.* 287:781–87.
62. Cohn, J.N., Limas, C.J., and Guiha, N.H. 1974. Hypertension and the heart. *Arch. Intern. Med.* 133:969–79.
63. Fries, E.D. 1960. Hemodynamics of hypertension. *Physiol. Rev.* 40:27–54.
64. Lund-Johnson, P. Hemodynamics in essential hypertension. *Clin. Sci.* 59, supp. 343s–354s.
65. Borer, J.S.A., Jason, M. Devereux, R.B., Fisher, J., Green, M.V., Bacherach, S.L., Pickering, J. and Taragh, J.H. 1983. Function of the hypertrophying left ventricle at rest and during exercise. *Am. J. Med.* 75, Suppl. 3A:34.
66. Inouye, I., Massie, B., Loge, D., Topic, N., Silverstein, D., Simpson, P., and Tubau, J. 1984. Abnormal left ventricular filling: an early finding in mid to moderate systemic hypertenson. *Am. J. Cardiol.* 53:120–25.
67. Tubau, J.F., Szlachcic, J., Braun, S., Henderson, S., Vollmer, C., and Massie, B.M. 1986. Is there abnormal contractile reserve in hypertensive patients with left ventricular hypertrophy? *J. Am. Coll. Cardiol.* 7:24A.
68. Shapiro, L.M., and McKenna, W.J. 1984. Left ventricular hypertrophy: relation of structure to diastolic function in hypertension. *Br. Heart J.* 51:637–42.
69. Fouad, F.M., Slominski, J.M., and Tarazi, R.C. 1984. Left ventricular diastolic function in hypertension: relation to left ventricular mass and systolic function. *Am. J. Coll. Cardiol.* 3:1500–06.
70. Mirsky, J.F., Pfeffer, J.M., Pfeffer, M.A. 1983. Mechanical properties of normal and hypertrophied myocardium: is there a relationship between diastolic and systolic function? In *Myocardial Hypertrophy and Failure*, N.R. Alpert, ed. New York: Raven Press.
71. Pinsky, W.W., Lewis, R.M., Hartley, C.J., and Entman, M.L. 1979. Permanent changes of ventricular contractility and compliance in chronic volume overload. *Am. J. Physiol.* 237:H575–83.

72. Bing, O.H., Sen, S., Conrad, C.H., and Brooks, W.W. 1984. Myocardial function, structure, and collagen in the spontaneously hypertensive rat: progression from compensated hypertrophy to haemodynamic impairment. *Eur. Heart J.* 5:43–52.
73. Hess, O.M., Schneider, J., Koch, R., Bamert, C., Grimm, J., and Krayenbuehl, H.P. 1981. Diastolic function and myocardial structure in patients with myocardial hypertrophy. *Circulation* 63:360–71.
74. Eichorn, P., Grimm, J., Koch, R., Hess, O.M., Carroll, J., and Krayenbuehl, H.P. 1982. Left ventricular relaxation in patients with left ventricular hypertrophy secondary to aortic valve disease. *Circulation* 65:1395–1404.
75. Tubau, J., Szlachcic, J., Hirsch, A., Henderson, S., Vollmer, C., and Massie, B. 1985. Left ventricular function in hypertensive patients with left ventricular hypertrophy. *J. Am. Coll. Cardiol.* 5:414.
76. Tubau, J.F., Szlachcic, J., Massie, B.M., Henderson, S., and Vollmer, C. 1986. Improvement of diastolic filling following hypertrophy reversal. *J. Am. Coll. Cardiol.* 7:112A
77. Frohlich, E.D., Tarazi, R.C., and Dustan, H.P. 1971. Clinical-physiological correlations in the development of hypertensive heart disease. *Circulation* 56:446–55.
78. Mueller, T.M., Marcus, M.L., Kerber, R.E., Young, J.A., Barnes, R.W., and Abboud, F.M. 1978. Effect of renal hypertension and left ventricular hypertrophy on the coronary circulation in dogs. *Circ. Res.* 42:543–49.
79. Bache, R.J., Vrobel, T.R., Arentzen, C.E., and Steves Ring, W. 1981. Effect of maximal coronary vasocilation on transmural myocardial perfusion during tachycardia in dogs with left ventricular hypertrophy. *Circ. Res.* 49:742–50.
80. Marcus, M.L., Mueller, T.M., Eastham, C.L. 1981. Effects of short- and long-term left ventricular hypertrophy on coronary circulation. *Am. J. Physiol.* 241:H358–62.
81. Wangler, R.D., Peters, K.G., Marcus, M.L., and Tomanek, R.J. 1982. Effects of duration and severity of arterial hypertension and cardiac hypertrophy on coronary vasodilator reserve. *Circ. Res.* 51:10–18.
82. Tomanek, R.J., Searls, J.C., and Lachenbruch, P.A. 1982. Quantitative changes in the capillary bed during developing, peak, and stabilized cardiac hypertrophy in the spontaneously hypertensive rat. *Circ. Res.* 51:296–304.
83. Wicker, P., Tarazi, R.C., and Kobayashi, K. 1983. Coronary blood flow during the development and regression of left ventricular hypertrophy in renovascular hypertensive rats. *Am. J. Cardiol.* 51:1744–49.
84. Kobayashi, K., Tarazi, R.C., Lovenberg, W., and Rakusan, K. 1984. Coronary blood flow in genetic cardiac hypertrophy. *Am. J. Cardiol.* 53:1360–64.
85. Bache, R.J., Arentzen, C.E., Simon, A.B., and Vrobel, T.R. 1984. Abnormalities in myocardial perfusion during trachycardia in dogs with left ventricular hypertrophy: metabolic evidence for myocardial ischemia. *Circulation* 69:409–17.
86. Marcus, M.L., Doty, D.B., Hiratzka, L.F., Wright, C.B., and Eastham, C.L. 1982. Decreased coronary reserve: a mechanism for angina pectoris in patients with aortic stenosis and normal coronary arteries. *N. Eng. J. Med.* 307:1362–6.
87. Strauer, B.E. 1979. Ventricular function and coronary hemodynamics in hypertensive heart disease. *Am. J. Cardiol.* 44:999–1006.
88. Nichols, A.L., B., Sciacca, R.R., Weiss, M.B., Blood, D.K., Brennan, D.L., and Cannon, P.J., 1980. Effect of left ventricular hypertrophy on myocardial blood flow and ventricular performance in systemic hypertension. *Circulation* 62:329–340.
89. Pichard, A.D., Gorlin, R., Smith H., Ambrose, J., and Meller, J. 1981. Coronary flow studies in patients with left ventricular hypertrophy of the hypertensive type. *Am. J. Cardiol.* 47:547–54.
90. Opherk, D., Mall, G., Zebe, H., Schwarz, F., Weihe, E., Manthey, J., and Kübler, W. 1984. Reduction of coronary reserve: a mechanism for angina pectoris in patients with arterial hypertension and normal coronary arteries. *Circulation* 69:1–7.
91. Legrand, V., Hodgson, J., MCcB, Bates, E.R., Aueron, F.M., Mancini, J., Smith, J.S., Gross, M.D., and Vogel, R.A. 1985. Abnormal coronary flow reserve and abnormal radionuclide exercise test results in patients with normal coronary angiograms. *J. Am. Coll. Cardiol.* 6:1245–53.
92. Koyanagi, S., Eastham, C.L., Harrison, D.G., and Marcus, M.L. 1982. Increased size of

myocardial infarction in dogs with chronic hypertension and left ventricular hypertrophy. *Circ. Res.* 50:56–62.

93. Koyanagi, S., Eastham, C., and Marcus, M.L. 1982. Effects of chronic hypertension and left ventricular hypertrophy on the incidence of sudden cardiac death after coronary artery occlusion in conscious dogs. *Circulation* 65:1192–97.

94. Shimamoto, N., Goto, N., Tanabe, M., Imamoto, T., Fujiwara, S., and Hirata, M. 1982. Myocardial energy metabolism in the hypertrophied hearts of spontaneously hypertensive rats. *Basic Res. Cardiol.* 77:359–71.

95. Ingwall, J.S. 1984. The hypertrophied myocardium accumulates the MB-creatine kinase isozyme. *Eur. Heart J.* 5:129–39.

96. Sen, S. 1983. Regression of cardiac hypertrophy: experimental animal model. *Am. J. Med.* 75 (Suppl. 3A):87–93.

97. Rushoaho, H. 1984. Regression of cardiac hypertrophy with drug treatment in spontaneously hypertensive rats. *Med. Biol.* 62:263–276.

98. Tarazi, R.C. 1983. Regression of left ventricular hypertrophy by medical treatment: present status and possible implications. *Am. J. Med.* 75 (Suppl. 3A):80–86.

99. Panidis, I.P., Kotler, M.N., Ren, J-F., Mintz, F.S., Ross, J., and Kalman, P. 1984. Development and regression of left ventricular hypertrophy. *J. Am. Coll. Cardiol.* 3: 1309–20.

100. Sen, S., Tarazi, R.C., and Bumpus, F.M. 1976. Biochemical changes associated with development and reversal of cardiac hypertrophy in spontaneously hypertensive rats. *Cardiovasc. Res.* 10:154–261.

13. THE REGRESSION OF CARDIAC HYPERTROPHY: FUNCTIONAL, ANATOMIC, AND HEMODYNAMIC CONSIDERATIONS

GEORGE COOPER, IV

Hemodynamic overloads, if substantial and progressive, inevitably lead to the deterioration of initially compensatory cardiac hypertrophy into congestive heart failure and death. As our ability to relieve these overloads by surgical and pharmacological interventions improves, it becomes increasingly important to know at what stage in this process the cardiac response to hemodynamic overloads is reversible and how much of a return to normal cardiac structure and function can be expected.

Following the initial experimental documentation of the anatomical reversibility of cardiac hypertrophy in response to pressure- [1] or volume-overload [2], similar descriptions based on experimental and clinical observations [3–5] have appeared. While it was clear from these studies that anatomical reversal of cardiac hypertrophy in response to either pressure or volume overload is possible, it was not known whether the functional deterioration associated with some forms of cardiac hypertrophy returned towards normal during the regression of the anatomical enlargement.

On a more basic level, it was not known whether the contractile dysfunction, frequently associated with cardiac hypertrophy, as related to the hypertrophy process itself or was instead caused by the type of hemodynamic stress which induced the hypertrophy. In addition, it was not known whether cardiac hypertrophy and its reversal were a primary response to the imposition and the removal of the increased load or were instead a result of concomitant changes in factors which accompany hemodynamic challenges, such as sympathetic nervous system activation and other neural and hormonal changes.

275

For these reasons, there has been a great deal of interest in three questions: first, whether there are demonstrable functional abnormalities as a necessary concomitant of cardiac hypertrophy; second, whether both the functional and the anatomical abnormalities are fully reversible when the hemodynamic overload is removed; and third, whether such cardiac changes in response to differing hemodynamic states are a primary response to the load alteration itself, or whether they are instead related to secondary factors which accompany the load alteration. Each of these three questons will be addressed briefly.

CONTRACTILE FUNCTION OF HYPERTROPHIED MYOCARDIUM

Adequate pump performance by hypertrophied myocardium is typically maintained for variable periods of time during at least the initial course of hemodynamic overloads of gradual onset. In attempting to explain the frequent eventual deterioration of pump performance in the intact organism, it seemed possible that the increase in pump mass might be sustaining performance at the same time that the contractile performance per unit mass of that pump was gradually deteriorating. If this deterioration were progressive, one would expect that as the metabolic limits of structural hypertrophy were approached, the gradual reduction in contractile performance per unit mass of hypertrophying myocardium would eventually lead to decreased overall cardiac performance. An early study employing papillary muscles removed from the hypertrophied right ventricle of the cat allowed in vitro contractile performance per unit mass of myocardium to be characterized in terms of the velocity and extent of isotonic contractions as well as in terms of the active tenion generated during isometric contractions [6]. It was found that contractile performance per unit mass of myocardium hypertrophying in response to a pressure overload was indeed distinctly reduced. We later confirmed this finding in another study utilizing the same basic model [7]. In view of the question of whether the abrupt, fixed afterload increment employed in this particular experimental model is of relevance to the more gradual afterload increases seen in most human disease states, we more recently have repeated this study using a gradually progressive pressure overload of the cat right ventricle [8]. Despite the fact that cardiac performance in the intact cat was well maintained, the decrement in contractile performance per unit mass of hypertrophied myocardium was clear and appeared to be progressive with time.

Even when the question was confined to this particular experimental model, we found that contractile dysfunction was not related to hypertrophy itself, but to the type of hemodynamic overload which caused the hypertrophy. That is, when we employed a volume overload as opposed to a pressure overload to stress the cat right ventricle, we found that for an identical degree and duration of hypertrophy, the marked in vitro contractile abnormalities, observed in response to a pressure overload, were not seen to any extent in response to a volume overload [9]. In a recent attempt to explain this difference, we performed a structural analysis of right ventricular myocardium from these two feline models, where the pressure overload was imposed by banding the pulmonary artery, and the volume overload was imposed by creating an atrial septal defect [10]. The single structural difference found between these two types of hypertrophied myocardium was a decrease in the proportion of muscle tissue and an increase in the proporton of interstitial tissue found in pressure-overloaded but not in volume-overloaded myocardium. Given the critical importance of these two tissue components to both systolic and diastolic cardiac function, these data seemed to provide a potential structural basis for at least some of the functional abnormalities observed in the model of pressure-overload hypertrophy but not in the model of volume-overload hypertrophy.

For the cat right ventricle, therefore, it would appear that it is the nature of the inducing stress rather that the hypertrophy process itself which is responsible for the abnormal contractile performance noted in response to a pressure overload. This gradual deterioration of contractile performance per unit mass of hypertrophied myocardium at a time when the heart in the intact organism is well compensated would seem to provide an attractive experimental basis for the clinically observed deterioration of initially compensatory hypertrophy into the congestive heart failure state. However, this suggestion must be made with some caution in terms of its generality in view of the fact that most clinical disease states affect the left rather than the right ventricle, and the response of left ventricular myocardium to pressure and volume overloads may well be quite different from that observed for right ventricular myocardium, either in experimental models or in the clinical setting.

FUNCTIONAL AND ANATOMICAL HYPERTROPHY REVERSAL

In an early attempt to determine whether the functional and anatomical abnormalities described above for cat right ventricular myocardium, which had hypertrophied in response to a pressure overload, are fully reversible when this hemodynamic overload is relieved, we developed a technique which allowed a band that had been placed around the pulmonary artery to be removed [11]. Coincident with band removal, right ventricular hemodynamics returned to normal. As is shown in figures 13–1 and 13–2, within a month after the removal of this abnormal afterload, there had been a return to contractile normality when defined in terms of standard isotonic and isometric contractile indices for papillary muscles excised from these right ventricles [12]. That is, the marked contractile defects which had been found in right ventricular papillary muscles of the banded group had returned to normal in the unbanded group. We also found during this study that the structural hypertrophy was fully reversible, both on the level of right ventricular mass and on the level of right ventricular muscle cell dimensions. Thus, this study demonstrated for the first time not only that full structural reversal of pressure

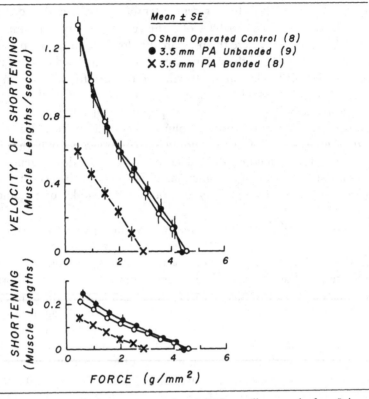

Figure 13–1. *Upper panel*: average force-velocity values ± SE for papillary muscles from 8 sham-operated control cats, 9 cats with hypertrophy reversal, and 8 cats with presure overload hypertrophy. *Lower panel*: extent of shortening versus force. (From Cooper et al. [12], with permission.)

overload induced hypertrophy is possible, but there is also a concomitant return to normal of the structural abnormalities associated with this cardiac muscle state.

In this initial study of hypertrophy reversal, we employed an abruptly applied pressure overload which was of fixed extent until its removal. However, not only does such a model bear only rather tenuous relevance to most clinical pathophysiology, but two subsequent studies [13, 14] found acute functional and structural cardiac injury after the imposition of this type of pressure overload. Thus, our finding of reversible cardiac dysfunction, along with reversible cardiac hypertrophy, may have been, to an unknown extent, a description of functional cardiac recovery from an acute injury. In our more recent work described in the previous section of this chapter [8], we had characterized the structure and function of a pathophysiologically more appropriate model of cardiac hypertrophy, that is, chronic progressive pressure overload of the cat right ventricle. Despite the fact that no myocardial injury was apparent at the light or electron microscopic level, a progressive

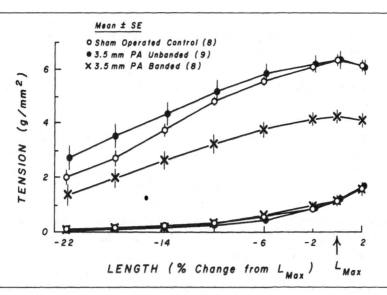

Figure 13-2. Average length-tension values ± SE for the same papillary muscles whose data is shown in figure 13-1. The upper set of curves shows active tension, and the lower set of curves shows passive tension. (From Cooper et al. [12], with permission.)

decrement in contractile function and increases in stiffness and collagen concentration were found in this hypertrophied but nonfailing myocardium.

In a recent study [15], we sought to determine whether the structural cardiac hypertrophy and the associated functional abnormalities produced by this chronic progressive pressure overload were reversible. At one-half year after initial placement of the pulmonary artery band, the band was removed; the return of normal right ventricular hemodynamics was documented, and the animals were allowed to recover for a further five months. The structure, composition, and function of this myocardium were characterized about one-half year after band removal. There was no difference between the right ventricular myocardium from these unbanded cats and their concurrently studied sham-operated controls. With respect to systolic contractile function, the findings essentially duplicated those shown earlier in figures 13-1 and 13-2 for the reversal of an acute pressure overload. Of particular interest, both the abnormal diastolic compliance and the increased collagen content, which had been observed during hypertrophy, were also found to return to normal when the pressure overload was removed. Three conclusions may be drawn from these studies of cardiac hypertrophy reversal. First, both the cardiac hypertrophy and the associated functional abnormalities produced by a pressure overload are fully reversible when the pressure overload is removed from a nonfailing ventricle. Second, this reversibility does not represent functional cardiac recovery from an acute injury, since we had shown [8] for a chronic progressive pressure overload that no apparent injury is produced and that progression of, rather than recovery from, cardiac abnormalities occurs when the pressure overload is left in place. Third, while it might be expected that the progressive increases in collagen concentration and passive stiffness that we observed with this model would remain as fixed features of the tissue, both of these factors returned to normal when the pressure overload was relieved.

The most compelling rationale for these experimental studies of hypertrophy reversal is the need for basic information about the extent to which pathological cardiac hypertrophy in man, with its associated abnormalities of systolic contractile function and diastolic compliance, can be returned towards normal following surgical or pharmacological interventions.

With respect to structural hypertrophy and the attendant systolic abnormalities, recent clinical observations of hypertrophy induced by either volume [16] or pressure [17] overloads show that only partial rather than full anatomical regression of ventricular enlargement follows replacement of an abnormal cardiac valve. The functional abnormalities associated with each hemodynamic overload also show only a partial reversal [18, 19]. While this partial return to normal structure and function may be due to the residual gradients left by most prosthetic valves, it should be noted that asymptomatic patients are not commonly submitted to surgical valve replacement, and when initially compensatory hypertrophy progresses to frank clinical congestive heart failure, the potential for anatomical or functional reversal is even more limited. [20].

An experimental basis for these clinical observations has become available over the past decade. Following our initial demonstration [12] that both the structural and functional abnormalities produced by an abrupt, fixed pressure overload are reversed when the pressure overload is removed, and our more recent demonstration [15] of the same basic findings with respect to a chronic progressive pressure overload, similar observations were made for an abrupt, fixed volume overload [21]. When each hemodynamic abnormality was allowed to progress to heart failure, both pressure [22] and volume [23] overloads were found to produce irreversible abnormalities. Indeed, we have found recently [24] that a severe acute afterload increase produces largely irreversible hypertrophy even before the progression to heart failure has occurred. Thus, it would seem that the extent of the reversibility of structural hypertrophy, and any associated systolic contractile defects, is a function of the severity of the inducing hemodynamic stress, whether the process has eventuated in congestive heart failure, and the extent to which hemodynamic normality can be restored.

With respect to the myocardial fibrosis and attendant diastolic abnormalities which may accompany hypertrophy, relief of a hemodynamic overload resulting in improved systolic performance may be of little benefit if decreased myocardial compliance persists. Valve replacement in man for volume or pressure overloads may result in improved, but not necessarily normal, myocardial compliance [25]. Indeed, there is some reason to think that anatomical interstitial fibrosis, as opposed to functionally impaired relaxation, may be irreversible [26]. This is in contrast to our experimental findings in the cat right ventricle [15], where there was a full regression of the increased tissue collagen concentration accompanying the anatomical regression of hypertrophy. To the extent that it may be applicable to humans, the clinical implication of this finding is that in pressure overload prior to the development of massive hypertrophy or congestive heart failure, the increase in interstitial connective tissue and the diastolic abnormalities can be reversed if the pressure overload is fully relieved. Nonetheless, since the experimental pressure-overload removal was always complete, no direct insight is provided into why, in the clinical situation, there is so much variability in the myocardial response to the variety of interventions used to treat pathological pressure overloads.

REGULATION OF CARDIAC MASS IN THE ADULT

Apart from the above descriptive studies of cardiac hypertrophy and its reversal, a more basic question is, which causative mechanisms are responsible for regulating cardiac mass in the adult. This question becomes particularly interesting in view of the fact that, at least in the case of the muscular component of the heart, one is dealing with terminally differentiated cells, such that changes in cardiac mass are based necessarily on changes in the volume of these cells rather than on any change in their number.

The question that we wished to address was whether changes in cardiac mass are based on a primary response of the heart muscle cell (cardiocyte) to the variations in loading conditions which it experiences or whether instead these changes in cardiac mass are based on secondary factors which accompany load alterations, such as changes in sympathetic tone or in other trophic factors.

In our initial work in this area, we developed a model that allowed the load on a particular segment of ventricular myocardium to be changed without any concomitant alteration in the local blood supply, innervation, or frequency of contraction. We transected the chordae tendinae of a single cat right ventricular papillary muscle in order to remove the external load from this tissue. Following two studies [27, 28], in which the response of such papillary muscles to a reduced load was characterized, we further defined the response of such previously unloaded tissue to a restoration of normal load after the transected chordae tendinae were reattached to the tricuspid valve apparatus during a second operative procedure [29, 30]. These studies can be seen as a mirror image of the research in cardiac hypertrophy and its reversal, with two major differences: first, the myocardial response to a reversible reduction in load was characterized, and second, this was done without occasioning any hemodynamic change in the organism as a whole. We found that, following

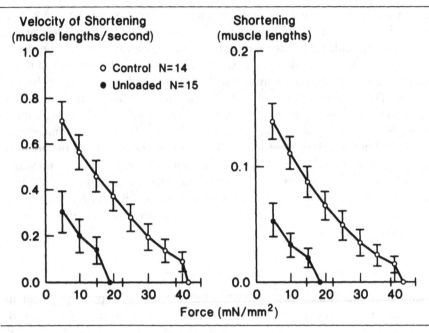

Figure 13-3. *Left panel:* average force-velocity values ± SE for 14 control papillary muscles and 15 unloaded papillary muscles. *Right panel:* extent of shortening versus force. (From Cooper and Tomanek [28], with permission.)

this load reduction, there were rapid ultrastructural changes in the sarcomeres, which included disorientation and lysis of contractile filaments as well as a loss of Z-line substance. Cardiocyte cross-sectional area decreased to two-thirds of the control value at three days after the operation . As is shown in figures 13-3 and 13-4, isotonic and isometric contractile function was markedly depressed in the unloaded muscles as early as one day after unloading, with a negative shift of the entire force-velocity and the active length-tension relationships. There was a major increase in the passive stiffness of the unloaded muscle as the proportion of myocardial connective tissue increased. We found that when papillary muscles were reloaded one week after they had been unloaded, both the cardiocyte cross-sectional area and ultrastructural organization of the papillary muscles returned to normal within one week. As is shown in figures 13-5 and 13-6, the contractile function of the papillary muscles returned fully to normal after two weeks of reloading. We also found that there were disproportionate losses of contractile proteins during cardiac atrophy, which were again fully reversible upon cardiac reloading. Thus, this series of studies demonstrated that adult mammalian myocardium responds to unloading with a marked loss of cellular differentiation, organization, and function—all of which are fully reversible with reloading. In view of the fact that other factors thought to potentially regulate cardiac mass had not changed appreciably in these animals, we felt that these data suggested that load may be the primary

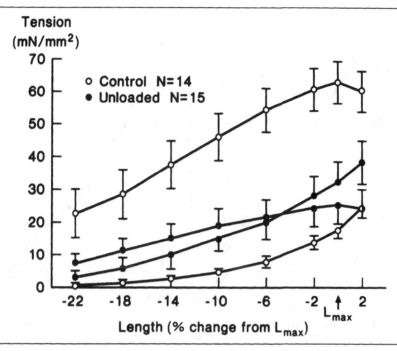

Figure 13–4. Average length-tension values ± SE for the same papillary muscles whose data is shown in figure 13–3. The convex pair of lines, beginning on the left with the upper pair of points nearest the ordinate, represents active tension. The concave pair of lines, beginning on the left with the lower pair of lines nearest the ordinate, represents resting tension. (From Cooper and Tomanek [28], with permission.)

determinant of myocardial structure, and ultimately of myocardial function.

In a further series of studies designed to evaluate hemodynamic versus adrenergic control of cardiac mass [31], we imposed differential loading on the cat right ventricle, where the ventricle as a whole was pressure overloaded by banding the pulmonary artery, while a constituent papillary muscle was unloaded by transecting its chordae tendinae. This model was used to see whether any endogenous or exogenous substance caused uniform hypertrophy, or whether instead locally appropriate load responses caused ventricular hypertrophy with papillary muscle atrophy. The latter result obtained, both when each aspect of differential loading was simultaneous and when a previously hypertrophied papillary muscle was unloaded in a pressure-overloaded right ventricle. We also employed epicardial denervation followed by pressure overload to assess the role of local neurogenic catecholamines in the genesis of hypertrophy. The degree of hypertrophy caused by these procedures was the same as that caused by pressure overload alone. In a third and fourth series of experiments, beta-adrenoceptor or alpha-adrenoceptor blockade was produced before and maintained during pressure overload. The hypertrophic response did not differ in either case from that caused by pressure overload

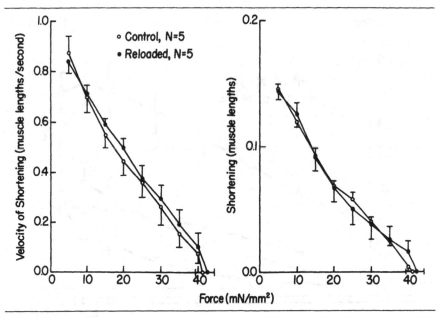

Figure 13–5. *Left panel:* average force-velocity values ± SE for 5 control papillary muscles and 5 reloaded papillary muscles. *Right panel:* extent of shortening versus force. (From Thompson et al. [29], with permission.)

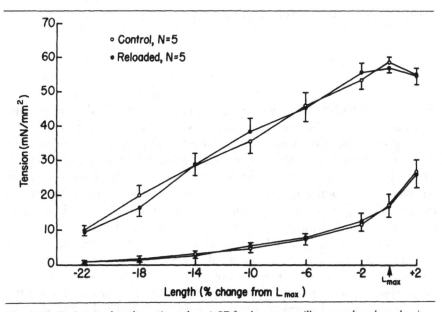

Figure 13–6. Average length-tension values ± SE for the same papillary muscles whose data is shown in figure 13–5. The convex pair of lines, beginning on the left with the upper pair of points nearest the ordinate, represents active tension. The concave pair of lines, beginning on the left with the lower pair of lines nearest the ordinate, represents resting tension. (From Thompson et al. [29], with permission.)

without adrenoceptor blockade. We felt that these experiments demonstrated the following: first, cardiac hypertrophy is a local response to increased load, so that any factor serving as a mediator of this response must be either locally generated or selectively active only in those cardiocytes in whch load is increased; second, catecholamines are not that mediator, in that adrenergic activation does not significantly affect the cardiac hypertrophic response to an increased hemodynamic load.

Apart from the identification of load as the primary regulator of cardiac structure and function in these studies, the means by which changing hemodynamic loads serve as the primary stimulus to cardiac mass changes is of considerable interest. Elucidating the mechanism(s) by which changing load is transduced into changing mass in adult mammalian myocardium remains as one of the most important problems to be addressed in normal and abnormal cardiac physiology.

CONCLUSION

The most remarkable finding of this series of studies is the extraordinary plasticity exhibited in terms of structure and function by the terminally differentiated cardiac muscle cells of the adult mammal. Across a spectrum ranging from overloading, through normal loading, to reduced loading, adult heart muscle responds with a directionally appropriate change in mass. Functionally, it appears that heart muscle may well contract optimally when "normally" loaded. Within the bounds of degree and duration imposed by the experimental models which we have employed, the marked structural and functional changes induced by either overloading or underloading appear to be fully reversible upon the restoration of normal loading, although this would clearly not continue to hold true if these bounds were greatly exceeded.

In basic terms, the manner in which load alterations serve to regulate the biology of adult heart muscle is of fundamental interest and forms the focus of our ongoing research in this area. In clinical terms, an understanding of the factors which limit the potential reversibility of load-induced changes in adult myocardium is becoming increasingly important as therapeutic interventions bearing less risk to the patient, and therefore the promise of earlier beneficial usage, become available.

REFERENCES

1. Patton, H.S., Page, E.W., and Ogden, E. 1943. The results of nephrectomy on experimental renal hypertension. *Surg. Gynecol. Obstet.* 76:493–497.
2. Drury, A.N. 1944. Observations relating to cardiac hypertrophy produced in the rabbit by arterio-venous anastomosis: The effect of closure of the anastomosis. *J. Exp. Physiol.* 33: 107–112.
3. Hall, O., Hall, C.E., and Ogden, E. 1953. Cardiac hypertrophy in experimental hypertension and its regression following reestablishment of normal blood pressure. *Am. J. Physiol.* 174: 175–178.
4. Engle, M.A., Holswade, G.R., Goldberg, H.P., Lukas, D.S., and Glenn, F. 1958. Regression after open valvotomy of infundibular stenosis accompanying severe valvular pulmonic

stenosis. *Circulation* 17:862–873.

5. Beznak, M., Korecky, B., and Thomas, G. 1969. Regression of cardiac hypertrophies of various origin. *Can. J. Physiol. Pharmacol.* 47:579–586.

6. Spann, J.F., Buccino, R.A., Sonnenblick, E.H., and Braunwald, E. 1967. Contractile state of cardiac muscle obtained from cats with experimentally produced ventricular hypertrophy and heart failure. *Circ. Res.* 21:341–354.

7. Cooper, G., Satava, R.M., Harrison, C.E., and Coleman, H.N. 1973. A mechanism for the abnormal energetics of pressure-induced hypertrophy of cat myocardium. *Circ. Res.* 33: 213–223.

8. Cooper, G., Tomanek, R.J., Ehrhardt, J.C., and Marcus, M.L. 1981. Chronic progressive pressure overload of the cat right ventricle. *Circ. Res.* 48:488–497.

9. Cooper, G., Puga, F.J., Zujko, K.J., Harrison, C.E., and Coleman, H.N. 1973. Normal myocardial function and energetics in volume-overload hypertrophy in the cat. *Circ. Res.* 32:140–148.

10. Marino, T.A., Kent, R.L., Uboh, C.E., Fernandez, E., Thompson, E.W., and Cooper, G. 1985. Structural analysis of pressure-versus volume-overload hypertrophy of cat right ventricle. *Am. J. Physiol.* 249:H371–H379.

11. Cooper, G., and Satava, R.M. 1974. A method for producing reversible long-term pressure overload of the cat right ventricle. *J. Appl. Physiol.* 37:762–764.

12. Cooper, G., Satava, R.M., Harrison, C.E., and Coleman, H.N. 1974. Normal myocardial function and energetics after reversing pressure-overload hypertrophy. *Am. J. Physiol.* 226:1158–1165.

13. Williams, J.F., and Potter, R.D. 1974. Normal contractile state of hypertrophied myocardium after pulmonary artery constriction in the cat. *J. Clin. Invest.* 54:1266–1272.

14. Bishop, S.P., and Melsen, L.R. 1976. Myocardial necrosis, fibrosis and DNA synthesis in experimental cardiac hypertrophy induced by sudden pressure overload. *Circ. Res.* 39: 238–245

15. Cooper, G., and Marino, T.A. 1984. Complete reversibility of cat right ventricular chronic progressive pressure overload. *Circ. Res.* 54:323–331.

16. Clark, D.B., McAnulty, J.H., and Rahimtoola, S.H. 1980. Valve replacement in aortic insufficiency with left ventricular dysfunction. *Circulation* 61:411–420.

17. Henry, W.L., Bonow, R.O., Borer J.S., Kent, K.M., Ware, J.H., Redwood, D.R., Itscoitz, S.B., McIntosh, C.L., Morrow, A.G., and Epstein, S.E. 1980. Evaluation of aortic valve replacement in patients with valvular aortic stenosis. *Circulation* 61:814–825.

18. Kennedy, J.W., Doces, J., and Stewart, D.K. 1977. Left ventricular function before and following aortic valve replacement. *Circulation* 56:944–950.

19. Pantely, G., Morton, M., and Rahimtoola, S.H. 1978. Effects of successful, uncomplicated valve replacement on ventricular hypertrophy, volume, and performance in aortic stenosis and aortic incompetence. *J. Thorac. Cardiovasc. Surg.* 75:383–391.

20. Dodge, H.T., Frimer, M., and Stewart, D.K. 1974. Functional evaluation of hypertrophied heart in man. *Circ. Res.* 34/35 (suppl II):122–127.

21. Papadimitriou, J.M., Hopkins, E.B., and Taylor, R.R. 1974. Regression of left ventricular dilation and hypertrophy after removal of volume overload. *Circ. Res.* 35;127–135.

22. Coulson, R.L., Yazdanfar, S., Rubio, E., Bove, A.A., LeMole, G.M., and Spann, J.F. 1977. Recuperative potential of cardiac muscle following relief of pressure-overload hypertrophy and right ventricular failure in the cat. *Circ. Res.* 40:41–49.

23. Newman, W.H., Webb, J.G., and Privitera, P.J. 1982. Persistence of myocardial failure following removal of chronic volume overload. *Am. J. Physiol.* 243:H876–H883.

24. Wisenbaugh, T., Allen, P., Cooper. G., O'Connor, W.N., Mezaros, L., Streter, F. Bahinski, A., Houser, S., and Spann, J.F. 1984. Hypertrophy without contractile dysfunction after reversal of pressure overload in the cat. *Am. J. Physiol.* 247:H146–H154.

25. Schwarz, F., Flameng, W., Schaper, J., and Hehrlein, F. 1978. Correlation between myocardial structure and diastolic properties of the heart in chronic aortic valve disease. Effects of corrective surgery. *Am. J. Cardiol.* 42:895–903.

26. Perloff, J.K. 1982. Development and regression of increased ventricular mass. *Am. J. Cardiol.* 5:605–611.

27. Tomanek, R.J., and Cooper, G. 1981. Morphological changes in the mechanically unloaded myocardial cell. *Anat. Rec.* 200:271–280.

28. Cooper, G., and Tomanek, R.J. Load regulation of the structure, composition, and function of mammalian myocardium. *Circ. Res.* 50:788–798.
29. Thompson, E.W., Marino, T.A., Uboh, C.E., Kent, R.L., and Cooper, G. 1984. Atrophy reversal and cardiocyte redifferentiation in reloaded cat myocardium. *Circ. Res.* 54:367–377.
30. Kent, R.L., Uboh, C.E., Thompson, E.W., Gordon, S.S., Marino, T.A., Hoober, J.K., Cooper, G. 1985. Biochemical and structural correlates in unloaded and reloaded cat myocardium. *J. Mol. Cell. Cardiol.* 17:153–165.
31. Cooper, G., Kent, R.L., Uboh, C.E., Thompson, E.W., and Marino, T.A. 1985. Hemodynamic versus adrenergic control of cat right ventricular hypertrophy. *J. Clin. Invest.* 75: 1403–1414.

14. REGRESSION OF LEFT VENTRICULAR HYPERTROPHY: CLINICAL CONSIDERATIONS

ANTHONY P. GOLDMAN AND MORRIS N. KOTLER

Left ventricular hypertrophy (LVH) is an important adaptive response to pressure or volume overload of the left ventricle. The presence of LVH is most accurately detected by echocardiography or cardiac angiography [1, 2], and has important implications with regard to the prognosis of the underlying heart disease. Left ventricular hypertrophy is initially a physiological adaptive response, but with time this physiological response becomes pathological, and may be associated with impaired contractility and irreversible myocardial dysfunction. The point at which this transition from physiological to pathological hypertrophy occurs is unknown. Regression of LVH has been shown to occur in animals and humans. The evidence for left ventricular regression and the significance of this regression and its relationship to myocardial function, as well as the prognostic implications, form the basis of this chapter.

DEFINITION

Left ventricular hypertrophy is defined as an increase in the size of existing myocardial fibers, resulting in increased wall thickness and left ventricular mass [3]. Normal left ventricular mass ranges up to 141 gms in adult women and 175–203 gms in adult men. It may be slightly higher (±220 gms) with chronic exercise and in people with large body size [1, 4–6]. The main cause of increased left ventricular mass is LVH, although it can also occur with infiltrative myocardial disorders.

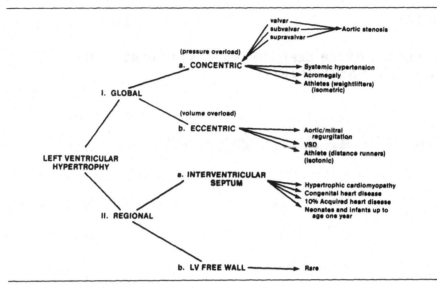

Figure 14–1 Causes of left ventricular hypertrophy

Left ventricular hypertrophy may be global (diffuse), involving all walls equally, or regional, where the wall thickening is disproportionate. The classification of LVH and its main causes are presented in figure 14–1. The development of LVH and its physiological significance has been discussed in detail elsewhere in this book.

EVIDENCE FOR LEFT VENTRICULAR REGRESSION

Animal Experimentation

Most of the animal work on regression of LVH has been done with spontaneously hypertensive rats (SHR) [7–11] or rats rendered hypertensive by means of reno-vascular hypertension utilizing a clip placed on one renal artery [12–14]. Other investigators have used progressive pressure-loading by banding the aorta or the pulmonary artery [15–16]. The animal studies have been hampered by difficulties in quantifying LVH. The initial studies of reversible cardiac hypertrophy involved the surgical cure of the lesion imposed, i.e., nephrectomy in renovascular hypertension [17]. Cutiletta et al. [15] described reduction in ribonucleic acid (RNA) and reduced weight of the heart after removal of the aortic band that had produced cardiac hypertrophy. Beznak et al. [18] reported regression of hypertrophy in Deoxycorticosterone (DOC) hypertensive rats following removal of the implanted DOC pellet. In those studies, however, only animals with short-lived hypertrophy had regressed by unloading the heart.

In many studies, the use of antihypertensive drugs produced regression of

LVH, but the effects of these different types of antihypertensive drugs on LVH in SHR have been quite diverse and contradictory [7–11, 19, 29]. It has been shown that the degree of LVH in SHR did not correlate with systolic blood pressure levels as it did with renovascular hypertension in rats [12]. The use of methyldopa reduced ventricular weight with moderate blood pressure control [7, 18, 19, 24]. Methyldopa has also been shown to prevent the development of cardiac hypertrophy in young SHR. The vasodilator hydralazine was associated with no change in ventricular weight [7, 24], whereas minoxidil [24] in fact increased ventricular weight despite blood pressure control. Vaughan-Williams et al. [22] used beta-blockers in normotensive animals and showed up to a 30% decrease in cardiac weight, whereas others showed only a moderate change or no change. In another study, using propranolol, there was no significant influence on cardiac weight in SHR despite effective adrenergic blockade [24]. On the other hand, some investigators found that propranolol caused a reduction in left ventricular mass without reducing blood pressure [30]. In a different study, hypertension in the SHR was lowered by the beta-blocker oxprenolol, whereas hydralazine alone, had no effect. However, the accompanying ventricular hypertrophy was reversed by both drugs [9]. Studies with a converting enzyme inhibitor captopril have shown that it can reverse cardiac hypertrophy in SHR, and that improved cardiac function and reversal of cardiac hypertrophy may also occur without blood pressure control [10, 26].

These animal studies indicate that other factors besides pressure load modulate the hypertrophic response of the myocardium in hypertension. The varying effects of these drugs on hypertension and regression of hypertrophy may be explained by the differences in duration of therapy, and the varied effects on the neurohumoral mechanisms and blood volume, thereby in turn altering blood flow and vascular resistance and ultimately systemic arterial pressure.

Biochemical factors

The constituents within the muscle cells are normally within a state of dynamic equilibrium, constantly undergoing degradation and regeneration. The half-life of myofibrillar proteins is about 7–10 days [31]. Thus, contractile proteins renew themselves almost completely every month. Hypertrophic stimuli have been shown to provoke an increase in concentration and the amount of actomyocin within hypertrophied cells [32].

A positive correlation exists between the degree of hypertrophy and elevation of RNA [33]. Both concentration and total RNA are significantly reduced to normal in rats with medical or surgical reversal of hypertrophy [7, 12]. Ventricles which have hypertrophied, due to pressure overload contain more collagen than normal and therefore more hydroxyproline. It has been shown, however, that regression of hypertrophy may be associated with increased concentrations of hydroxyproline. In contrast, other studies have shown reduction of total ventricular hydroxyproline after reversible hypertrophy with angiotensin-converting enzyme inhibitors. The presence of hydroxyproline, which indicates collagen, makes reversal of hypertrophy more difficult because, once formed, collagen fibers are not as accessible for removal as the intracellular components [34]. Sen et al. [35] have also shown in rats that early administration of methyldopa could prevent the increase in collagen, whereas there were no reversible changes when the methyldopa was given for six weeks to hypertensive rats.

These biochemical changes help confirm that regression does take place, but more studies are needed in relation to the functional significance of these changes and the mechanism of regression.

FACTORS MODULATION REGRESSION

In the initial studies of regression of LVH in animals, it appeared that this regression was merely a function of unloading the heart. Later studies indicated that there is a wide spectrum of responses of ventricular mass to reduction in pressure load and that more factors influence reversal of cardiac hypertrophy than control of blood pressure alone. The factors that modulate left ventricular regression have not been adequately studied but there are a number of important known influences, particularly in relation to systemic hypertension.

Blood Pressure Control

There are a number of controversies concerning whether regression of LVH correlates with blood pressure control [36–48]. In most studies, there is a good correlation between blood pressure control and regression of LVH [42–48]. But in many studies associated with reversal of LVH, there was no correlation between the degree of blood pressure reduction and the decrease in left ventricular mass [36, 39, 41]. Regression of hypertrophy that is unassociated with a concomitant decrease in blood pressure is undesirable, as it will result in an increased wall stress by decreasing the compensatory hypertrophy needed for the high pressure [3].

The reversal of hypertrophy also did not occur in all patients treated by the same antihypertensive agents [36–38]. The factors determining this diversity of response are not clear. However, there may be obvious reasons for this such as poor patient compliance or coexisting cardiac disease such as valvular or coronary disease. Differences in the degree of blood pressure control is another possible explanation. Continuous blood pressure monitoring techniques were used in some studies and in these studies there was a closer correlation between average diurnal blood pressure levels, rather than single recordings, and reduction in left ventricular mass in both treated and untreated hypertensive patients.

Catecholamines

Catecholamines play a large role in the development of cardiac hypertrophy. In animal studies catecholamine stimulation is a potent factor in preventing reversal of LVH despite adequate blood pressure control. If the vasodilators are used, for example hydralazine alone, there is a reflex increase in catecholamines that required additional doses of beta-blocking drugs to produce regression of LVH. In the study by Tarazi et al. [11], propranolol produced regression of LVH when added to 30 mg/l of hydralazine, but it did not reduce cardiac weight when added to 80 mg/l of vasodilator, although the latter dose did lead to blood pressure control. A possible explanation for this is that a larger dose of propranol was probably needed to overcome the increase in catecholamines induced by hydralazine for regression of LVH to occur. The increase in cardiac mass induced by catecholamines is significantly less when beta-blockers are given concurrently with vasodilators. It appears that the degree of interferences with adrenergic drive, the side effects of the drug, and the stage and evolution of hypertension, may all influence the response of ventricular hypertrophy to reduction of blood pressure.

Renin-Angiotensin System

The renin-angiotensin system is another possible neurohumeral modulator of left ventricular hypertrophy reversal. Angiotensin-converting enzyme inhibitors can cause regression of LVH, without the need for beta-blockade or sympatholytic drugs, as they can lower blood pressure without inducing a hyperadrenergic state [10, 49]. The role of angiotensin II inhibition in the reversal of hypertrophy may be related to a direct inhibition of angiotensin II itself or indirectly to inhibition of the potentiation of sympathetic activity centrally or peripherally. There is also inhibition of myocardial protein synthesis caused by angiotensin II, which may be another factor.

Associated Cardiac Disorders

The presence of valvular heart disease with hypertension may compound the problem and interfere with regression of hypertrophy or set up a vicious cycle to maintain the hypertrophy.

Coronary artery disease may result in decreased flow through the hypertrophied myocardium as well as decreased coronary vascular reserve. This may result in fibrosis which may cause permanent irreversible changes and hence prevent reversal of hypertrophy.

Genetic Factors

It is possible that LVH initiated early in life can only be reversed to a fairly minor extent or prevented by an intervention late in life. Part of the explanation may be a substantial contribution of myocardial hyperplasia in association with a genetically linked predisposition to structural cardiovascular adapatation, either inherent in the patient, and/or caused by trophic influences of a hormone.

CLINICAL IMPLICATIONS OF REGRESSION

Studies in Athletes

In athletes, the left ventricle responds to sustained exercise by the development of LVH [50–58]. This increase in ventricular mass provoked by pressure or volume overload as a result of training appears to be a desirable adaptive response that permits the heart to function normally at greater work loads, i.e., the athletic heart is the prototype of physiological hypertrophy.

The adaptive response to training remains controversial. Athletes engaged in isometric exercise (weight lifters, wrestlers, shot putters, etc.) have mainly concentric hypertrophy, of the type seen with chronic pressure overload. Athletes engaged in isotonic exercise (long-distance runners, swimmers, cyclists, basketball players, etc.) have mainly eccentric hypertrophy similar to the type seen with chronic volume overload [50, 51].

It has recently been shown that cyclists have features of both i.e., a mixed eccentric-concentric type of hypertrophy, due to a combination of isotonic exercise of the legs and isometric exercise of the arms, causing both pressure and volume overload [54]. Some investigators have shown left ventricular hypertrophy to be related to the duration of exercise and not the type of exercise. This discrepancy can be partially explained by runners lifting weights and weight lifters doing some running. Systolic left ventricular function has clearly been shown to be normal in athletes. There is limited knowledge about the diastolic filling properties of athletic hearts. Shapiro et al [55] reported a 30% increase in posterior wall thickness without any detectable changes in relaxation or diastolic function as determined by digitized echocardiography. In another study of trained marathon runners, despite significant left ventricular hypertrophy, there was a trend to improved diastolic filling rates [57]. These changes imply that increased left ventricular mass is not invariably associated with impaired diastolic filling. This is further evidence that LVH in athletes is truly physiological, as diastolic abnormalities can be detected in most other disorders associated with LVH.

In animal experiments, myocardial function has been shown to increase in rats after training by swimming [59] and in dogs after treadmill training [60]. Regression of exercise-induced hypertrophy occurs rapidly in rats. i.e., two weeks after the cessation of training. The structural alterations typical of LVH also regress substantially, and the light microscopic findings are almost indistinguishable from that of normal rats [61].

In humans, left ventricular regression has been shown to be rapid within months following cessation of physical activity [56, 58]. However, in one reported study, left ventricular regression was found to be incomplete during an abstinence period of a few months, but probably would have been complete if the athletes continued to abstain [56].

Patients with Systemic Hypertension

Numerous studies have shown regression of cardiac hypertrophy in hypertensive patients treated with various antihypertensive medications [36, 37, 41–48, 62–70] (Table 14–1). This regression of hypertrophy has been assessed initially by a reduction in serial electrocardiographic voltage and subsequently by means of M-mode and two-dimensional echocardiography. The latter studies demonstrated reduction in LV mass and decrease in the interventricular septal and posterior wall thickness.

In the earlier reported studies [62, 63, 71], a reduction in electrocardiographic voltage correlated with successful control of hypertension. However, electrocardiographic voltage criteria depend on age, weight, and distance of the left ventricle from the chest wall and therefore do not allow accurate quantification of alterations in left ventricular mass.

Different forms of cardiac hypertrophy have been described in hypertension including concentric, eccentric, and predominant septal hypertrophy. Regression of hypertrophy has occurred in all forms. It is uncertain however, whether the regression occurs preferentially in some parts of the left ventricle. Von Bibra et al. [72] have reported early reduction in interventricular septal thickness during antihypertensive therapy with little or no concomitant change in the thickness of the posterior wall. Septal hypertrophy is reported to be particularly common in patients with early or borderline hypertension. Preferential hypertrophy of the septum may be explained by susceptibility of the interventricular septum to adrenergic stimuli and to a locally higher wall stress as a result of its flatter configuration [73]. In most studies where left ventricular mass had been reduced by blood pressure control, the ratio of the interventricular septum to the posterior wall did not change significantly.

The time period required for left ventricular regression is of obvious clinical importance. In animal experiments the biochemical processes of hypertrophy appear within hours of an added load and structural changes can be demonstrated within two weeks [74]. In humans, Wollam [65] showed reduction in left ventricular posterior wall-thickening at end-diastole as early as one month after arterial pressure was controlled and Weinstein [48] showed that regression was apparent after three weeks of therapy. The rapid, early reduction in left ventricular mass then appears to stablize at a new level during treatment [39]. However, there is a continued reduction in left ventricular wall thickness even after one year following therapy [75, 76].

There have been three groups of antihypertensive agents that have been reported to induce regression of LVH when used as single therapy. These include: the sympatholytic drugs particularly methlydopa and reserpine [36, 45, 46, 48, 63, 65, 66], the beta blockers, particularly propranolol, nadolol,

Table 14–1. Reported studies of regression of left ventricular hypertrophy in hypertension.

Reference (first author)	Patients (no.)	Treatment	Method	Results	Follow-up
Fouad (36)	11	Methyldopa (2 pts); Methyldopa, HCTZ (9 pts)	Echo	35% ↓ LVM (4 pts)	9 mo
Ibrahim (37)	17	Atenolol	Echo	12% ↓ LVM ↓ IVS-PW	8 wk
Nakashimay (41)	7	Enalapril	Nuclear	107–95% ↓ LVM	7 mo
Sonotani (42)	34	Combination (HCTZ, methyldopa, blockers)	Echo	↓ IVS-PW, ↓ LV mass	1 to 2 yr
Hill (43)	14	Nadoldol or Propranolol	Echo	↓ IVS-PW	12 wk
Dunn (44)	22	Combination	Echo	↓ IVS-PW, 19% ↓ LVM	9 mo
Corea (45)	7	Methyldopa	Echo	→ IVS-PW	16 to 18 mo
Reichek (46)	27	HCTZ (15 pts); HCTZ, methyldopa (12 pts)	Echo	→ IVS-PW, 18% ↓ LVM	11 mo
Rowlands (47)	25	Combination	Echo	↓ LVM	12 ± 7 mo
Weinstein (48)	21	Combination methyldopa, HCTZ Amiloride	Echo	12–17% ↓ LVM	3–8 wk
Ibrahim (62)	50	Not given	ECG	↓ Voltage	9 yr
Poblete (63)	137	Combination (HCTZ, methyldopa, B-blockers)	ECG	↓ Voltage	2.9 yr
Schlant (64)	68	Not given	Echo	21% ↓ LVM	5 yr
Wollam (65)	29	HCTZ (7 pts); methyldopa (6 pts); both (16 pts)	Echo, ECG	12–16% ↓ LVM	1 to 12 mo
Drayer (66)	23	HCTZ, methyldopa	Echo	↓ IVS-PW	4 wk
Rowlands (67)	9	Timolol	Echo	10% ↓ LVM	16 wk
Drayer (68)	20	HCTZ	Echo	IVS ↑ (9 pts) IVS ↑ or-(11 pts)	6 wk
Corea (70)	8	Timolol	Echo	IVS-PW ↓ ↓ 16% LVM	16–18 mo

ECG = electrocardiogram; Echo = M-mode echocardiography; HCTZ = hydrochlorothiazide; IVS = interventricular septum; LVM = left ventricular mass; pts = number of patients; PW = posterior wall; — = unchanged; ↓ = decreased; ↑ = increased atenolol and timolol [37, 43, 67, 70], and the converting enzyme inhibitors captopril [69] and enalapril [41]. The use of the vasodilators and diuretics when used alone as single therapy for hypertension have generally been found to be ineffective in causing left ventricular regression, despite adequate blood pressure control [66, 68]. Combinations of antihypertensive therapies that have lead to regression of LVH have usually included either a sympatholytic or a beta-blocker. In many of the studies, however, multiple therapy has been employed so that the interpretation of the effects of individual drugs is difficult.

Diuretics when used alone have been associated with a decrease, increase, or no change, in left ventricular wall thickening [40, 46, 68], but the addition of a small dose of methyldopa to diuretics has lead to significant reduction in left ventricular mass with little or no change in arterial blood pressure [36]. Of the vasodilators, minoxidil in particular, was found to cause an increase in LV mass despite blood pressure control [10]. Possible reasons for the failure of diuretics and vasodilators as single therapy may be increased activity of the sympathetic nervous system and elevated norepinephrine levels or possibly stimulation of the renin-angiotensin system.

The reversibility of LVH is also related to the size of left ventricular mass prior to treatment. The greater the left ventricular mass, the more reduction in mass after treatment [37, 39, 43]. This raises the question as to whether a heart with normal mass can be reduced with antihypertensive therapy. Using a beta-blocker, Rowlands et al. did show a decreased left ventricular mass in hypertensive patients who had no evidence of increase in mass or wall thickness prior to treatment [77]. These data have not been confirmed by other investigators.

Patients with Aortic Regurgitation

Reduction in LV mass has been reported in patients with aortic regurgitation treated with arterial vasodilators such as hydralazine [76], but it was a short-term study, so that little is known about the long-term effects. Following aortic valve replacement, reduction in left ventricular mass as assessed by electrocardiography, echocardiography, and angiography, has been demonstrated in patients with chronic aortic regurgitation from 6 months to 3 years see table 14–2 [79–92].

Most of the electrocardiographic voltage changes occurred within one year of valve replacement and studies after this period revealed stable voltage measurements [81, 88, 90]. The majority of patients with aortic regurgitation achieve a normal left ventricular end-diastolic dimension 1–2 weeks after surgery and subsequently, over the next 6–9 months, a significant regression of LV hypertrophy occurs [92]. In the late postoperative period, some patients have persistent LVH. There are thus three possible outcomes following aortic valve replacement for aortic regurgitation.

Table 14–2. Reported studies of regression of left ventricular hypertrophy in aortic valve disease

Reference (first author)	Heart Disease	Patients (no.)	Method	% Decrease LVM	Follow-up
Panidis (3)	AS	10	Echo	34	6 to 84 mo
Henry (79)	AS	42	Angio, Echo	15	6 mo
Cody (80)	AS	12	Echo	35	3 to 5 wk
Carroll (81)	AR	25	ECG	↓ voltage	6 mo
Schuler (82)	AR	16	Echo	37	15 (9 to 35) mo
Bodem (83)	AR	33	Echo	36	6 mo
Carroll (84)	AR	23	Echo	20 to 28% ↓ CSA	9 to 12 mo
Schwartz (85)	AS, AR or both	23	Echo	24 to 43	6 mo
Pantely (86)	AS, AR	18	Angio	42 to 46	15 to 20 mo
Kennedy (87)	AS, AR, or both	24	Angio	32	19 mo
Gaasch (88)	AR	19	Echo	40	6 mo
Fioretti (89)	AR	42	Echo	16–26% ↓ CSA	12 mo–3 yr
Donaldson (90)	AR	67	ECG	↓ voltage	6 mo–3 yr
Toussaint (91)	AR	18	Echo	32% ↓ CSA	8–27 mo
Gaasch (92)	AR	32	Angio	21% ↓ LV volume	24 mo–5 yr
			Echo	23% ↓ CSA	

Angio = angiography; AR = aortic regurgitation; AS = aortic stenosis; CSA = cross-sectional area; ECG = electrocardiogram; Echo = M-mode echocardiography; LV = left ventricle; LVM = left ventricular mass; ↓ = decrease.

1. A normal left ventricular end-diastolic dimension or volume and normal left ventricular mass.
2. A normal left ventricular end-diastolic dimension with incomplete regression of hypertrophy and
3. Persistent left ventricular enlargement with no reduction of LV mass [79–92].

The reasons for partial regression include myocardial fibrosis, residual gradient or leak from the prosthetic valve, associated systemic hypertension, the presence of other cardiac valvular lesions, and coronary artery disease. In the study by Donaldson et al. [92], 61% of patients with abnormal myocardial histology and histochemistry developed persistent dilatation and hypertrophy after surgery, but 39% of these cases with abnormal biopsies improved functionally and developed significant regression of hypertrophy. They also found a good correlation with loss of myofibrillar components from the hypertrophied myocardial cells and persistent ventricular dilatation. Extent of fibrosis is important; significant regression may be prevented by an extensive fibrotic framework.

The symptomatic patient with significant aortic regurgitation should be treated surgically. A major concern in patients with aortic regurgitation is the timing of surgery as irreversible myocardial dysfunction may be present prior to the development of significant symptoms. It was hoped that noninvasive testing might be able to identify a subgroup of patients that were at risk of developing irreversible left ventricular dysfunction. i.e., the group who would persist with left ventricular enlargement and no reduction in LV mass. Henry et al. [93] reported a high-risk group that either died during or after surgery from congestive heart failure. In the group that died, 9 of 13 had a preoperative left ventricular end-systolic dimension greater than 55 millimeters. Similarly Kumpuris et al. [94] found values greater than 50 mm were signs of irreversible cardiac dilatation. On the other hand, Fioretti et al. [95] studied 47 consecutive patients who underwent aortic valve replacement for isolated aortic regurgitation. Of the 27 patients with preoperative end-systolic dimension >55 mm, and 20 patients with preoperative end-systolic dimension <55 mm/Hg, there were no preoperative or postoperative deaths in a late follow-up averaging 41 months. In both groups, the left ventricular end-systolic dimension decreased. These results were confirmed by others who could not confirm irreversible dysfunction from preoperative data. Unfortunately, most of the reported data on postoperative left ventricular function have not been obtained serially, but it is still not known whether postoperative regression of left ventricular hypertrophy has significant functional consequences, i.e., it is uncertain whether the patients with complete regression of LVH have a better functional result than those with incomplete regression of hypertrophy.

Patients with Aortic stenosis

Reduction of LVH as assessed by echocardiography and angiography has been reported for aortic stenosis after aortic valve replacement (table 14–2) This has been observed as early as 3–5 weeks following aortic valve replacement and at 6 months after surgery. In the series reported by Panidis et al. [3], 10 patients were studied by M-mode echocardiograph preoperatively, in the early postoperative period (less than 6 months), and in the late postoperative period (more than 6 months). There was a 34% reduction in LV mass only during the late postoperative period. There was also a decrease in the left ventricular posterior wall and interventricular septal thickness. In some patients with mixed aortic valve disease (stenosis and regurgitation), the increased left ventricular mass and abnormal left ventricular function persisted even after successful surgery, as it has in cases of isolated aortic regurgitation.

It is not clear if this difference in reversibility of LVH and left ventricular function between aortic stenosis and regurgitation is real, or occurs as a result of different methods of assessment. It is possible that aortic stenosis may be present for a shorter time before it produces symptoms requiring surgical intervention, while patients with aortic regurgitation are less symptomatic so that surgery is delayed for a longer time, resulting in irreversible fibrosis.

It is not clear whether primary depression of myocardial contractility is greater, and hypertrophy therefore more detrimental to left ventricular function, in patients with volume overload than in patients with pressure load of the left ventricle.

Patients with Cardiomyopathy

Regression of LVH has not been well studied in the cardiomyopathies, but regression of cellular hypertrophy has been documented in patients with idiopathic dilated cardiomyopathy treated with vasodilators [96]. In the study by Unverferth et al. [96], there was actual decrease in myocardial cell size after treatment with isorbide dinitrate and hydralazine. In addition, biochemical changes such as reversal to normal of RNA content occurred. These changes were also associated with improved left ventricular function, but it is unknown whether this improvement in myocardial function will be maintained over the long term, and whether it will be associated with a decreased mortality.

In hypertrophic cardiomyopathy, prolonged medical treatment has not been associated with regression of septal hypertrophy, but in this condition, the pathophysiology of the hypertrophy is much more complicated and, unlike systemic hypertension or aortic valve disease, the primary overload has not been removed [97, 98]. However, disproportionate septal thickening in infants of diabetic mothers regresses spontaneously within the first 12 months of life [99].

FUNCTIONAL SIGNIFICANCE OF REGRESSION

The effects of reduction in LV mass on LV function have still not been completely elucidated. Analysis of the functional consequences of a reduced left ventricular mass has mainly concerned systolic or pump function. A broader approach is needed as this is a complex issue since diastolic abnormalities may be detected with normal systolic function in patients with increased left ventricular mass. There are also biochemical alterations and changes in coronary flow that my influence the functional significance of regression.

In patients with LVH due to pressure overload, the increase in wall thickness compensates for the increased systolic pressure and maintains a constant normal left ventricular wall stress and thus, a normal stroke volume against a high resistance, i.e., normal left ventricular function. In volume overload, there is a proportionate increase in left ventricular end-diastolic radius and wall thickness, thus maintaining a normal chamber wall thickness ratio and allowing the left ventricle to eject an augmented stroke volume against a normal or reduced resistance. This is appropriate hypertrophy, and abnormalities in left ventricular function occur when this becomes inappropriate.

Systolic Function

Studies of animals with hypertension indicate that regression of hypertrophy was associated with improved systolic left ventricular function with methyldopa in renovascular rats [13, 100]. But these results must be carefully assessed in order to differentiate between the effects of a reduction in left ventricular mass on ventricular function and the impact of the concomitant reduction in arterial pressure.

Most of the studies of hypertensive human patients have relied on determinations of left ventricular ejection fraction, fractional shortening, and cardiac output [39, 41, 65, 70, 101–104]. None of these indices have decreased at rest after regression of hypertrophy, but as with experimental studies, it is difficult to dissociate the effects of blood pressure reduction from those of regression of LVH. Some studies have examined left ventricular function in relation to left ventricular end-systolic stress to avoid the effect of altered afterload on ventricular performance [41]. In all these studies, reduction in left ventricular mass has not been associated with a deterioration in systolic function relative to afterload. Another major consideration in assessing the functional signficance of regression on systolic left ventricular function is that baseline measurements were generally within normal limits, and available data document no change in systolic function. There is no precise information on hypertensive patients who already had systolic dysfunction prior to reversal of ventricular hypertrophy, but animal studies suggest improvement in systolic function in these cases [12, 25, 100]. Theoretically, reduction of left ventricular mass may be deleterious, if hypertension recurs after reversal of hypertrophy, as a sudden increase in systolic pressure, without the protective adaptation of a gradual increase in myocardial mass, could result in markedly increased wall stress and may precipitate acute heart failure.

In the early period after aortic valve replacement, many patients have some temporary left ventricular dysfunction, but persistent postoperative hypertrophy after aortic valve replacement is usually associated with persistent left ventricular dysfunction. In the first 6–9 months after aortic valve replacement there is often a gradual improvement in left ventricular function, which is due, in part, to gradual reversal of hypertrophy. Regression of LVH in aortic valve disease, however, does not necessarily assume normalization of left ventricular function, and failure of regression does not necessarily mean that function is abnormal.

Diastolic Function

Left ventricular systolic function remains normal in most patients with mild to moderate hypertension. Congestive heart failure is a common and lethal complication of chronic systemic hypertension. Recently, with the aid of a variety of echocardiographic techniques, abnormalities of diastolic filling have been described in the presence of normal systolic left ventricular function in most patients [105–112]. See table 14–3.

These echocardiographic features include left atrial enlargement and flattening of the E-F slope, which are indirect signs of altered diastolic compliance. Evaluation of the posterior aortic wall to assess the rapid and slow phases of left ventricular diastolic filling, and computer digitization methods whereby various phases of the cardiac cycle can be studied, may be a more accurate method of detecting abnormalities in relaxation and filling.

Diastolic abnormal filling in hypertension is related to left ventricular mass, in that the more marked the hypertrophy the greater the diastolic dysfunction [107]. Moreover, these diastolic abnormalities have been detected in the absence of left ventricular hypertrophy by electrocardiogram and, in some cases, without increased left ventricular mass by echocardiography. The causes of abnormal diastolic function are thought to be related to increased collagen deposition and/or interstitial fibrosis which causes changes in myocardial elastic properties and alters myocardial stiffness and compliance [103]. Reduced diastolic compliance has also been demonstrated in other hypertrophic states, such as hypertrophic cardiomyopathy [113]. Abnormal diastolic function has not been associated with the physiological hypertrophy of athletes [57].

To date, there have been no studies of diastolic function after reversal of hypertrophy. The changes in diastolic function occur early in patients with hypertension and may be the cause of irreversible change, if fibrosis is a major factor in the etiology. Further studies are needed to evaluate diastolic function,

Table 14–3. Reported studies on diastolic function in left ventricular hypertrophy

Author (1st Author)	No. of Patients	Cause of LVH	Abnormal Systolic Function	Abnormal Diastolic Function	Method of Assessment
EcheveRia (105)	20	H/T	10% (2 pts)	35% (7 pts)	Echo
Inouye (106)	39	H/T	5% (2 pts)	84% (32 pts)	Echo Angio
Smith (107)	50	H/T	12% (3 pts)	88% (22 pts)	Echo Nuclear
Fouad (108)	33	H/T	0	All pts had abn diastolic function as a group vs control	Echo Nuclear
Dreslinkski (109)	31	H/T	0	Diastolic function abn detected as a group vs control	Echo
Hanrath (110)	76	H/T Aortic Valve Disease Dilated Cardiomyopathy	0	Diastolic function abn detected in all pts as a group vs control	Echo

Abn = abnormality; HT = hypertension; Pts = patients

as this may be a major factor contributing to heart failure, morbidity, and mortality in hypertension. Early treatment may be needed to reverse these diastolic filling abnormalities in hypertension.

Effects on Coronary Circulation

Coronary blood flow, when expressed per unit weight of myocardial mass, is normal at rest in hypertrophied ventricles [114–115]. Coronary vascular reserve, however, is probably also normal in the presence of LVH, but there is some controversy as some studies confirm this and others do not [116]. Effects of antihypertensive therapy and associated regression depends mainly on the status of the coronary arteries, the effects of the drugs on the coronary arteries, and changes in flow as a result of the hypertrophic process itself.

If the pressure load on the heart, the degree of LVH, and the driving pressure of the coronary circulation are closely related, then coronary vascular reserve is usually normal. But if there is dissociation between coronary driving pressure (systemic pressure) and the degree of hypertrophy, then major consequences of coronary vascular reserve may occur. The functional significance of this is that coronary vascular reserve remains normal if the decrease in blood pressure, following antihypertensive medication, parallels regression of hypertrophy. If treatment normalizes blood pressure, but not left ventricular mass, this will result in a marked decrease in coronary reserve and possible deleterious consequences. This of course will be aggravated by the presence of coronary artery disease, which is frequently associated with systemic hypertension.

LIMITATIONS OF STUDIES SHOWING REGRESSION

Most of the studies demonstrating regression of LVH in patients with hypertension or aortic valve disease included only a small number of patients and utilized M-mode echocardiography to estimate left ventricular mass. M-mode echocardiography has several limitations in measuring wall thickness and estimating left ventricular mass, especially when serial changes are assessed. Furthermore changes in LV wall thickness, although significant, were in the range from 1–2 mm, and ventricular mass usually decreased by less than 20% in patients who were treated for hypertension. Thus, conflicting results have been reported concerning the relation of blood pressure control and regression of hypertrophy, as well as the ability of various antihypertensive drugs to induce regression. Studies of aortic valve disease were performed at various intervals and utilize different methods. In the studies of the effects of drug therapy on LV regression in many cases multiple therapeutic regimens have generally been employed, making interpretation of the effects of individual drugs difficult. Electrocardiographic, echocardiographic, and angiographic techniques are unable to distinguish muscle from connective tissue or scar tissue and, therefore, a decrease in left ventricular mass by these techniques does not differentiate whether it is a decrease in muscle mass or a loss of connective tissue.

CONCLUSION

There is substantial evidence that regression of left ventricular hypertrophy occurs in treated patients with systemic hypertension, aortic valve disease, and in patients with cardiomyopathy. This regression is modified by numerous factors, including control of pressure or volume overload, catecholamines, renin-angiotensin system, associated cardiac diseases, and genetic factors. In systemic hypertension, regression of LVH is related not only to blood pressure control, but also to the type of antihypertensive agents used. Vasodilators and diuretics used alone do not seem to result in regression of hypertrophy, but sympatholytic agents, beta-blockers, and angiotensin-converting enzyme inhibitors are associated with regression of hypertrophy. Following aortic valve replacement, regression of hypertrophy occurs in most patients, but is usually incomplete. In systemic hypertension, after regression of hypertrophy occurs, systolic left ventricular function is not altered, but little is known about the consequences of diastolic dysfunction following reversal of hypertrophy. Diastolic abnormalities are frequently detected early in systemic hypertension before systolic dysfunction occurs. In aortic valve disease, following reversal of hypertrophy, left ventricular function improves in the majority of cases provided that left ventricular dysfunction was not severe prior to surgery. In asymptomatic patients with severe aortic valve disease, there is no clinical echocardiographic or angiographic variable that can predict which patients will develop irreversible left ventricular dysfunction. Coronary vascular reserve is essentially normal following regression of hypertrophy provided the blood pressure and regression occur concomitantly. If the blood pressure is controlled and regression does not occur at the same time, deleterious effects may occur. More studies are needed with regard to assessing the functional significance of regression of hypertrophy in relation to diastolic left ventricular function.

REFERENCES

1. Devereux, R.B., and Reichek, N. 1980. Left ventricular hypertrophy. *Cardiovasc. Rep.* 1:5–68.
2. Reichek, N., and Devereux, N.B. 1979. Left ventricular hypertrophy: Relationship of anatomic, echocardiographic, and electrocardiographic findings. *Circulation* 63:1058–1065.
3. Panidis, I.P., Kotler, M.N., Ren, J., Mintz, G.S., Ross, J., and Kalman, P. 1984. Development and regression of left ventricular hypertrophy. *J. Am. Coll. Cardiol.* 3:1309–1320.
4. McFarland, T.M., Goldstein, A.M., Pichard, S.D., and Stein, P.D. 1978. Echocardiographic diagnosis of left ventricular hypertrophy. *Circulation* 57:1140–1144.
5. Wahr, D., Wang, Y.S., Skioldebrand, C., Schiller, E., Lipton, and Schiller, N.B. 1983. Clinical quantitative echocardiography. III. Left ventricular mass in a normal adult population (abstract) *Clin. Res.* 30:23A.
6. Devereux, R.B., Casale, P.N., and Kligfield, P. 1983. Normalization of left ventricular anatomic measurements (abstract) *Clin. Res.* 31:128A.

7. Sen, S., Tanazi, R.C., Khalrallah, P.A., and Bumpus, F.M. 1974. Cardiac hypertrophy in spontaneous hypertensive rats. *Circ. Res.* 35:775–781.

8. Tomanek, R.J., Davis J.W., and Anderson, S.C. 1979. The effects of alpha-methyldopa on cardiac hypertrophy in spontaneously hypertensive rats: Ultrastructural stereological and morphometric analysis. *Cardiovasc. Res.* 13:173–182.

9. Idikio, H., Fernandez, P.G., Triggle, C.R., and Kim, B.K. 1983. Regression of left ventricular hypertrophy and control of hypertension in the spontaneously hypertensive rat (SHR): Oxprenolol versus hydrochlorthiazide. *Clinical and Investigative Medicine* 6:43–48.

10. Pfeffer, J.M., Pfeffer, M.A., Minsky, I., and Braunwald, E. 1983. Prevention of the development of heart failure and the regression of cardiac hypertrophy by captopril in the spontaneously hypertensive rat. *European Heart Journal* 4:(supplement A) 143–148.

11. Sen, S., Tarazi, R.C., and Bumpas, F.M. 1983. Regression of myocardial hypertrophy and influence of adrenergic system. *Am. J. Physiol.* 244:97–101.

12. Sen, S., Tarazi, R.C., and Bumpas, F.M. 1981. Reversal of cardiac hypertrophy in renal hypertensive rats: Medical vs. surgical therapy. *Am. J. Physiol.* 240:H408–H412.

13. Kuwajima, I., Kardon, M.B., Pegram, B.L., Sesoko, S., and Frolich, E.D. 1982. Regression of left ventricular hypertrophy in two-kidney, one clip Goldblatt hypertension. *Hypertension* 4:(Suppl. II) II-113–II-118.

14. Wicker, P., Tarazi, R.C., and Kobayashi, K. 1983. Coronary blood flow during the development and regression of left ventricular hypertrophy in renovascular rats. *Am. J. Cardiol.* 51:1744–1749.

15. Cutiletta, A.F. 1982. Regression of myocardial hypertrophy: III. Alterations in left ventricular performance. *J. Mol. Cell Cardiol.* 14:695–701.

16. Jouannot, P., and Hatt, P.Y. 1975. Rat myocardial mechanisms during pressure-induced hypertrophy development and reversal. *Am. J. Physiol.* 229:355–364.

17. Hall, O., Hall, C.E., and Ogden, E. 1953. Cardiac hypertrophy in experimental hypertension and its regression following re-establishment of normal blood pressure. *Am. J. Physiol.* 174:175–178.

18. Beznak, M., Karecky, B., and Thomas, G. 1969. Regression of cardiac hypertrophy of various organs. *Can. J. Physiol. Pharmacol.* 47:579–586.

19. Pegram, B.L., Ishıse, S., and Frohlich, E.D. 1982. Effect of methyldopa, clonidine, and hydrallazine on cardiac mass and haemodynamics in Wistar Kyoto and spontaneously hypertensive rats. *Cardiovasc. Res.* 16:40–46.

20. Caspari, P.G., Gibson, K., and Harris, D. 1975. Changes in myocardial collagen in normal development and after β-blockade: Recent advance studies on cardiac structure. *Metabolism* 7:99–104.

21. Ferrandes, M., Onesdi, G., Fiorentini, R., Kim, K.E., and Swartz, S. 1976. Effect of chronic administration of propranolol on the blood pressure and heart weight in experimental renal hypertension. *Life* SU 18:867–870.

22. VaughanWilliams, E.M., Raine, A.E.G., Caberera, A.A., and Whyte, J.M. 1979. The effects of prolonged B adreno-receptor blockade on heart weight and cardiac intracellular potentials in rabbits. *Cardiovasc. Res.* 9:579–582.

23. Pfeffer, M.A., Pfeffer, J.M., Weiss, A.K., and Frolich, E.D. 1977. Development of SHR hypertension and cardiac hypertrophy during prolonged beta-blockade. *Am. J. Physiol.* 232:H639–H644.

24. Sen, S., Tarazi, R.C., and Bumpus, F.M. 1977. Cardiac hypertrophy and antihypertensive therapy. *Cardiovasc. Res.* 11:427–433.

25. Pfeffer, J.M., Pfeffer, M.A., Flecher, P., Fishbein, M., and Braunwald, E. 1982. Favorable effects of therapy on cardiac performance in spontaneously hypertensive rats. *Am. J. Physiol.* 242:H776–H784.

26. Koike, H., Ito, K., Miyamoto, M., and Nishino, H. 1980. Effects of long-term blockade of angiotensin-converting enzyme with captopril (SQ 14, 225) on hemodynamics and circulation blood volume in spontaneously hypertensive rats. *Hypertension* 2:299–303.

27. Wicker, P., and Tarazi, R.L. 1982. Coronary blood flow in left ventricular hypertrophy: A review of experimental data. *Eur. Heart J.* 3:111–118.

28. Motz, W. and Strauer, B.E. 1984. Regression of structural cardiovascular changes by antihypertensive therapy. *Hypertension* 6:(Suppl. III) III-133–III-139.

29. Tarazi, R.C., Sen, S., Fouad, F.M., and Wicker, P. 1983. Regression of myocardial hypertrophy: Conditions and sequelae of reversal in hypertensive heart disease. Perspectives

in cardiovascular research. In: *Myocardial hypertrophy and failure*. Alpert, N.R., ed., pp. 637–651. New York: Raven Press.

30. Yamori, Y., Tarazi, R.C., and Ooshima, A. 1980. Effect of β-receptor-blocking agents on cardiovascular structural changes in spontaneous and nonadrenaline-induced hypertension in rats. *Clin. Sci.* 59(Suppl. 6) 457s–460s.

31. Rabinowitz, M. 1974. Overview on pathogenesis of cardiac hypertrophy. *Circ. Res.* 34, 35:Suppl. II:II-3–II-11.

32. Frederiksen, D.W., Hoffnung, J.M., Frederiksen, R.T., and Williams, R.B. 1978. The structural proteins of normal and diseased human myocardium. *Circ. Res.* 42:459–466.

33. Rabinowitz, M., and Zak, R. 1972. Biochemical and cellular changes in cardiac hypertrophy. *Ann. Rev. Med.* 23:245–262.

34. Cutiletta, A.F. 1975. Regression of myocardial hypertrophy II. RNA synthesis and RNA polymerase activity. *J. Mol. Cell. Cardiol.* 7:761–780.

35. Sen, S., and Bumpus, F.M. 1979. Collagen synthesis in development and reversal of cardiac hypertrophy in spontaneously hypertensive rats. *Am. J. Cardiol.* 44:954–958.

36. Fouad, F.M., Nakashima, Y., Tarazi. R.C., and Salcedo, E.E. 1982. Reversal of left ventricular hypertrophy in hypertensive patients treated with methyldopa: Lack of association with blood pressure control. *Am. J. Cardiol.* 49:795–801.

37. Ibrahim, M.M., Madkour, M.A., and Mossalam, R. 1981. Factors influencing cardiac hypertrophy in hypertensive patients. *Clin. Sci.* 61:(Suppl. 7) 1055–1085.

38. Drayer, J.M. Weber, M.A., Gardin, J.M., and Lipson, J.L. 1983. Effect of long-term antihypertensive therapy on cardiac anatomy in patients with essential hypertension. *Am. J. Med.* 75 (Suppl 3A):116–120.

39. Tarazi, R.C., and Fouad, F.M. 1984. Reversal of cardiac hypertrophy in humans. *Hypertension* 6:(Suppl. III) III-140–III-146.

40. Devereux, R.B., Savage, D.D., Sach, S.I., and Laragh, J.H. 1980. Effect of blood pressure control on LV hypertrophy and function in hypertension. *Circ.* 62:(Suppl. II:II-36.) (abstr.).

41. Nakashima, Y., Fouad, F.M., and Tarazi, R.C. 1984. Regression of left ventricular hypetrophy from systemic hypertension by Enalapril. *Am. J. Cardiol.* 53:1044–1049.

42. Sonotani, N., Kubo, S., Nishioka, A., and Takatsu, T. 1981. Electrocardiographic and echocardiograhic changes after one to two years' treatment of hypertension. Analyses of voltages ($SV_1 + RV_5$), wall thickness, cavity, mass, and hemodynamics of the left ventricle. *Jpn. Heart J.* 22:325–33.

43. Hill, L.S., Monaghan, M., and Richardson, P.J. 1979. Regression of left ventricular hypertrophy during treatment with antihypertensive agents. *Br. J. Clin. Pharmacol.* 7 (Suppl. 2):255s–60s.

44. Dunn, F.G., Bastian, B., Lawrie, T.D., and Lorimer, A.R. 1980. Effect of blood pressure control on left ventricular hypertrophy in patients with essential hypertension. *Clin. Sci.* 59 (Suppl. 6):441s–3s.

45. Corea, L., Bentivolglio, M., and Verdecchia, P. 1981. Reversal of left ventricular hypertrophy in essential hypertension by early and long-term treatment with methldopa. *Clin. Trials. J.* 18:380–94.

46. Reichek, N., Franklin, B.B. Chandler, T., Muhammad, A., Plappert, T., and Sutton, M.S.J. 1982. Reversal of left ventricular hypertrophy by antihypertensive therapy. *Eur. Heart J.* 3 (Suppl. A):A–1–65–9.

47. Rowlands, D.B., Glover, D.R., Ireland, M.A., McLeay, R.A., Stallard, T.J., and Littler, W.A. Assessment of left ventricular mass and its response to antihypertensive treatment. *Lancet* 2:467–70.

48. Weinstein, M., Hilewitz, H., and Rogel, S. 1984. The effect of single-dose methyldopa and diuretic on blood pressure and left ventricular mass. *Arch. Intern. Med.* 144:1629–1632.

49. Lombardo, M., Zaini, G., Pastori, F., Fusco, M., Pacini, S., and Foppol, C. 1983. Left ventricular mass and function before and after antihypertensive treatment. *Hypertension* 1:215–219.

50. Roeske, W.R., O'Rourke, R.A., Klein, A., Leopold, G., and Karliner, J.S. 1976. Noninvasive evaluation of ventricular hypertrophy in professional athletes. *Circulation* 53:286–292.

51. Morganroth, J., Maron, B.J., Henry, W.L., and Epstein, S.E. 1975. Comparative left ventricular dimensions in trained athletes. *Ann. Intern. Med.* 82:521–524.

52. Oakley, D. 1984. Cardiac hypertrophy in athletes. *Br. Heart J.* 52:121–123. (Editorial)

53. Shapiro, L.M. 1984. Physiological left ventricular hypertrophy. *Br. Heart J.* 52:130–135.
54. Fagard, R., Aubert, A., Staessen, J., Eynde, E.V., Vanhees, L., and Amery, A. Cardiac structure and function in cyclists and runners. Comparative echocardiograhic study. *Br. Heart J.* 52:124–129.
55. Shapiro, L.M., and Smith, R.G. 1983. Effect on training on left ventricular structure and function: An echocardiographic study. *Br. Heart J.* 50:534–539.
56. Nishimura, T., Yamada, Y., and Kawai, C. 1976. Echocardiographic evaluation of long-term effects of exercise on left ventricular hypertrophy in professional athletes. *Circulation* 53:286–292.
57. Shapiro, H.R., Katz, A.M., and Riba, A.L. 1985. Rapid ventricular filling in left ventricular hypertrophy: I. Physiologic hypertrophy. *J. Am. Coll. Cardiol.* 95:862–868.
58. Ehsani, A.A., Hagberg, J.M., and Hickson, R.C. 1978. Rapid changes in left ventricular dimensions and mass in response to physical conditioning and deconditioning. *Am. J. Cardiol.* 42:52–56.
59. Penpargkul, S., and Scheuer, J. 1970. The effect of physical training upon the mechanical and metabolic performance of the rat heart. *J. Clin. Invest.* 49:1859–1868.
60. Riedhammer, H.H., Rafflenbeul, W., Weihe, W.H., and Krayenbuhl, H.P. 1976. Left ventricular contractile function in trained dogs with cardiac hypertrophy. *Basic Res. Cardiol.* 71:297–308.
61. Krayenbuehl, H.P., Hess, O.M., Schneider, J., and Turina, M. 1983. Physiologic or pathologic hypertrophy. *European Heart J.* 4:(Suppl. A) 29–34.
62. Ibrahim, M.M., Tarazi, R.C., Dustan, H.P., and Gifford, R.W. Jr. 1977. Electrocardiogram in evaluation of resistance to antihypertensive therapy. *Arch. Intern. Med.* 56:416–23.
63. Poblete, P.F., Kyle, M.C., Pipberger, H.V., and Freis, E.D., 1973. Effect of treatment on morbidity in hypertension. Veterans Administration Cooperative Study on Antihypertensive Agents: effect on the electrocardiogram. *Circulation* 48:481–90.
64. Schlant, R.C., Felner, J.M., Blumenstein, B.A., Shulman, N.B., Heynsfield, S.B., Hall, W.D., and Wollam, G.L. 1982. Echocardiograhic documentation of regression of left ventricular hypertrophy produced by the treatment of essential hypertension. *Am. J. Cardiol.* 49:951. (abstr.).
65. Wollam, G.L., Hall, W.D., Douglas, M.B., Blumenstein, B.A., Knudtson, M.L., Felner, J.M., and Schlant, R.C. 1982. The time course of regression of left ventricular hypertrophy in treated hypertensive patients. *Am. J. Cardiol.* 49:951. (abstr.).
66. Drayer, J.I.M., Gardin, J.M., Weber, M.A., and Aronow, W.S. 1982. Changes in cardiac anatomy and function during therapy with alpha-methyldopa: An echocardiographic study. *Curr. Ther. Res.* 32:856–65.
67. Rowlands, D.B. Ireland, M.A., Glover, D.R., McLeay, R.A.B., Stallard, T.J., and Littler, W.A. 1981. The relationship between ambulatory blood pressure and echocardiographically assessed left ventricular hypertrophy. *Clin. Sci.* 61 (Suppl.7):101s–3s.
68. Drayer, J.I.M., Gardin, J.M., Weber, M.A., and Aronow, W.S. 1982. Changes in ventricular septal thickness during diuretic therapy. *Clin. Pharmacol. Ther.* 32:283–8.
69. Mijais, S.K., Tarazi, R.C., Fouad, F.M., and Bravo, E.L. 1983. Reversal of left ventricular hypertrophy with captopril. *Clin. Cardiol.* 6:595–602.
70. Corea, L., Bentivoglio, M., Verdecchia, P., Providenza, M., and Motolese, M. 1984. Left ventricular hypertrophy regression in hypertensive patients treated with metoprolol. *Int. J. Clin. Pharmacol.* Therapy and Toxicology 22:363–370.
71. Dunn, R.A., Zenner, R.J., and Pipberger, H.V. 1977. Serial electrocardiograms in hypertensive cardiovascular disease. *Circulation* 56:416–23.
72. Von Bibra, H., and Richardson, P.J. 1979. Left ventricular hypertrophy in patients with moderate essential hypertension: An echocardiographic study. In *Left ventricular hypertrophy in hypertension*, Robertson, J.S. and Caldwell, A.D.S., eds., New York: Academic Press and Grune and Stratton. pp. 47–54.
73. Safar, M.E., Lehner, J.P., Vincent, M.I., Plainfosse, M.T., and Simon, A.C. 1979. Echocardiograhic dimensions in borderline and sustained hypertension. *Am. J. Cardiol.* 44:930–935.
74. Sasayama, S., Ross, J. Jr., Franklin, D., Bloor C.M., Bishop C., and Dilley R.B. 1976. Adaptations of the left ventricle to chronic pressure overload. *Circ. Res.* 38:172–178.
75. Drayer, J.I.M. 1985. Does left ventricular mass decrease during antihypertensive therapy. *Arch. Intern. Med.* 145:1583–1584. (editorial).

76. Trimarco, B., and Wikstrand, J. 1984. Regression of cardiovascular structural changes by antihypertensive treatment.
77. Rowlands, D.B., Glover, D.R., Stallard, T.J., and Littler, W.A., 1982. Control of blood pressure and reduction of echocardiographically assessed left ventricular mass with once-daily Timolol. *Br. J. Clin. Pharmcol.* 14:89–95.
78. Greenberg, B.H., and Rahimtoola, S.H. 1980. Long-term vasodilator therapy in aortic insufficiency. Evidence for regression of left ventricular dilatation and hypertrophy and improvement in systolic pump function. *Ann. Intern. Med.* 93:440–2.
79. Henry, W.L., Bonow, R.O., Borer, J.S., Kent K.M. Ware, J.H., Redwood, D.R., Itscoitz, S.B., McIntosh, C.L., Morrow, A.G., and Epstein, S.E. 1980. Evaluation of aortic valve replacement in patients with valvular aortic stenosis. *Circulation* 61:814–25.
80. Cody, R.J. Jr., Stephens, D.D., Walker, H.J., and Boucher, C.A. 1981. Early postoperative changes in left ventricular dimensions and mass following valve replacement in adults with aortic stenosis. *J. Cardiovas. Surg.* 22:19–27.
81. Carroll, J.D., Gaasch, W.H., Naimi, S., and Levine, H.J. 1982. Regression of myocardial hypertrophy: Electrocardiographic-echocardiograhic correlations after aortic valve replacement in patients with chronic aortic regurgitation. *Circulation* 65:980–7.
82. Schuler, G., Peterson, K.L., Johnson, A.D., Francis, G., Ashburn, W., Dennish, G., Daily, P.O., and Ross, J. Jr. 1979. Serial noninvasive assessment of left ventricular hypertrophy and function after surgical correction of aortic regurgitation. *Am. J. Cardiol.* 44:585–94.
83. Bodem, R., Mehmel, H.C., and Storch, H.H. 1978. Regression of hypertrophy and contractile function of the left ventricle after aortic valve replacement for aortic regurgitation. *Circulation* 57, 58 (suppl. II):II–190.
84. Carroll, J.D., Gaasch, W.H., Zile, M.R., and Levine, H.J. 1981. Serial changes in left ventricular function after correction of chronic aortic regurgitation; dependence on early changes in preload and subsequent regression of hypertrophy in hypertensive patients. *Clin. Sci.* 61 (suppl. 7):105s–8s.
85. Schwartz, F., Flameng, W., Thormann, J., Sesto, M., Langebartels, F., Hehrlein, F., and Schlepper, M. 1978. Recovery from myocardial failure after aortic valve replacement. *J. Thorac. Cardiovasc. Surg.* 75:854–64.
86. Pantely, G., Morton, M., and Rahimtoola, S.H. 1978. Effects of successful, uncomplicated valve replacement on ventricular hypertrophy, volume, and performance in aortic stenosis and in aortic incompetence. *J. Thorac. Cardiovas. Surg.* 75:383–91.
87. Kennedy, J.W., Doces, J., and Stewart, D.K. 1977. Left ventricular function before and following aortic valve replacement. *Circulation* 56:944–50.
88. Gaasch, W.H., Andrias, C.W., and Levine, H.J. 1978. Chronic aortic regurgitation: The effect of aortic valve replacement on left ventricular volume, mass, and function. *Circulation* 58:825–836.
89. Fioretti, P., Roelandt, J., Mariagrazia, S., Domenicucci, S., Haalebos, M., Bos, E., and Hugenholtz, P.G. 1985. Postoperative regression of left ventricular dimensions in aortic insufficiency: A long-term echocardiographic study. *J. Am. Coll. Cardiol.* 5:856–861.
90. Donaldson, R.M., Florio, R., and Olsen, E. 1984. Left ventricular mass, volume, and biopsy analysis in prediction of ventricular function after surgery for chronic aortic regurgitation. *Herz* 9:333–340.
91. Toussaint, C., Cribier, A. Cazor, J.L., Soyer, R., and Letac, B. Hemodynamic and angiographic evaluation of aortic regurgitation 8 and 27 months after aortic valve replacement. *Circulation* 3:456–463.
92. Gaasch, W.H., Carroll, J.D., Levine, H.J., and Criscitiello, M.G. 1983. Chronic aortic regurgitation: Prognostic value of left ventricular end-systolic dimension and end-diastolic radius/thickness ratio. *J. Am. Coll. Cardiol.* 1:775–782.
93. Henry, W.L., Bonow, R.O., Borer, J.S., Ware, J.H., Kent, K.M., Redwood, D.R., McIntosh, C.L., Morrow, A.G., and Epstein, S.E. 1980. Observations on the optimum time for intervention for aortic regurgitation. I. Evaluation of the results of aortic valve replacement in symptomatic patients. *Circulation* 61:471–483.
94. Kumpuris, A.G., Quinones, M.A., Waggoner, A.D., Kanon, D.J., Nelson, J.G., and Miller, R.R. 1982. Importance of preoperative hypertrophy, wall stress, and end-systolic dimension as echocardiographic predictors of normalization of left ventricular dilatation after valve replacement in chronic aortic insufficiency. *Am. J. Cardiol.* 49:1094–1100.
95. Fioretti, P., Roelandt, J., Bos, R.J. et al. 1983. Echocardiography in chronic aortic

insufficiency. Is valve replacement too late when left ventricular end-systolic dimension reaches 55 mm? *Circulation* 67:216–221.

96. Unverfeth, D.V., Mehegan, J.P., Magorien, R.D., Unverferth, B.J., and Leier, C.V. 1983. Regression of myocardial cellular hypertrophy with vasodilator therapy in chronic congestive heart failure associated with idiopathic dilated cardiomyopathy. *Am. J. Cardiol.* 51:192–1398.

97. Murgo, J.P. 1982. Does outflow obstruction exist in hypertrophic cardiomyopathy? *N. Engl. J. Med.* 307:1008–1009.

98. Goodwin, J.F. 1980. An appreciation of hypertrophic cardiomyopathy. *Am. J. Med.* 68:797–80.

99. Way, G.L. Wolfe, R.R., Eshaghpour, E., Bender, R.L., Jaffee, R.B., and Ruttenberg, H.D. 1979. The natural history of hypertrophic cardiomyopathy in infants of diabetic mothers. *J. Pediatr.* 95:1020–1025.

100. Ferrario, C.M., Spech, M.M., Tarazi, R.L., and Doi, R. 1979. Cardiac pumping ability in rats with experimental renal and genetic hypertension. *Am. J. Cardiol.* 44:979–985.

101. Perloff, J.K. 1982. Development and regression of increased ventricular mass. *Am. J. Cardiol.* 50:605–611.

102. Messerli, F.H. 1983. Clinical determinants and consequences of left ventricular hypertrophy. *Am. J. Med.* 75:51–56.

103. Massie, B.M. 1983. Myocardial hypertrophy and cardiac failure. A Complex interrelationship. *Am. J. Med.* 75:67–74.

104. Tarazi, R.C. 1984. Regression of left ventricular hypertrophy: Partial answers for persistent questions. *J. Am. Coll. Cardiol.* 3:1349–1351.

105. Echeverria, H.H., Bilsker, M.S., Myerburg, R.J., and Kessler, K.M. Congestive heart failure: Echocardiographic insights. *Am. J. Med.* 75:750–755.

106. Inouye, I., Massie, B., Loge, D., Topic, N., Silverstein, D., Simpson, P., and Tubau, J. 1984. Abnormal left ventricular filling: An early finding in mild to moderate systemic hypertension. *Am. J. Cardiol.* 53:120–126.

107. Smith, V., Schulman, P., Karimeddini, M.K., Wite, W.B., Meeran, M.K., and Katz, A.M. 1985. Rapid ventricular filling in left ventricular hypertrophy: II Pathologic hypertrophy. *J. Am. Coll. Cardiol.* 5:869–874.

108. Fouad, F.M., Slominski, J.M., and Tarazi, R.C. 1984. Left ventricular diastolic function in hypertension: Relation to left ventricular mass and systolic function. *J. Am. Coll. Cardiol.* 3:1500–1506.

109. Dreslinski, G.R., Frohlich, E.D., Dunn, F.G., Messerli, F.H., Suarez, D.H., and Reisin, E. 1981. Echocardiograhic diastolic ventricular abnormality in hypertensive heart disease: Atrial emptying index. *Am. J. Cardiol.* 47:1087–1091.

110. Hanrath, P., Mathey, D.G., Siegert, R., and Bleifeld, W. 1980. Left ventricular relaxation and filling pattern in different forms of left ventricular hypretrophy: An echocardiographic study. *Am. J. Cardiol.* 45:15–23.

111. Hess, O.M., Schneider, J., Koch, R., Bamert, C., Grimm, J., and Krayenbuehl, H.P. 1981. Diastolic function and myocardial structural in patients with myocardial hypertrophy. Special reference to normalized viscoelastic data. *Circulation* 62:360–371.

112. Grossman, W., Mclaurin, L.P., and Stefadouros, M.A. 1984. Left ventricular stiffness associated with chronic pressure and volume overloads in man. *Circ. Res.* 35:793–800.

113. Goodwin, J.F. 1978. Left ventricular relaxation and filling in hypertrophic cardiomyopathy. An echocardiographic study. *Br. Heart J.* 40:596–601.

114. Bing, R.J., Hammond, M.M. Handelsman, J.C., Powers, S.R., Spencer, F.C., Eckenhoff, J.E., Goodale, W.T., Hafkenschiel, J.H., and Kety, S.S. 1949. The measurement of coronary blood flow, oxygen consumption and efficiency of the left ventricle in man. *Am. Heart J.* 38:1–24.

115. Marcus, M.L., Mueller, T.M., Gascho, J.A., and Kerber, R.E. 1979. Effects of cardiac hypertrophy secondary to hypertension on the coronary circulation. *Am. J. Cardiol.* 44:1023–1028.

116. Wicker, P., Tarazi, R.C., and Kobayashi, K. 1983. Coronary blood flow in the development and regression of left ventricular hypertrophy in renovascular hypertensive rats. *Am. J. Cardiol.* 51:1744–1749.

15. THE CARDIOCYTE IN SENESCENCE

ROBERT J. TOMANEK

Cardiac pathology is common among the elderly and has long received attention. Despite the high incidence of some heart diseases in old age, the role of biological aging in cardiovascular diseases is not well established. Aging in its broadest sense is regarded as a process spanning the time from conception to death. In this chapter, however, the term "aging" will be limited to the period between middle age and death. This definition excludes changes associated with maturation.

Several problems inherent in aging research have limited scientific findings. Longitudinal studies involve long periods of time to accumulate data and usually suffer from a lack of adequate controls. On the other hand, cross-sectional studies require large sample sizes in order to minimize individual or animal variability. The dissociation of underlying disease and biological aging is always a challenge, especially in humans. While several species have provided data which may be useful in understanding aging and the heart, the most widely used animals have been rodents. Their relatively short lifespan and resistance to coronary atherosclerosis has made them a convenient model for aging studies on the heart.

This review focuses on the cardiocyte during senescence and examines possible components of biological aging. Experimental data are discussed with regard to alterations in myocardial function during the aging process. Also

Supported by NIH grants HL-18629 and HL-14388.

discussed are reviews of the effects of aging on the heart and cardiovascular system, which have been published during the last decade [2–6].

CARDIAC PERFORMANCE

Before addressing specific age-related structural, biochemical, and contractile changes in the cardiocyte, a more global assessment of cardiac performance is appropriate. Such a consideration is important in determining whether more specific changes lead to altered ventricular performance. A decline in cardiac output in middle age and thereafter has been cited as an indicator of declining cardiac function [3]. Aging in rats is reportedly characterized by decrements in cardiac output, cardiac index, and stroke volume [7–9]. These data, however, are based on basal conditions and therefore do not provide an indicator of ventricular pumping ability. A lower cardiac output in senescence, compared to the young adult, could be related to lower basal metabolic rates and may not indicate inadequate perfusion of the tissues. Clinical studies have revealed some age-related changes in subjects who did not exhibit hypertension and cardiovascular disease [6]. However, these differences (a slower ventricular diastolic filling, and an increase in diastolic aortic root dimension in the older group) do not indicate altered performance. Importantly, the old subjects did not differ from the young group in left ventricular ejection time, velocity of circumferential fiber shortening, or ventricular systolic and diastolic cavity dimensions.

To unmask the more subtle changes of aging, ventricular performance needs to be assessed under stress conditions, e.g., enhanced preload or afterload. This approach provides a test of the ventricle's ability to respond to enhanced functional demand. Other approaches which may provide greater insights into ventricular performance are the use of isolated hearts and interventions such as cholinergic and adrenergic blockade. Such experimental conditions provide an avenue for the dissociation of myocardial changes from those secondary to extrinsic factors. Finally, the evaluation of cardiac performance in studies which are aimed at exploring specific properties of the myocardium are of great advantage in evaluating cardiac function, since specific biochemical, pharmacological, contractile, and structural properties may be considered with regard to their effect on cardiac function.

GENERAL STRUCTURAL CHANGES

Contrary to the belief that the heart atrophies during sensescence, data from many studies in man [2] as well as those from rats [10, 11], and dogs [12] suggest that heart mass increases slightly in senescence. The left ventricle in aged male rats is relatively dilated, compared to that of younger rats [13]. While cardiocytes in aged rats are more irregular in shape with some exhibiting degenerative changes [14], there is no morphological evidence of widespread degeneration of cardiocytes in senescence. Histopathological examination of hearts from Fischer 344 rats, used in gerontological studies, indicates that aging is not associated with consistent structural abnormalities and diseases at the light microscopic level [15]. However, the fact that myocardial mass increases with age, in spite of the focal degeneration of some cells, suggests that other cardiocytes may grow late in life.

Several studies have examined intracellular structures in an attempt to provide a structural basis for possible impairment of ventricular function. Investigations on rats are in agreement: myofibrillar volume density [11, 16] and mitochondrial volume density [11, 17] are not altered during senescence. In contrast, cardiocyte mitochondrial volume density was found to increase in hamsters [18] and decrease in mice [19] during late life. Qualitative alterations in mitochondria from old animals have been observed consistently. The frequency of mitochondrial profiles exhibiting degenerative changes (i.e., translucent matrix and disrupted cristae) increases during senescence [11, 14, 20, 21]. However, the vast majority of mitochondria in senescent hearts exhibits normal ultrastructure. Other consistent focal changes include increases in the number of sarcolemmal vesicles, dense accumulations of small mitochondrial profiles and enhancement of the Golgi apparatus components [14]. Dilatations of the nonspecialized junctions of the intercalated discs are also common.

Clearly, the major morphological characteristic of cardiocytes from old animals is the widespread occurrence of residual bodies (lipofuscin pigment). An age-related accumulation of these structures has been described in humans, cats, dogs, rats, guinea pigs, and mice [14, 18, 21–25]. Residual bodies, which contain residues of autophagy, increase sharply after 18 months of age in the rat [21]. This increase is also characteristic of senescence in atrial cells [26]. Thus, senescence is characterized by rather specific subcellular morphological changes.

AUTOLYSIS AND PROTEIN TURNOVER

Studies on mice from one laboratory have shown that protein synthesis in isolated perfused hearts decreases during the aging process [27, 28]. These data are in agreement with a study on rat hearts which showed that protein synthesis was lower in senescent (two-year-old) rats than it was in young adult (3–4-month-old) rats [29]. This decline was attributed to both a fall in ribosome concentration and a decreased rate of translation, caused by a drop in transfer RNA. Protein degradation was also reduced in the senescent group—a finding which conflicts with another study on rats which reported a sharp increase in autolytic degradation of sarcoplasmic proteins between 15 and 25 months of age [30]. In contrast, cardiocyte mitochondrial turnover in old (24 months) and adult (12 months) rats was shown to be virtually identical [31].

As noted in the previous section, morphological evidence for an accumulation of the products of autolysis is clearly an age-related event. Hochschild [32] suggested that peroxidation of membrane lipids damages lysosomes enabling leakage of hydrolytic enzymes which degrade DNA, RNA, and other macromolecules. However, the accumulation of residual bodies with time does not necessarily indicate a biochemical defect in the lysosomal system, but could be due instead to the cardiocyte's limited ability to remove the products of autolysis via exocytosis. Yet, an increase in the total activities of three hydrolytic enzymes (N-acetyl-β-D-glucosaminidase, β-glucuronidase and arylsulfatase) was found to occur in mouse heart during aging [25]. In contrast, acid phosphase activity was not altered with age. These authors suggested that a temporal relationship may exist between lipofuscin pigment (residual body) accumulation and increases in certain lysosomal enzyme activities. In view of all these data, a firm conclusion concerning the effects of aging is not warranted. A decrease in protein synthesis, coupled with an increase in autolysis, should result in cardiocyte atrophy. Yet ventricular mass has been shown to increase slightly during aging. Moreover, the finding that mito-chondrial turnover is not altered with aging is inconsistent with morphological evidence of more frequently observed mitochondria undergoing degenerative changes in senescent rats. One possible explanation of this finding and the well-documented increase in residual bodies with age is that, regardless of the rate of autophagy in senescence, its products simply increase as a function of time. Alternatively, the cardiocyte's ability to eliminate the products of autophagy may decline with age.

CONTRACTILITY

A number of studies have compared the heart's contractile properties in adult and old rats. Both the force developed by cardiac muscle during isometric contractions and the maximum rate of force production are similar for the two age groups, even when Ca^{2+} concentration in the perfusate is varied [33–35]. Moreover, age does not appear to affect the potentiation of force development to continued paired stimulation [33]. In contrast, the duration of isometric contraction has been repeatedly shown to be prolonged in cardiac muscle of senescent compared to adult rats [5]. Similar data have been derived from studies on humans [36], guinea pigs [37], and dogs [38]. Consistent with this finding is a prolongation of both time-to-peak tension [39] and the half time of relaxation [34]. More recently Capasso et al. [40] evaluated the mechanical performance under isometric and isotonic conditions of isolated papillary muscles from rats aged 3, 6, 12, and 24 months. Their findings, based on L_{max} muscle length, indicate a progressive prolongation of time-to-peak tension and time-to-peak rate of tension over the lifespan. However, half time of relaxation and time-to-peak rate of tension fall were prolonged only between 3 and 6 months but not between 12 and 24 months. Thus, the change in relaxation cannot be attributed to senescence but rather to development and maturation. Weisfeldt [6] has noted that electromechanical restitution requires a longer period in senescent than in adult heart. This was demonstrated by progressively decreasing the interval between stimuli and noting when the muscle failed to contract. He concluded that the excitation-contraction cycle in the aged heart is impeded by a prolonged contraction time.

Sarcoplasmic reticulum, which releases and sequesters Ca^{2+}, has been implicated in age-associated changes which may effect contractility. Microsomes obtained from cardiocytes of 24 month old rats accumulate Ca^{2+} at slower rates, over a 0.5–2.0 μM range, than cardiocytes from 6 month old rats [41]. Moreover, both the volume density as well as the membrane area per myofibrillar mass, as evaluated morphometrically, has been shown to be lower in old (555 days), than it was in young (250–300 days) hamster cardiocytes [18]. Considering these findings, it would appear that cardiocytes of senescent animals may have two liabilities that could affect contractility: 1) the rate of Ca^{2+} sequestration and 2) the amount of sarcoplasmic reticulum available for Ca^{2+} release and sequestration. During reoxygenation subsequent to hypoxia, contraction duration was longer in 25 month-than in 6-month-old rats [3]. This recovery period imposes a stress on Ca^{2+} sinks and therefore is considered to be a functional test of the sarcoplasmic reticulum.

An age-related decrease in myofibrillar ATPase has been shown by several groups of investigators. Chesky and co-workers found that ATPase and creatine phosphorylase fell in rat hearts between the ages of 2 and 16 months [42, 43]. In reviewing data on the age-related decline in myofibrillar ATPase, Lakatta and Yin [5] noted that the decline occurred primarily during the maturation period, rather than during senescence. However, more recently Capasso et al. [40] demonstrated a significant decline in actomyosin ATPase activity between 12 and 24 months in rats.

While it is evident that several mechanical and biochemical parameters of cardiac muscle change with age, not all can be attributed to senescence since they occur prior to 12 or 16 months in the rat. Importantly, both maximum force development and maximum rate of force development are similar in senescent and adult rats.

CARDIAC NERVES AND BIOGENIC AMINES

Because catecholamines are important activators of contractile responses, their role in aging has been considered in several laboratories. Norepinephrine content has been shown to decrease during the course of aging in all four chambers of rat hearts [9]. Using ultrastructural cytochemical techniques to label noradrenergic vesicles of sympathetic nerve terminals in rat heart atria, McLean et al. [26] found no age-related changes in the vesicle population of intact nerve terminals. However, a significant sympathetic axonal degeneration occurred between 3 and 24 months. They concluded that the decline in norepinephrine content in the heart with age may be due to axonal degeneration.

The effect of aging on the cardiocyte's contractile response to catecholamines has also been examined. In old rats the maximal rate of tension development in response to norepinephrine and isoproterenol was significantly less than in adult rats [5]. A subsequent study by this group showed that cylic AMP levels and protein kinase activity elevations after isoproterenol were similar in adult and old rats [44]. However, the rate of force development (dF/dt) of cardiac muscle was considerably greater in the adult group than in the senescent animals when dibutyryl cyclic AMP was administered. Since dibutyryl cyclic AMP enhances contraction independent of β-receptors, the authors noted that the limited response of senescent hearts to catecholamines is not due to changes at the receptor level. They found that β-receptor number and affinity were similar in the two age groups. Accordingly, they concluded that aging affects some mechanism(s) distal to protein kinase activation.

In vivo experiments in several species have examined the heart's response to neural stimulation [45]. The threshold stimulation of sympathetic nerves required to cause significant hemodynamic changes was approximately twofold higher in old, compared to young, rabbits. Similarly, the voltage necessary to induce bradycardia via vagal stimulation was significantly higher in senescent rats, cats, and rabbits than in their adult counterparts. When acetylcholine was administered, a smaller dose was required to induce bradycardia in old, compared to adult, rabbits, but no difference between these age groups was found in rats. These findings suggest that neural alterations occur during senescence which may affect myocardial function. The increased sensitivity to acetylcholine in aged rabbits is seen as an adaptation or compensatory change since acetylcholine synthesis is decreased.

CONTRIBUTION OF AND RESPONSE TO STRESS

Two aspects of stress could be of importance with regard to aging. First, long-term cardiac function may in itself lead to age-related alterations in the myocardium. Second, the capacity of the cardiocyte to respond in increased functional demand (stress) may become compromised with time.

The possible relationship between stress and the accumulation of the products of autolysis has some support. Studies on spontaneously hypertensive rats in my laboratory indicate that accumulation of residual bodies and degenerative structures is accelerated in the hypertrophied left ventricle of spontaneously hypertensive rats [11, 46]. Cytochemical data indicate that lysosomes, autolysosomes, and degenerative structures become more numerous and widespread in cardiocytes of SHR than in normotensive WKY of the same age [46]. These differences became marked by the age of 15 months which is relatively late in the lifespan of SHR and WKY. Others have also demonstrated that cardiac hypertrophy due to aortic constriction [47], or isoproterenol administration [48], is characterized by an increase in lysosomes. Meerson and associates [29] proposed the idea that "wear and tear" of enhanced cellular work is responsible for ultrastructural changes seen during aging. While there is evidence of age-related alterations in protein synthesis and degradation, and an accumulation of the by-products of the latter, these changes do not in themselves imply functional impairment.

The observation that heart mass increases into senescence has led to speculation that some of the alterations corresponding to aging could be due to the effect of cardiac hypertrophy rather than to biological aging. For example, prolonged contraction time is a common finding in cardiac hypertrophy [49–52] and, as noted earlier in this chapter, certain ultrastructural features of aging are accelerated in spontaneously hypertensive rats that, predictably, develop left ventricular hypertrophy. Yin and associates [53] have considered the relationship between hypertrophy and aging. They induced the same magnitude of LVH by aortic constriction in 15 as is present in 24 month old rats. While contraction duration was prolonged, the magnitude of the increase was only about 30% of that which occurred in normotensive rats between 15 and 24 months. They pointed out that contraction duration is also prolonged in the right ventricle which does not hypertrophy and that hearts which atrophy, due to transplantation into the abdominal cavity, also have a prolonged contraction time by the twenty-fourth month. Further evidence against the hypothesis that hypertrophy contributes to age-related functional changes is provided by a recent study [54]. Contractile protein ATPase activity, studied under a wide range of conditions, did not differ in age-matched SHR and WKY. However, in both groups, ATPase activity showed a decline between 5 and 52 weeks. Myosin isoenzyme distributions were also similar in the two strains. Therefore, the development and persistence of cardiac hypertrophy and hypertension did not alter the decrease in myosin ATPase activity nor the increase in myosin isoenzyme V_3 characteristic of normotensive rats.

The underlying cause of LVH during aging is not clear, but it should be noted that its magnitude is small, i.e., about 15%, between midlife and senescence in the rat [5]. Weisfeldt [55] suggested that in man, LVH may compensate for a presumed increased impedence to LV ejection permitting a normal ejection fraction in healthy elderly subjects. Accordingly, this modest increase in heart mass may be a useful biological adaptation that enables adequate pump function in senescence.

Little is known about the heart's ability to respond to acute stress, such as may be imposed by abrupt increases in afterload, hypoxia, or exercise. A comparison of elderly (mean age = 68.5 years) and young (mean age = 29.6 years) men revealed that at rest they did not differ with regard to heart rate, blood pressure, left ventricular systolic dimension, or velocity of contractile element shortening [56]. Moreover, these parameters were similar in the two groups when systolic blood pressure was raised by about 30 mm Hg either by phenylephrine or hand grip exercise. However, when phenylephrine was given to raise blood pressure after β-blockade with propanolol, left ventricular diastolic dimension was increased by 2.3 ± 0.6 mm in the old subjects but only by 1.0 ± 0.05 mm in the young group. These data suggest that the older individuals utilize the Frank-Starling mechanism in order to meet the demands of enhanced overload. Thus, under conditions of β-blockade, a difference between young and old subjects became evident.

SUMMARY AND CONCLUSIONS

Aging of the cardiocyte is characterized by several morphological changes, most of which are discernable with electron microscopy. An accumulation of residual bodies and membrane fragments are hallmarks of aging; some other consistent changes include dilatations of the intercalated discs and increases in the number of sarcolemmal vesicles. Yet, widespread cell degeneration does not typify senescence, and the structural changes that occur during aging do not necessarily imply decrements in cell function. While altered rates of protein turnover have been reported during aging, there is no evidence of impaired cardiocyte organelle renewal or limitations in growth.

In vitro experiments have demonstrated that senescence is assoicated with a prolongation of contraction time, and time-to-peak tension. Associated with these alterations are:

1. a slower rate of Ca^{2+} sequestration and
2. a decrease in volume density and membrane area per myofibrillar mass of sarcoplasmic reticulum.

Myofibrillar ATPase activity also appears to decline during aging. Cardiocytes have been shown to undergo a decreased sensitivity to catecholamines late in life. This impairment appears to occur distal to protein kinase activation, rather than at the level of the receptor.

Although some structural and functional changes are common to both aging and cardiac hypertrophy, a causal relationship between stress and myocardial aging has not been established. While it has been observed that stress associated with hypertension-induced left ventricular hypertrophy accelerates some structural changes characteristic of aging, other parameters are not affected by long-term hypertension and cardiac hypertrophy. The mild cardiac hypertrophy observed during senescence does not appear to impair ventricular function but may instead constitute a favorable compensatory mechanism.

Finally, although we know that the myocardium is affected by aging, interpretation of the observed changes with regard to ventricular pumping ability is at best controversial. Because there is evidence of an age-associated decrement in cardiac function in response to stress, future studies need to design experiments which adequately stress the heart. It is quite plausible that aging may impair the cardiocyte's ability to respond to enhanced workloads, particularly for prolonged periods of time.

REFERENCES

1. Pomerance, A. 1981. Cardiac pathology in the elderly. *Cardiovas. Clin.* 12:9–54.
2. Lakatta, E.G. 1979. Alterations in the cardiovascular system that occurs in advanced age. *Fed.*

Proc. 38:163–167.

3. Baskin, S.I., Kendrick, Z.V., Roberts, J., and Tomanek, R.J. 1981. The cardiovascular system. *Aging and Cell Structure* 1:305–331.
4. Weisfeldt, M.L., ed. 1980. *The Aging Heart. Its Function and Response to Stress* (Aging, Vol. 12). New York: Raven Press.
5. Lakatta, E.G., and Yin, F.C. 1982. Myocardial aging: functional alterations and related cellular mechanisms. *Am. J. Physiol.* 242:H927–H941.
6. Weisfeldt, M.L. 1985. The Aging Heart. *Hosp. Pract.* 20:115–120, 125–130.
7. Rothbaum, D.A., Shaw, D.J., Angell, C.S., and Shock, N.W. 1973. Cardiac performance in the unanesthetized senescent male rat. *J. Gerontol.* 28:287.
8. Lee, J.C., Karpelis, L.M., and Downing, S.E. 1972. Age-related changes of cardiac performance in male rats. *Am. J. Physiol.* 222:432.
9. Roberts, J., and Goldberg, P.B. 1976. Changes in basic cardiovascular activities during the lifetime of the rat. *Exp. Aging. Res.* 2:487–517.
10. Yin, F.C.P., Spurgeon, H.A., Rakusan, K., Weisfeldt, M.L., Lakatta, E.G. 1982. Use of tibial length to quantify cardiac hypertrophy. *Am. J. Physiol.* 243:H941–H947.
11. Tomanek, R.J., and Hovanec, J.M. 1981. The effects of long-term pressure overload and aging on the myocardium. *J. Mol. Cell Cardiol.* 13:471–488.
12. Munnel, J.F., and Getty, R. 1968. Nuclear lobulation and amitotic division associated with increasing cell size in the aging canine myocardium. *J. Geront.* 23:363–369.
13. Shreiner, T.P., Weisfeldt, M.L., and Shock, N.W. 1969. Effects of age, sex, and breeding status on the rat heart. *Am. J. Physiol.* 217:176–180.
14. Tomanek, R.J. and Karlsson, U.L. 1973. Myocardial ultrastructure of young and senescent rats. *J. Ultrastruct. Res.* 42:201–220.
15. Goldberg, P.B. 1978. Cardiac function of Fischer 344 rats in relation to age. In *The Aging Heart. Its Function and Response to Stress.* (Aging Vol. 6) G. Kaldor and W.J. DiBatlista, eds. pp. 87–99. New York: Raven Press.
16. Frenzel, H., and Feimann, J. 1984. Age-dependent structural changes in the myocardium of rats. A quantitative light- and electron-microscopic study on the right and left chamber wall. *Mech. Aging Dev.* 27:29–41.
17. Kmet, A., Leibetseder, J., and Burger, H. 1966. Gerontologische Untersuchung und Rattenberzmitochondrien. *Gerontologia* 12:193–199.
18. Sachs, H.G., Colgan, J.A., and Lazarus, M.L. 1977. Ultrastructure of the aging myocardium: A morphometric approach. *Am. J. Anat.* 150:63–72.
19. Herbener, G.H.A. 1976. A morphometric study of age-dependent changes in mitochondrial populations of mouse liver and heart. *J. Gerontol.* 31:8–12.
20. Feldman, M.L., and Navaratnam, V. 1981. Ultrastructural changes in atrial myocardium of the aging rat. *J. Anat.* 133:7–17.
21. Travis, D.F., and Travis, A. 1972. Ultrastructural changes in the left ventricular rat myocardial cells with age. *J. Ultrastructure Research* 39:124–148.
22. Fawcett, D.W., and McNutt, N.S. 1969. Ultrastructure of cat myocardium. I. Ventricular papillary muscle. *J. Cell Biol.* 42:1–45.
23. Jamieson, J.D. 1963. Secretory granules and lipofuscin pigments in mammalian atria. *J. Cell Biol.* 19:36A.
24. Malkoff, D.B., and Strehler, B.L. 1963. The ultrastructure of isolated and in situ human cardiac age pigment. *J. Cell Biol.* 16:611.
25. Traurig, H.H., and Papka, R.E. 1980. Lysosomal acid hydrolase activities in the aging heart. *Exp. Geront.* 15:291–299.
26. McLean, M.R., Goldberg, P.B., and Roberts, J. 1983. An ultrastructural study of the effects of age on sympathetic innervation and atrial tissue in the rat. *J. Mol. Cell Cardiol.* 15:75–92.
27. Geary, S., and Florini, J.R. 1972. Effect of age on rate of protein synthesis in isolated perfused mouse hearts. *J. Gerontol.* 27:325–332.
28. Florini J.R., Saito, Y., and Manowitz, E.J. 1973. Effect of age on thyroxine-induced cardiac hypertrophy in mice. *J. Gerontol.* 28:293–297.
29. Meerson, F.Z., Javich, M.P., and Lerman, M.I. 1978. Decrease in the rat of RNA and protein synthesis and degradation in the myocardium under long-term compensatory hyperfunction and on aging. *J. Mol. Cell Cardiol.* 10:145–159.
30. Mohan, S., and Radha, E. 1978. Age-related changes in muscle protein degradation. *Mech. Age Develop.* 7:81–87.
31. Menzies, R.A., and Gold P.H. 1971. The turnover of mitochondria in a variety of tissues of

young adult and aged rats. *J. Biol. Chem.* 246:2425.

32. Hochschild, R. 1971. Lysosomes, membranes, and aging. *Exp. Geront.* 6:153–166.

33. Gerstenblith, G., Spurgeon, H.A., Froehlich, J.P., Weisfeldt, M.L. and Lakatta, E.G. 1979. Diminished inotropic responsiveness to ouabain in aged rat myocardium. *Circ. Res.* 44:517–523.

34. Lakatta, E.G., Gerstenblith, G., Angell, C.S., Shock, N.W., and Weisfeldt, M.L. 1975. Prolonged contraction duration in aged myocardium. *J. Clin. Invest.* 55:61–68.

35. Spurgeon, H.A., Thorne, P.R., Yin, F.C.P., Shock, N.W., and Weisfeldt, M.L. 1977. Increased dynamic stiffness of trabeculae carneae from senescent rats. *Am. J. Physiol.* 232:H373–H380.

36. Harrison, T.R., Dixon, K., Russell, R.O., Bidwai, P.S., and Coleman, H.N. 1964. The relation of age to the duration of contraction, ejection, and relaxation of the normal human heart. *Amer. Heart J.* 67:189–199.

37. Rumberger, E. and Timmermann, J. 1976. Age-changes of the force frequency relationship and the duration of action potential isolated papillary muscles of guinea pig. *Eur. J. Appl. Physiol. Occup. Physiol.* 34:277–284.

38. Templeton, G.H., Willerson, J.T., Platt, M.R., and Weisfeldt, M. 1978. Contraction duration and diastolic stiffness in aged canine left ventricle. In *Recent Advances in Studies on Cardiac Structure and Metabolism*. Heart Function and Metabolism, T. Koybayashi, T. Sano, and N.S. Dhalla, eds, pp. 169–173. Baltimore MD: University Park.

39. Alpert, N.R., Gale, H.H., and Taylor, N. 1967. The effect of age on contractile protein ATPase activity and the velocity of shortening. *Factors Influencing Myocardial Contractility.* R.D. Tans, F. Kavaler, J. Roberts, eds. New York: Academic Press.

40. Capasso, J.M., Malhotra, A., Remily, R.M., Scheuer, J., and Sonnenblick, E.H. 1983. Effects of age on mechanical and electrical performance of rat myocardium. *Am. J. Physiol.* 245:H72–H81.

41. Froehlich, J.P., Lakatta, E.G., Beard, E., Spurgeon, H.A., Weisfeldt, M.L., and Gerstenblith, G. 1978. Studies of sarcoplasmic reticulum function and contraction duration in young adult and aged rat myocardium. *J. Mol. Cell. Cardiol.* 10:427–438.

42. Chesky, J.A. and Rockstein, M. 1977. Reduced myocardial actomyosin adenosine triphosphatase activity in the aging male Fischer rat. *Cardiovas. Res.* 11:242–246.

43. Chesky, J.A., Rockstein, M., and Lopez, T. 1980. Changes with age of myocardial creatine phosphokinase in the male Fischer rat. *Mechanisms of Aging and Development* 12:237–243.

44. Guarnieri, T., Filburn, C.R., Zitnik, G., Roth, G.S., and Lakatta, E.G. 1980. Contractile and biochemical correlates of β-adrenergic stimulation of the aged heart. *Am. J. Physiol.* 239:H501–H508.

45. Frolkis, V.V., Shevtchuk, V.G., Verkhratsky, N.S., Stupina. A.S., Karpova, S.M., and Lakiza, T.Y.U. 1979. Mechanisms of neurohumoral regulation of heart function in aging. *Experimental Aging Research* 5:441–477.

46. Tomanek, R.J., Trout, J.J., and Lauva, I.K. 1984. Cytochemistry of myocardial structures related to degenerative processes in spontaneously hypertensive and normotensive rats. *J. Mol. Cell Cardiol.* 16:227–237.

47. Breisch, E.A. 1982. Myocardial lysosomes in pressure-overload hypertrophy. *Cell Tissue Res.* 223:615–625.

48. Hibbs, R.G., Ferrans, V.J., Walsh, J.J., and Burch, G.E. 1965. Electron microscopic observations on lysosomes and related cytoplasmic components of normal and pathological cardiac muscle. *Anat. Rec.* 153:173–186.

49. Alpert, N.R., Hamrell, B.B., and Halpern, W. 1974. Mechanical and biochemical correlates of cardiac hypertrophy. *Circ. Res.* 34 & 35 Suppl. II: 71–82.

50. Bassett, A.L. and Gelband, H. 1973. Chronic partial occlusion of pulmonary artery in cats: change in ventricular action potential configuration during hypertrophy. *Circ. Res.* 32:15–26.

51. Bing, O.H.L., Fanburg, B.L., Brooks, W.W., and Matsushita, S. 1978. The effects of the lathyrogen β-amino proprionitrile (BAPN) on the mechanical properties of experimentally hypertrophied rat cardiac muscle. *Circ. Res.* 43:632–637.

52. Jouannot, P. and Hatt, P.Y. 1975. Rat myocardial mechanics during pressure-induced hypertrophy development and reversal. *Am. J. Physiol.* 229:355–364.

53. Yin, F.C.P., Spurgeon, H.A., Weisfeldt, M.L, and Lakatta, E.G. 1980. Mechanical properties of myocardium from hypertrophied rat hearts. A comparison between hypertrophy induced

by senescence and by aortic banding. *Circ. Res.* 46:292–300.

54. Sharma, R.V., McEldoon, J.P., and Bhalla, R.C. Age-dependent changes in myosin ATPase activity in the myocardium of spontaneously hypertensive rats. *Cardiovas. Res.* in press.

55. Weisfeldt, M.L. 1980. Left ventricular function. In *The Aging Heart* (Aging, Vol. 12). ML Weisfeldt, ed. pp. 297–314. New York: Raven Press.

56. Yin, F.C.P. 1978. Guarnieri, T., Spurgeon, H.A., Lakatta, E.G., Fortuin, N.J., and Weisfeldt, M.L. 1978. Age-associated decrease in ventricular response to hemodynamic stress during beta-adrenergic blockade. *Br. Heart J.* 40:1349–1355.

16. STRESS AND SUDDEN DEATH

EDWARD M. DWYER JR.

Sudden death has been the subject of considerable interest throughout recorded history. Currently, the medical community's understanding of sudden death has been heightened by our increased knowledge of the pathophysiology of coronary artery disease, gained over the past 20 years. There has been a substantial scientific effort to categorize subsets of those who die suddenly, to accurately predict those persons at risk of sudden death, to delineate those factors that trigger the event, and to develop medical approaches that provide a rapid access to treatment for those who experience sudden cardiac arrest.

Estimates of the incidence of sudden death vary considerably depending on how it is classified and whether noncardiac disease is included as a cause. It is probably safe to estimate that 200,000–300,000 persons die suddenly from cardiac causes each year, and most of those die without benefit of medical assistance. The vast number (approximately 80%) of these deaths are due to coronary artery disease. We know from the Framingham study [1] that over 50% of persons dying suddenly are experiencing this event as the first manifestation of their disease.

Intertwined through the multiple etiologies of sudden death is a common thread of stress which appears to be an important factor in many sudden deaths, or, at the very least, an important "trigger" mechanism. There is substantial historical background, as well as current clinical and experimental data to implicate psychological, emotional, and physical stress as mechanisms which may affect a rapid change in cardiac rhythm or coronary artery tone, resulting in sudden death.

Historical accounts begin with Hippocrates who observed the importance of the relationship between chest pain and sudden death, commenting that "the frequent recurrence of cardialgia in an elderly person, announces sudden death [2]. In the early seventeenth century, Lancisi in his work *Desubitaneis Mortibus*, described, observations from a population study which showed the link between recurrent chest pain, obesity, advanced age, and sudden death [3].

More interesting to us were those early descriptions which linked sudden death and emotional stress. Fothergill, in 1776, described a patient with angina pectoris who "in a sudden and violent transport of anger, (he) fell down and expired immediately" [4]. A contemporary report of John Hunter's death [5] recounts how his sudden demise occurred during a heated exchange with several of his colleagues. Prior to his death, he had described the occurrence of angina during emotional outbursts and predicted that his death might follow such a pattern. In an excellent article, Engel [6] reviews accounts of sudden death attributed to, or precipitated by, severe emotional stress. He cites examples of emotional stress and sudden death following news of the death of a loved one; during periods of acute grief, during profound life changes, and the mysterious "voodoo deaths" in primitive tribes after the "hex" is placed on the individual by the tribal witch doctor.

There are similar chronicles of sudden death associated with the stress of strenuous physical activity. One of the earliest and most famous examples is the death of Pheidippides in 490 BC [7]. Pheidippides was the messenger chosen to run the 25 mile distance from Marathon to Athens to alert the Athenians that the battle with the Persians at Marathon had been won by the Greeks. After gasping out the message of the victory, he fell to the ground, dead. In a more recent vein, the news media are replete with articles reporting the sudden death of a young man participating in an athletic event or of a middle-aged man jogging in the park.

The data and research methodology are not available to quantify the importance of emotional or physical stress in the genesis of sudden death. It is our hope to provide in this chapter a framework of sudden death and to delineate the role of emotion, psychological factors, and physical activities in that event.

SUDDEN DEATH: SCOPE AND DEFINITION

Although multiple causes of sudden death exist, coronary artery disease is unquestionably the primary cause of sudden death in our country. Considerable confusion in the definition of sudden death has existed for many years because of

1. differing definitions of time from symptoms to death;
2. frailty and variability in the reliability of reporting systems throughout the country and

3. the substantial number of unwitnessed deaths.

In numerous studies, the time interval has varied from one to twenty-four hours while other reports have focused on instantaneous deaths. The World Health Organization [8], attempting to standardize research in this area, suggested death within a twenty-four hour period after the onset of symptoms as the appropriate definition of sudden death. In recent years, a consensus has been developing to define sudden death as a witnessed death within one hour of the onset of symptoms. This definition tends to focus research efforts on resuscitation and prevention as well as directing efforts toward a more homogeneous group of patients.

An additional consideration in the analysis of sudden death data is the presence or absence of a reliable witness as well as the availability of a discerning, skillful and knowledgeable interviewer of that witness. Data are generally gathered in a retrospective manner through interviews with the deceased's family or friends who were present at the time of death. The ability to establish mechanisms responsible for sudden death depends heavily on the ability of the interviewer to elicit prodromal and acute symptoms related to the death. Such information is vital in determining the importance of emotional and physical stress in sudden death. A new calssification, devised by Hinkle and Thaler [9], depends primarily on detailed retrospective interviews. In a recent prospective postinfarction study (MPIP) [10], which relied on the Hinkle classification and the detailed review of the circumstances of death, it was observed that approximately one-third of the deaths were unwitnessed. In stress-related sudden deaths, instantaneous death is the rule. This observation suggests the presence of a subset of the sudden death population which has a specific mechanism (arrhythmia) and a treatment (early identification and prevention).

MECHANISMS OF SUDDEN DEATH

The pathophysiologic mechanisms which result in sudden death have intrigued physicians for centuries, but little light has been shed on the event until the development of the electrocardiographic monitor, coronary care unit, mobile care unit, coronary arteriography, Holter monitoring and modern-day electrophysiologic experimental studies over the past 20 years. With an increased focus on sudden death in the past decade, the role of emotional and physical stress has come under increasing scrutiny. The mechanisms by which stress may trigger a sudden death are important, not only in understanding the role of stress, but in understanding the more global issue of sudden death.

Terminal arrhythmias

Early reports recognized the importance of both ventricular fibrillation and asystole as the final electrical event at the time of death. The development of mobile care units, pioneered by Pantridge [11] in Northern Ireland, provided the opportunity to determine the relative frequency of the terminal rhythm at the time of cardiac arrest. In addition, recent reports of Holter recordings have documented the terminal rhythm during sudden death [12]. Ventricular fibrillation was the terminal rhythm in the vast majority (88%) of patients, reported by Liberthson et al. [13] with the Miami mobile care system, while an incidence of 95% was observed in a larger series reported by Goldstein et al. [14] from several mobile units throughout the Midwest.

Bradyarrhythmias are commonly observed at or around a cardiac arrest in the form of sinus bradycardia or AV block. These arrhythmias are most commonly associated with inferior infarction, where increased vagal tone results presumably from stimulation or necrosis of a large network of cholinergic ganglion and post-ganglionic fibers which are present in the posterior wall of the left ventricle. In general, these rhythm disturbances are easily managed. On the other hand, the presence of asystole at the time of cardiac arrest is not usually responsive to resuscitative efforts, which suggests extensive and irreversible damage to the left ventricle or a total disruption of the His conduction system with inadequate response of lower pacemakers.

Role of Ischemia

In 80% of persons dying suddenly, coronary artery disease is the etiology. In these patients, there is an inescapable, as well as confusing, relationship between ischemia and arrhythmia. The reasons they cannot be separated are several. It has been recognized for some time that both acute infarction and transient ischemia could occur without symptoms. The incidence of patients with a deficient warning system appears to be between 20–25% of patients with coronary artery disease. In a recent report by Goldstein et al [14], of their resuscitative experience in over 2000 cardiac arrests, they observed that 22% of resuscitated patients with subsequently documented acute infarction had no prodromal symptoms preceding collapse. Similar observations were made by Hinkle et al. [15] in a prospective study of high-risk patients.

The presence of silent ischemia or infarction followed by ventricular fibrillation will be perceived, even when witnessed by the most experienced observer, as a primary arrhythmic event. The presence of substantial numbers of unwitnessed deaths further confounds the evaluation of any group of patients dying suddenly. Ischemia, in its symptomatic form, occurs in approximately two thirds of witnessed deaths. This finding has been described by Hinkle et al. [15], using both clinical and pathologic evidence. Confirmation of this high incidence of ischemia preceding sudden death has been provided in a prospective post-infarction (MPIP) study [10] and Goldstein et al. [14] in his large series of resuscitated patients by mobile care teams in several Midwestern counties.

In persons dying suddenly with prodromal ischemia (overt or silent), ischemia leads eventually to either circulatory collapse or an arrhythmia as the final mode of death. Death with circulatory collapse within one hour is decidedly uncommon, occurring in 1–8% in two studies that have used this classification. On the other hand, an arrhythmic death following symptomatic evidence of ischemia is quite common. There is considerable experimental evidence linking ischemia to ventricular fibrillation. Increased automaticity can result from hypoxia. There is a large experimental experience which not only establishes the relationship between acute ischemia and ventricular arrhythmias but describes plausible mechanisms for the genesis of the arrhythmias. Han and Moe [16] have demonstrated that, in the presence of ischemia, disparate rates of depolarization may occur. This is result in a circus or reentry mechanism which may lead to the development of ectopic beats and ventricular tachyarrhythmias.

Ischemia and psychological stress

Emotional stress may trigger sudden death by

1. inducing an ischemic state,
2. initiating a ventricular arrhythmia or
3. exaggerating a preexisting ventricular arrhythmia.

Psychological stress, when acute and severe, may increase myocardial oxygen requirements by initiating (a) tachycardia and/or hypertension, or may impair coronary blood flow by vasoconstriction [17] or frank spasm with total occlusion [18]. Platlet aggregation has been implicated in sudden death due to coronary artery disease, either through initiating a spasm or participating in the development of a thrombotic occlusion of a diseased coronary artery [19]. Stress is known to cause a tenfold increase in the concentration of epinephrine, which may activate platlets and stimulate aggregation [20].

Ischemia and physical stress

Physical stress produces an ischemic state in patients with impaired coronary blood flow. Under usual circumstances, the ischemic state is quickly reversible with cessation of physical activity, and it leaves no lasting effects. In spite of this observation, physical stress has been observed to frequently produce serious problems in patients with both ischemic and non-ischemic cardiac disorders. Certain subsets of patients demonstrate high grade ventricular arrhythmias during exercise—which, when combined with sustained or uncontrolled physical activity, may produce severe ischemia associated with a serious ventricular arrhythmia, each affecting the other in an adverse manner. A frequent observation at post mortem examination in sudden death is plaque rupture [21], which might be initiated by excessive hypertension associated with physical stress. In most cases of patients with coronary artery disease, physical activity is advised. In spite of this advice, physical activity may prove detrimental in a subset of patients somewhere along the course of their disease.

Role of arrhythmia

Ventricular fibrillation has been the central theme of any discussion dealing with the cause of sudden death. The primary role of ventricular fibrillation has been reinforced by the presence of high-grade ventricular arrhythmias in many patients succumbing to sudden death. In addition, the vast majority of sudden death victims are found to have ventricular fibrillation at the time of their cardiac arrest. However, as outlined in the previous section dealing with ischemia, the data suggest that most patients dying suddenly experience ischemia first, followed by ventricular fibrillation. There are still subgroups of patients who likely develop ventricular fibrillation without prior ischemia. These patients include young people (< 35 years) who have severe valvular disease, hypertrophic or dilated cardiomyopathy, congenital QT syndrome, congenital anomalies of the coronary arteries and myocarditis. In patients over 35, the etiology is almost always coronary artery disease. Within the over 35 group, there is a subset of patients with idiopathic ventricular fibrillation; some of these have either an emotional or physical stress trigger to their arrhythmia. Lown et al. [22] has clearly demonstrated the trigger potential of severe psychological stress in precipitating serious ventricular arrhythmias.

Role of autonomic nervous system in sudden death

Recent data summarized by Schwartz and Stone [23] propose an important role of the autonomic nervous system in sudden death. Myocardial ischemia can simultaneously excite the autonomic nervous system and be adversely affected by that same neural activity. In addition, the autonomic nervous system can destabilize cardiac electrical activity in non-ischemic hearts.

Myocardial ischemia activates both sympathetic and vagal afferent cardiac fibers which, in turn, elicit severe reflex responses. Within a few seconds of ischemia, cardiac sympathetic sensory endings are activated. This activation elicits an excitatory cardiocardiac reflex. This efferent sympathetic activity appears to travel preferentially through left-sided nerves and the left stellate ganglion. In addition, the cardiocardiac sympathetic activity can selectively inhibit the activity of efferent vagal fibers. This reflex may generate excessive sympathetic activity, which may be responsible for, or increase, the early ventricular arrhythmias associated with myocardial ischemia. Experimental interruption of this reflex is capable of suppressing ventricular arrhythmias associated with coronary occlusion.

In infarction of the posterior wall of the left ventricle, vagal hyperreactivity is commonly observed. Some enhancement of vagal tone may be beneficial; vagal activity may suppress ventricular arrhythmias and blunt excessive increases in heart rate. Excessive vagal activity, as with excessive sympathetic activity, may produce serious adverse events i.e., hypotension, bradycardia, or asystole. An appropriate balance between sympathetic and vagal activity may be the key to the prevention or suppression of ventricular arrhythmias.

Sympathetic activity, elicited by ischemia, not only affects electrical stability in the heart but can reduce coronary blood flow through vasoconstriction of coronary arteries [24]. This reflex vasoconstriction can be eliminated in experimental animals by removal of the left stellate ganglion. In spite of an increase in myocardial metabolic demand, reflex sympathetic activity can increase ischemia and exacerbate serious ventricular arrhythmias.

A number of observations suggest that within the sudden death population (both ischemic and nonischemic), there is a subset of persons who have hearts "too good to die," yet develop ventricular fibrillation. Studies examining out-of-hospital resuscitation demonstrate that most defibrillated patients have no recurrence of ventricular fibrillation and only a small percentage (20%) have evidence of an acute infarction. These resuscitated patients are a small and highly select group but the observations indicate that cardiac arrest can occur without extensive permanent damage to the left ventricle.

These data suggest a major role of the sympathetic nervous system in the genesis of ventricular arrhythmias. Ischemia-generated reflexes and emotional input via higher centers of the brain appear to be the transient triggers which may initiate serious ventricular arrhythmias or move an electrically unstable myocardium into ventricular fibrillation.

EMOTIONAL STRESS AND SUDDEN DEATH

Although much of the data on the causal relationship of psychological stress and sudden death is anecdotal, the myriad of such reports poses the need for a serious inquiry into the question. Death coming suddenly during severe emotional stress such as anger, frustration, or cute grief has been the subject of numerous folktales or more recently, newspaper articles.

As described in the previous section, there is a clear anatomic and physiologic substrate to explain the interrelationship of emotional stress perceived by higher regions of the brain and sudden death from ventricular fibrillation. Interactions through the limbic system exist between the frontal lobes, hypothalmus, and the autonomic effectors in the medulla. The "defense reaction" is an example of this reaction in action. Perceived danger is transformed immediately into alterations in the cardiovascular system, i.e., increased heart rate and blood pressure. Excessive vagal response to emotional stress may be mediated in the same fashion. Clinical examples include fainting with bradycardia and hypotension (vasodepressor syncope) during acute grief or psychologically stressful situations. The opossum exhibits a similar, but more profound, response when confronted with a "fight or flight" situation. Here the opossum becomes hypotensive, bradycardic, and apneic, feigning death.

Animal experimentation provides several additional examples of the interrelationship of psychological stress and adverse cardiac responses. Direct stimulation of the central nervous system can evoke ventricular arrhythmias or fibrillation [25]. Studies using various forms of environmental stress have also shown that such stress produces both myocardial damage and sudden death [26]. In settings of experimental ischemia or infarction, the threshold for ventricular fibrillation is reduced significantly by psychological stress [27]. Cholinergic stimulation and beta blockade severly blunt the adverse effects of emotional stress mediated through the sympathetic nervous system [28]. These experiments provide the framework for the proposition that psychological stress can alter electrical stability and increase the likelihood of ventricular fibrillation, particularly in a setting of acute ischemia.

Responses of humans to severe psychological stress may be quantitatively similar to that in animal investigations; unfortunately, we have no opportunity either to structure the stimuli or prospectively study the response. In spite of these limitations, several studies warrant further examination and comment. Psychological stress may be seen as having two forms. The first is "acute stress" such as sudden emotional outbursts in the form of anger, joy, acute grief, or fright; the second is "chronic stress" such as mourning over a protracted period, significant life changes or continued job or financial pressures.

Greene et al. [29] studied the emotional circumstances surrounding the sudden death of 25 men through interviews with close relatives. They estimated that at least 50% of the men were undergoing highly stressful situations at the time of their death, of which many were acute in nature. Meyers and Dewar [30], in a similar study of 100 men dying suddenly from coronary artery disease, found 23 who were experiencing intense emotional stress in the 30 minutes preceding death, e.g., notification of divorce, an attack by dogs.

In a Helsinki study by Rissanen et al. [31] both "acute" and "chronic" stress situations were evaluated in coronary disease related sudden death. Patients experiencing *acute* emotional stress were more likely to develop an instantaneous death from ventricular fibrillation. In a comprehensive review, Engel [6] summarized social and personal circumstances surrounding newspaper reports of 275 examples of sudden death. Acute emotional stress was present in nearly two-thirds of the group. These patients included 21% on hearing news of the collapse or death of a close person; 9% were experiencing the threat of immediate loss of such a person; 27% were involved in a situation of extreme personal danger or threat of injury; and 6% were in the excitement of reunion, triumph, or happy ending.

Reich et al. [32] identified emotional triggers to ventricular fibrillation in 21% of 117 patients who had been resuscitated from a cardiac arrest. A substantial (44%) percentage of the patients without any structural heart disease demonstrated psychological triggers to ventricular tachycardia or fibrillation. In a companion study Lown et al. [22] found a significant increase in PVCs during acute psychological stress testing in a similar group of survivors from cardiac arrest or life-threatening arrhythmias.

The concept of *chronic* psychosocial stresses playing an important role in the development of cardiovascular events has been under investigation for a considerable period of time. Rahe [33] has pioneered a method of quantifying life events to study the effect of accumulating various types of chronic psychosocial stresses such as divorce, death of a spouse, loss of job, etc. These life changes were measured retrospectively in sudden death victims in Helsinki. The investigators observed a marked increase in life changes during the six months prior to death, compared to one year earlier, in those same patients. Rees et al. [34] also found a 12% mortality in the first year in a group who had just experienced the loss of a close person. This finding was more dramatic in men than in women.

Depression has been demonstrated to have an important relationship to sudden death. Greene et al. [29] reported that victims of sudden death had a high incidence (76%) of depression in the weeks or months prior to death. The depression was usually secondary to a serious personal problem, e.g., separation, estrangement, or disappointment. Shortly before death, half of the group became increasingly depressed, while the other half became anxious or angry. Wolf and associates [35] studied and followed a series of 65 postinfarction patients. They attempted to predict which ten of the control and study group would die first. Based primarily on the degree of depression observed in the patients, they were able to prospectively predict the first ten individuals to die. Eight of the ten died suddenly.

Jenkins [36] as well as Friedman and Rosenman [37] have described a coronary prone behavior pattern or Type A personality who has a greater incidence of angina, myocardial, infarction, and sudden death. However, in a recent prospective study of postinfarction patients (MPIP) Case et al. [38], using a Jenkins personality assessment, failed to find an increased incidence of infarction, death, or sudden death in the Type A group in the year following the acute infarction. There are several studies [39] attempting to alter behavior patterns in Type A patients in the hope of decreasing subsequent infarction or death.

At the present time, the role of chronic stress, among other behavior patterns, in sudden death is uncertain and certainly has less background pathophysiologic data to support it than we demonstrated with acute emotional stress. Further investigation is needed in both areas of acute and chronic stress, particularly in the exploration of intermediate mechanisms which could give us insight into approaches to blunt the impact of psychosocial triggers of sudden death.

PHYSICAL STRESS AND SUDDEN DEATH

Our attitude toward physical stress in patients with coronary artery disease (who always carry the specter of sudden death) is nothing short of schizophrenic. Physical activity is widely recommended in both primary and secondary prevention of ischemic heart disease. On the other hand, the dramatic newspaper headline reporting the sudden death of a young man engaged in an athletic event or a middle-aged man while jogging creates concern and ambivalence in physicians with responsibility for rendering advice to the community. We will review only the evidence which establishes a relationship between physical stress and sudden death. It is outside the scope of this chapter to review the data showing the positive value of exercise in preventing death from coronary artery disease.

In the area of nonischemic heart disease, exercise, and sudden death, Maron et al. [40] analyzed the underlying cause and circumstances around the sudden death of highly conditioned competitive and recreational athletes. In those under the age of 35, sudden death was uniformly associated with nonischemic structural heart disease. The most common (50%) cause was a hypertrophic cardiomyopathy, followed by disorders such as aortic stenosis, myocarditis, anomalous coronary arteries, ruptured aortic aneurysm, and disorders of the conduction system. In contact sports, the additional factor of blunt injury must also be considered. There are numerous accounts of cardiac contusion, laceration or thrombosis of a coronary artery secondary to chest trauma. The solution to prevention of instantaneous (presumably arrhythmic) death in the young during exercise lies clearly in the area of early identification and heightened awareness of these uncommon disorders, particularly in those participating in competitive athletics.

Participation in sports or exposure to strenuous physical activities is, of course, not limited to the young. In groups over the age of 35, coronary artery disease becomes increasingly prevalent and this disease is the leading cause of sudden death. Jokl and Meltzer [41] reported 63 sudden deaths which occurred during physical work or participation in sports. Forty-three victims had ischemic cardiac disease as the underlying etiology.

Friedman et al. [42] reviewed clinical and autopsy findings in 59 people who died instantaneously from coronary artery disease. More than one-half occurred during or immediately following severe physical exertion. The deaths were probably caused by ventricular fibrillation, as most individuals had no prodromal symptoms, and pathological examination did not demonstrate any acute lesions. Cobb and Hallstrom [43] described a group of 25 patients who had a cardiac arrest while participating in a formal rehabilatation program. Such programs are usually composed largely of patients with coronary artery disease. The occurrence of sudden death in such closely monitored groups underlines the caution which must be exercised in less formal settings of apparently healthy middle-aged and elderly people. One must keep in mind the relatively high incidence of "silent" unidentified coronary patients within the population. Yater et al. [44] demonstrated that the frequency of sudden death during strenuous physical activity was more than double the proportion of time usually spent in those activities while the number of men stricken while asleep was but one-third of the expected incidence. In a very detailed and interesting report from Helsinki by Kala and associates, [46] the degree of physical activity prior to death was correlated with the time of death from the onset of symptoms. The only significant finding was that a very high percentage of instantaneous deaths occurred in individuals involved in strenuous exercise. All of this group who were autopsied had severe coronary artery disease. These findings suggest that physical stress may be an important trigger of ventricular fibrillation through simultaneous induction of ventricular arrhythmias, ischemia, and catecholamine infusion.

In the preceding pages we have attempted to review the relationship of stress to sudden death. Stress and sudden death, by their very nature, are both transient, uncontrolled, unpredictable, and nonreproducible phenomena in humans. For this reason, we must rely heavily on intuition, deduction, and experimental animal data to support any role of stress in sudden death. Using this approach, both emotional and physical stress appear to be important in a certain subset of those patients susceptible to sudden death. The critical subjects for future investigation will focus on the need to create improved methods of identifying those susceptible patients and to design more innovative methods of prevention.

REFERENCES

1. Gordon, T. and, Kannel, W.B. 1971. Premature mortality from coronary heart disease. The Framingham Study. *J. Am. Med. Assoc.* 215:1617–25.
2. Littre, E. *Oeuvres Complètes d'Hippocrates.* Traduction avec le texte Grec. Paris, Baillière 1839–1861. Coan Prenotions, Vol. V, 647, para 280.
3. Lancisi, G.M. 1707. *DeSubitaneis Mortibus.* Rome: Buagni.
4. Fothergill, J. 1776. Case of angina pectoris with remarks. *Med. Obsns. Inquir.* 5:233.
5. Hunter, J. 1794. *A Treatise on the Blood, Inflammation, and Gunshot.* London: Richardson.
6. Engel, G.L. 1978. Psychologic stress, vasodepressor (vasovagal) syncope, and sudden death. *Ann. Intern. Med.* 89:403–12.
7. Kent, J.H. 1966. Marathon, In World Book Encyclopedia. Chicago, Field Enterprises Educational Corp., p. 150.
8. WHO Scientific Group: The pathological diagnosis of acute ischaemic heart disease. 441:5, 1970.
9. Hinkle, L.E. and Thaler, H.T. 1982. Clinical classification of cardiac deaths. *Circulation* 65:457–64.
10. Marcus, F.I. (Personal communication)
11. Pantridge, J.F. and Geddes, J.S. 1967. A mobile intensive care unit in the management of myocardial infarction. *Lancet* 2:271.
12. Clark, M.B., Dwyer, E.M., and Greenberg, H.B. 1983. Sudden death during ambulatory monitoring: Analysis of six cases. *Am. J. Med.* 75:801–6.
13. Liberthson, R.R., Nagel, E.L., and Hirschman, J.C. 1974. Prehospital ventricular defibrillation: Prognosis and follow-up course. *N. Eng. J. Med.* 291:317–21.
14. Goldstein, S., Landis, J.R., Leighton, R., Ritter, G., Vasu, C.M., Lantis, A., and Serokman, R. 1981. Characteristics of the resuscitated out-of-hospital cardiac arrest victim with coronary artery disease. *Circulation* 977:977–84.
15. Hinkle, L.E. 1982. Short-term risk factors for sudden death. In *Sudden Coronary Death,* Greenberg, H.M. and Dwyer, E.M., eds. New York: Annals of the New York Academy of Sciences 382:22–37.
16. Han, J., and Moe, G.K. 1964. Nonuniform recovery of excitability in ventricular muscle. *Circ. Res.* 14:44–51.

17. Feigl, E.O. 1967. Sympathetic control of coronary circulation. *Circ. Res.* 20:262–71.
18. Maseri, A., Severi, S. Marzullo, P. 1982. Role of coronary arterial spasm in sudden coronary ischemic death. In Sudden Coronary Death, Greenberg, H.M. and Dwyer, E.M., eds. New York: Annals of the New York Academy of Sciences 382:204–17.
19. Haerem, J. 1972. Platelet aggregates in intramyocardial vessels of patients dying suddenly and unexpectedly of sudden coronary disease. *Atherosclerosis* 15:529–54.
20. Colman, R.W. 1982. The role of platelets in the genesis of ischemia. In *Sudden Coronary Death*, Greenberg, H.M. and Dwyer, E.M., eds. New York: Annals of the New York Academy of Sciences 382:190–203.
21. Davies, M.J., Thomas, A. 1985. Plaque-fissuring: The cause of acute myocardial infarction, sudden ischemic death and crescendo angina. *Brit. Heart J.* 53:363–73.
22. Lown, B., DeSilva, R.A. 1978. Roles of psychologic stress and autonomic nervous system changes in provocation of ventricular premature complexes. *Am. J. Cardiol.* 41:979–85.
23. Schwartz, P.J. and Stone, H.L. 1982. The role of the autonomic nervous system in sudden cardiac death, In Sudden Coronary Death, Greenberg, H.M. and Dwyer, E.M. eds. New York: Annals of the New York Academy of Sciences 382:162–79.
24. Mohrman, D.E. and Feigl, E.O. 1978. Competition between sympathetic vasoconstriction and metabolic vasodilation in the canine coronary circulation. *Circ. Res.* 42:79–86.
25. Johansson, G.L., Johnson, N., and Lannek, N. 1974. Severe stress-cardiopathy in pigs. *Am. Heart J.* 87:451–60.
26. Haft, J.I. 1979. Role of platelets in coronary artery disease. *Amer. J. Cardiol.* 43:1197–1206.
27. Corbalan, R., Verrier, R.L., and Lown, B. 1974. Psychologic stress and ventricular arrhythmia during myocardial infarction in the conscious dog. *Am. J. Cardiol.* 34:692–96.
28. De Silva, R.A. 1982. Central nervous system risk factors for sudden coronary death. In *Sudden Coronary Death*, Greenberg, H.M. and Dwyer, E.M., eds. New York: Annals of the New York Academy of Sciences 382:143–60.
29. Greene, W.A., Goldstein, S., and Moss, A.J. 1972. Psychosocial aspects of sudden death. *Arch. Intern. Med.* 129:725–31.
30. Myers, A. and Dewar, H.A. Circumstances attending 100 sudden deaths from 1975. Coronary artery disease with coroner's necropsies. *Brit. Heart. J.* 37:1133–40.
31. Rissenen, V., Romo, M., and Siltanen, P. 1978. Pre-monitory symptoms and stress factors preceeding sudden death from ischemic heart disease. *Acta Med. Scand.* 204:389–99.
32. Reich, P., DeSilva, R.A., Lown, B., and Murawski, B.J. 1981. Acute psychological disturbances preceeding life-threatening ventricular arrhythmias. *J. Amer. Med. Assoc.* 246:233–35.
33. Rahe, R.H., Romo, M., Bennett, L., and Siltanen, P. 1974. Recent life changes, myocardial infarction and abrupt coronary death. *Arch. Intern. Med.* 133:221–228.
34. Rees, W.D., Lutkins, S.G. 1957. Mortality of bereavement. *Br. Med. J.* 4:13–18.
35. Wolf, S. 1971. Psychosocial forces in myocardial infarction and sudden death, In *Soviety stress and Disease*, Levi L., ed. New York: Oxford University Press, Vol I., p. 324.
36. Jenkins, C.D. 1971. Psychologic and social precursors of coronary disease. *N. Engl. J. Med.* 284:244.
37. Friedman, M. and Rosenman, R.H. 1959. Association of specific overt behavior pattern with blood and cardiovascular findings. Blood cholesterol level, blood clotting time, incidence of arcus senilis, and clinical coronary artery disease. *J. Amer. Med. Assoc.* 169:1286–90.
38. Case, R.B., Heller, S.S., Case, N.B., and Moss, A.J. 1985. Type A behavior and survival after acute myocardial infarction. *N. Engl. J. Med.* 312:737–41.
39. Roseman, R.H. 1978. Role of type A behavior pattern in the pathogenesis of ischemic heart disease, and modification for prevention. In *Sudden Coronary Death*, Manninen, V., and Halonen, P.I., eds. Basel: S. Karger Vol. 25:35–46.
40. Moron, B.J., Roberts, W.C., and Epstein, S.E. 1982. Sudden death in hypertrophic cardiomyopathy: A profile of 78 patients. *Circulation* 35:1388–94.
41. Jokl, E. and Meltzer, L. 1971. Acute fatal nontraumatic collapse during work and sport. In *Medicine and Sport*, Jokl, E. and McClellan, J.T., eds. Baltimore. University Park Press, Vol. 5:12, 1971.
42. Friedman, M., Manwaring, J.H., Rosenman, R.H., Donlon, G., Ortega, P., and Grube, S.M. 1973. Instantaneous and sudden deaths: Clinical and pathological differentiation in coronary artery disease. *J. Amer. Assoc. Med.* 210:1319–25.

43. Cobb, L.A. and Hallstrom, A.P. 1982. Community-based cardiopulmonary resuscitation: What we have learned, In *Sudden Coronary Death*. Greenberg, H.M. and Dwyer, E.M., eds. New York: Annals of New York Academy of Sciences 382:330–41.

44. Yater, W.M., Traum, A.H., Brown, W.G., Fitzgerald, R.P., Geisler, M.A., and Wilcox, B.B. 1948. Coronary artery disease in men 18–39 years of age. *Amer. Heart J.* 36:334–40.

45. Kala, R., Romo, M., Siltanen, P., Halonen, P.I. 1978. Physical activity and sudden death. In *Sudden Coronary Death*, Manninen, V. and Halonen, P.I., eds. Basel: S. Karger Vol. 25:27–34.

INDEX